MENTAL HEALTH SCREENING
AND ASSESSMENT IN JUVENILE JUSTICE

Mental Health Screening and Assessment in Juvenile Justice

EDITED BY

THOMAS GRISSO
GINA VINCENT
DANIEL SEAGRAVE

THE GUILFORD PRESS
New York   London

Printed in the United States of America

This book is printed on acid-free paper.

Last digit is print number: 9 8 7 6 5 4 3 2 1

Library of Congress Cataloging-in-Publication Data

Mental health screening and assessment in juvenile justice / edited by Thomas Grisso, Gina Vincent, Daniel Seagrave.
    p. cm.
  Includes bibliographical references and index.
  ISBN 1-59385-132-4 (hardcover)
  1. Juvenile delinquents—Psychology. 2. Juvenile delinquents—Mental health services. I. Grisso, Thomas. II. Vincent, Gina. III. Seagrave, Daniel.
  HV9069.M46 2005
  364.36′01′9—dc22
                                                                    2004024044

About the Editors

Thomas Grisso, PhD, is Professor of Psychiatry, Director of Psychology, and Coordinator of the Law and Psychiatry Program at the University of Massachusetts Medical School in Worcester. His research, teaching, and clinical practice focus on forensic mental health evaluations and services. Dr. Grisso has received numerous awards, including the American Psychological Association's Award for Distinguished Contributions to Research in Public Policy, and has authored several books on psychology and juvenile justice. He is also a member of the MacArthur Foundation Research Network on Adolescent Development and Juvenile Justice.

Gina Vincent, PhD, is Assistant Professor in the Law and Psychiatry Program in the Department of Psychiatry at the University of Massachusetts Medical School. She is Co-Investigator of the National Norms for the MAYSI-2 project, funded by the William T. Grant Foundation, and Project Director of the Juvenile Adjudicative Competence project, funded by the MacArthur Foundation. Dr. Vincent has published and presented at over 25 international and national conferences in the areas of juvenile psychopathy, juvenile sex offending, violence risk assessment, and mental disorder in juvenile justice.

Daniel Seagrave, PsyD, is a clinical psychologist who holds a Diplomate in Forensic Psychology through the American Board of Professional Psychology. He is the former Director of the Forensic Division of the New Mexico State Hospital. Dr. Seagrave's private practice focused on forensic evaluations for both criminal and juvenile court, including competence to stand trial, mental state at the time of an offense, violence risk, and sexual offender risk. He is currently employed as a clinical psychologist with the Los Alamos National Laboratory where he primarily conducts fitness-for-duty evaluations of employees in nuclear-weapons-related positions. His research interests include juvenile violence risk assessment and the application of psychopathy concepts to juvenile offenders.

Contributors

Thomas Achenbach, PhD, Department of Psychiatry, University of Vermont, Burlington, Vermont

Amanda Anderson, BA, Drug Abuse Comprehensive Coordinating Office, Tampa, Florida

Robert P. Archer, PhD, Department of Psychiatry and Behavioral Sciences, Eastern Virginia Medical School, Norfolk, Virginia

Leena K. Augimeri, MEd, Child Development Institute, Toronto, Ontario, Canada

Emily M. Baker, PsyD, Department of Psychiatry and Behavioral Sciences, Eastern Virginia Medical School, Norfolk, Virginia

Robert Barnoski, PhD, Washington State Institute for Public Policy, Olympia, Washington

Patrick A. Bartel, PhD, Youth Forensic Psychiatric Services of British Columbia, Burnaby, British Columbia, Canada

Randy Borum, PsyD, Department of Mental Health Law and Policy, University of South Florida, Tampa, Florida

Jenine Boyd, PhD, Fort Bend County Juvenile Probation Department, Richmond, Texas

John Briere, PhD, Department of Psychiatry, University of Southern California, Los Angeles, California

Carl B. Clements, PhD, Department of Psychology, University of Alabama, Tuscaloosa, Alabama

Lois Oberlander Condie, PhD, Department of Psychiatry, Children's Hospital, Harvard Medical School, Boston, Massachusetts

Carla A. Counts, BS, Department of Psychology, Florida State University, Tallahassee, Florida

Joanne L. Davis, PhD, Department of Psychology, University of Tulsa, Tulsa, Oklahoma

Richard Dembo, PhD, Department of Criminology, University of South Florida, Tampa, Florida

Prudence Fisher, PhD, New York State Psychiatric Institute, Columbia University, New York, New York

Julian D. Ford, PhD, Department of Psychiatry, University of Connecticut Health Center, Farmington, Connecticut

Adelle E. Forth, PhD, Department of Psychology, Carleton University, Ottawa, Ontario, Canada

Naomi E. Sevin Goldstein, PhD, Department of Clinical and Health Psychology, Drexel University, Philadelphia, Pennsylvania

Thomas Grisso, PhD, Department of Psychiatry, University of Massachusetts Medical School, Worcester, Massachusetts

Samantha Harvell, BA, Department of Psychology, Georgetown University, Washington, DC

Kay Hodges, PhD, Department of Psychology, Eastern Michigan University, Ypsilanti, Michigan

Robert D. Hoge, PhD, Department of Psychology, Carleton University, Ottawa, Ontario, Canada

Rachel Kalbeitzer, MS, Department of Psychology, Drexel University, Philadelphia, Pennsylvania

Christopher J. Koegl, MA, Child Development Institute, Toronto, Ontario, Canada

David Lachar, PhD, Department of Psychiatry and Behavioral Science, University of Texas–Houston Medical School, Houston, Texas

Linda E. Lazowski, PhD, The SASSI Institute, Springville, Indiana

Anne-Marie R. Leistico, MA, Department of Psychology, University of Alabama, Tuscaloosa, Alabama

Kathryn S. Levene, MSW, Child Development Institute, Toronto, Ontario, Canada

Bryan R. Loney, PhD, Department of Psychology, Florida State University, Tallahassee, Florida

Christopher P. Lucas, MD, New York State Psychiatric Institute, Columbia University, New York, New York

Steven Markussen, BFA, Snohomish County Juvenile Court, Everett, Washington

Larkin S. McReynolds, PhD, New York State Psychiatric Institute, Columbia University, New York, New York

Franklin G. Miller, PhD, The SASSI Institute, Springville, Indiana

Jana Mullins, BA, Department of Psychology, University of Alabama, Tuscaloosa, Alabama

Elana Newman, PhD, Department of Psychology, University of Tulsa, Tulsa, Oklahoma

Judith C. Quinlan, BA, Department of Psychiatry, University of Massachusetts Medical School, Worcester, Massachusetts

Karen L. Salekin, PhD, Department of Psychology, University of Alabama, Tuscaloosa, Alabama

Randall T. Salekin, PhD, Department of Psychology, University of Alabama, Tuscaloosa, Alabama

Crystal L. Schrum, MA, Department of Psychology, University of Alabama, Tuscaloosa, Alabama

Gina Vincent, PhD, Department of Psychiatry, University of Massachusetts Medical School, Worcester, Massachusetts

Gail A. Wasserman, PhD, New York State Psychiatric Institute, Columbia University, New York, New York

Christopher D. Webster, PhD, Department of Psychology, Simon Fraser University, Burnaby, British Columbia, Canada, and Child Development Institute, Toronto, Ontario, Canada

Jennifer Meltzer Wolpaw, PhD, Department of Psychiatry, University of Connecticut Health Center, Farmington, Connecticut

Jennifer L. Woolard, PhD, Department of Psychology, Georgetown University, Washington, DC

Preface

At the time we were completing the editing of this volume, a U.S. House of Representatives subcommittee announced its review of a report on the incarceration of youths in our nation's juvenile pretrial detention centers. Unlike federal legislative reviews of juvenile justice issues in the early 1990s, this one did not focus on the escalation of youth violence and how to contain it. Instead, it affirmed that at least 15,000 youths annually are incarcerated upon their arrest not because they are especially dangerous, but because of their acute mental disorders. They are locked up in juvenile detention centers until someone can find psychiatric or community mental health resources to provide them treatment.

This report is only the latest evidence of a crisis in our nation's mental health services for children, and the impact of that crisis on delinquency and the juvenile justice system. It became apparent about a decade ago, and its necessary implications for juvenile justice policy are now fully acknowledged by federal agencies, state juvenile justice systems, and administrators of juvenile justice programs. The public safety and child welfare mandates of the juvenile justice system must attend to the extraordinary proportion of youths with mental disorders who are in the custody of our juvenile justice facilities. There is widespread agreement that it is bad policy to presume that the juvenile justice system must *become* our nation's mental health system for youths. But federal and state requirements have now made it clear that juvenile justice programs must be an active, affirmative, and effective part of the solution.

Two undeniable components in that mandate have arisen as clear obligations for the juvenile justice system. One is the obligation to *identify mental health needs* among youths in its custody. The other is to develop *emergency systems of care*—strategies for emergency mental health services, diversion, and collaboration with mental health agencies—to respond to youths' mental health needs as they enter the system, and to blend necessary mental health treatment with other delinquency rehabilitation programming for mentally disordered youths who remain in custody because of their serious delinquency.

This book is aimed at assisting the juvenile justice system to fulfill these new mandates by providing effective mental health screening and assessment of youths as they enter the juvenile justice system. Recognition of the crisis has resulted in a number of literature resources for juvenile justice personnel (which we describe in Chapter 1) that define the rising tide of youths with mental disorders in juvenile justice programs, describe their disorders, analyze necessary changes in juvenile justice policy, and call for reform. Yet the literature to date has provided few resources that offer specific guidance to assist juvenile justice personnel in translating the need for mental health screening and assessment into action. Offering such guidance is the purpose of this book.

During the past few years, we have served as consultants to policymakers, administrators, program managers, and mental health professionals in juvenile justice systems nationwide, assisting them in their struggle with the mandate to identify the mental health needs of youths in their custody. The difficulties that we have identified in this challenge have been largely problems of translating technology for a new application.

When juvenile justice programs take on mental health screening and assessment, they face the same challenges any organization faces in adopting a new technology. Often they are largely unfamiliar with the technology—that is, the screening and assessment tools that psychologists have recently developed for use in identifying youths' mental health needs. The test developers have been successful to varying degrees in configuring their tests for use specifically in juvenile justice settings, so different tests are likely to serve the needs of particular juvenile justice programs better or less well. Thus juvenile justice administrators and their clinicians must learn something about those tests in order to make their choices.

Yet, well beyond this, they must consider ways in which their own program operations must undergo modification when these tests are put in place. Mental health screening and assessment involve not only the tests themselves, but a process for administering them, training people to use them, deciding what to do with their results, and putting in place procedures that people will follow (e.g., diversion, emergency referral) when mental health needs are identified in this way. Like desktop computers when they were first introduced into commercial offices, screening and assessment tools are likely to be no more effective than the people who operate them and the office's procedures for maximizing their use. Moreover, staff members who are responsible for screening for mental health needs become more aware of those needs, and this itself can have an effect on the way that staffers carry out their obligations toward youths, their agency, and their special role in society.

Part I of this book consists of four chapters that fully explore the essential points to be considered in decisions to implement mental health screening and assessment in juvenile justice settings. It has been written for a wide range of juvenile justice personnel: administrators, program managers, mental health professionals who consult to juvenile justice settings, policymakers (e.g., legislators and federal or state juvenile justice planners), and judges and lawyers involved in juvenile justice endeavors. This audience includes students in training for any of these roles. Just as we do not need to know the circuitry and binary processes inside our desktop computers in order to use them effectively, these users of screening and assessment technology do not need to know the psychometric intricacies of test development. But they do need to know why, when, and how to use the technology to its greatest advantage. This was the aim that we had in mind as we made decisions about content and style of communication in these chapters.

However, we also envisioned that much of what these chapters convey would be of special interest as well to psychologists and psychiatrists (and their trainees) who develop screening and assessment methods for adolescents generally and for use in juvenile justice systems specifically. Test construction begins with measurement theory and a thorough knowledge of what one wishes to measure. But these things alone are unlikely to produce a useful test if one is not thoroughly familiar with the demands of the settings in which the test will eventually be used. The desktop computer would have been a failure if it had been developed only as a precise tool, without careful thought to the everyday demands of the offices that it was destined to serve. Similarly, these chapters provide psychometricians with a detailed, inside look at the enormously complex circumstances that arise when screening and assessment tools are put to work in nonclinical settings, often staffed by persons without clinical or psychometric training, where issues of public safety and due process create a very different set of demands from those of the mental health clinic or adolescent hospital ward.

The remaining sections of the book—Parts II through VI—provide reviews of some of the most promising tools currently available for use in juvenile justice programs to identify youths' mental health needs. Most of the instruments are relatively new, having been developed since 1990—an era in which the mental health assessment of adolescents (and of delinquent youths specifically) has experienced a surge, due to recent advances in theories of adolescent psychopathology itself. They were selected from a larger number of instruments on the basis of a few criteria: (1) Their manuals and other materials are available from commercial test publishers; (2) they were developed specifically for, or are often encountered in use in, juvenile justice settings; (3) they were developed with procedures that satisfy basic criteria for test construction; and (4) they are backed by enough research to have shown at least good promise of their reliability and validity for use in juvenile justice programs.

Each review is relatively brief, yet sufficiently complete to provide a thorough understanding of the utility of the instrument. Each instrument review follows precisely the same outline, which is helpful if one is comparing the content and utility of various instruments. In most cases, the reviewers of the instruments are the instruments' authors themselves, assuring that the information on each one provides the best insight into its development and the most recent information on its validation. The authors of the reviews have necessarily had to use some technical terms in describing the evidence for reliability and validity of their instruments. But we have been especially careful to prepare the reader for this in Chapter 4, which offers basic definitions of those terms in a manner that does not require any training in psychometrics and focuses only on the useful meanings of the terms and concepts in everyday application of the instruments.

Finally, we commend those who have decided to read this book and to place it on their bookshelves as a professional resource. You are doing so with the prospect of undertaking the difficult task of developing mental health screening and assessment in juvenile justice programs. You are not alone. It is an undertaking that has recently been recognized nationwide as essential to the welfare of our youths and the fulfillment of the system's mandate for public safety.

THOMAS GRISSO
GINA VINCENT
DANIEL SEAGRAVE

Contents

PART I

Preparing for Screening and Assessment in Juvenile Justice Programs

CHAPTER I

Why We Need Mental Health Screening and Assessment in Juvenile Justice Programs

Thomas Grisso

At a recent meeting of the states' administrators of juvenile correctional programs, the host asked one of them, "In your opinion, what are the three most pressing issues in juvenile justice facilities today?" The administrator answered without hesitation, "Mental health, mental health, and mental health."

He would probably have given a different answer if he had been asked the question 15 years ago. In the early 1990s, when the nation was facing a wave of juvenile homicides (Blumstein, 1995; Zimring, 1998), the most important issue on everyone's minds—the public's and juvenile justice administrators' as well—was "public safety, public safety, and public safety." That issue is still pressing. Yet only a decade or so later, the juvenile crime rate has subsided (Blumstein, Rivara, & Rosenfeld, 2000) while the issue of young offenders' mental disorders has grown, stirring enormous public attention and governmental efforts to respond to what is widely identified as a crisis.

This crisis is represented by the very high prevalence of mental disorders among youths in the juvenile justice system, verified only recently by adequate research studies (e.g., Teplin, Abram, McClelland, Dulcan, & Mericle, 2002; Wasserman, McReynolds, Lucas, Fisher, & Santos, 2002). Responses to this news by policymakers, legislators, administrators, and clinical professionals have been wide-ranging, calling for changes on four major fronts.

1. Youth advocates have stressed the need for more effective diversion of youths to mental health programs, in lieu of juvenile justice processing (e.g., Cocozza & Skowyra, 2000). Some youths with mental disorders who are arrested on minor or first-time offenses are likely to be better served by receiving mental health services in the community than by entering the juvenile justice process.

2. For youths who do enter the juvenile justice system, emergency mental health services need to be improved. This will facilitate immediate response to crisis conditions such as suicide risk, prevent the escalation of symptoms before they reach critical levels, and address high-risk consequences of alcohol or drug dependence (Wasserman, Jensen, & Ko, 2003).

3. The increasing proportion of youths with mental disorders in juvenile justice programs requires the development of rehabilitation plans that do more than seek "correctional" adjustments or general rehabilitation. When youths with mental disorders are delinquent, their delinquencies themselves are often related in some way to their disorders. Thus juvenile justice programming must include better resources and clearer plans for addressing youths' mental disorders as part of their rehabilitation, aimed at reducing recidivism.

4. Finally, juvenile advocates call for better treatment planning and more focused follow-up for delinquent youths with mental disorders as they reenter the community after incarceration (Burns & Hoagwood, 2002).

Moving toward these objectives is a complex process that requires diverse knowledge and resources. But one thing is clear. All of these proposed responses begin with a single, important requirement: *The juvenile justice system must be able to identify youths with mental health needs as they enter and reenter the system.* Diversion, emergency responses, and long-range treatment planning can occur only if we have reliable ways to identify which youths have serious mental health needs, what those needs really are, and how they can be described in ways that promote rational responses to the youths' clinical conditions.

Identification and description of youths' mental health needs are the objectives of mental health screening and assessment. The purpose of this book is therefore to provide juvenile justice personnel with critical, up-to-date information on mental health screening and assessment methods, in order to improve the juvenile justice system's identification of youths with mental health needs, and ultimately to improve its response through therapeutic interventions.

This chapter provides an overview of (1) the prevalence of mental disorders among youths in the juvenile justice system, (2) the nature of the system's obligation to respond to their disorders, (3) an introduction to mental health screening and assessment, and (4) a review of the contexts in which mental health screening and assessment are needed in juvenile justice programs.

The remainder of Part I (Chapters 2, 3, and 4) focuses on three types of information essential for understanding and selecting tools for mental health screening and assessment in juvenile justice settings. Chapter 2 describes features of adolescent personality and psychopathology from a developmental perspective; it focuses especially on the nature of mental disorders in adolescence and the challenges faced by those who develop tools to identify them. Chapter 3 discusses the practical demands of juvenile settings (the juvenile justice context), which must be considered when one is selecting tools to meet mental health screening and assessment objectives. Chapter 4 explains the specific properties of instruments that one needs to understand in order to evaluate them and select certain instruments for use in juvenile justice facilities and programs. With all this information as a background, Parts II through VI review individual tools that offer the field's current best efforts to assist the juvenile justice system to fulfill its objective to identify youths with special mental health needs.

WHAT DO WE KNOW ABOUT THE PROBLEM?

Only in recent years have we had reliable evidence regarding the prevalence of mental disorders among youths in juvenile justice custody. Studies before the 1990s were often performed in a single facility, using small samples, vague definitions of youths' disorders, and measures with questionable reliability (Otto, Greenstein, Johnson, & Friedman, 1992). They reported widely varying prevalence rates for mental disorders, and thus offered little guidance for national or local policymaking. The more recent studies discussed below have used larger samples across several jurisdictions, with clearer definitions of mental disorders and better measures of adolescent psychopathology than were available formerly. Some of these studies have employed psychiatric diagnoses as their focus, while others have examined alternative definitions of youths' clinical conditions.

Common Diagnoses in Juvenile Justice Programs

Studies of the prevalence of psychiatric diagnoses in juvenile justice programs begin with definitions of the domain of mental disorders that appear to be relevant for juvenile justice populations and objectives. This in itself is an important contribution, because it provides a common language with which juvenile justice policy makers and practitioners can address the issue. A recent comprehensive review (Grisso, 2004) indicates that the following are the most common disorders assessed in major studies of youths' mental disorders in juvenile justice programs:

- *Mood disorders*, such as major depression, dysthymia, bipolar disorder, and other depressive or bipolar disorders.
- *Anxiety disorders*, such as obsessive–compulsive disorder and posttraumatic stress disorder.

- *Substance-related disorders*, including disorders (i.e., abuse and dependence) related to chronic and serious drug or alcohol use.
- *Disruptive behavior disorders*, such as oppositional defiant disorder and conduct disorder.
- *Thought disorders*, such as schizophrenia or adolescent precursors of psychotic conditions.

Literature on child disorders and policy in juvenile justice often reveals skepticism about the inclusion of the disruptive behavior disorders as psychiatric diagnoses. These disorders are largely defined and identified by the *Diagnostic and Statistical Manual of Mental Disorders*, fourth edition (DSM-IV; American Psychiatric Association, 1994) and its text revision (DSM-IV-TR; American Psychiatric Association, 2000) on the basis of the presence of a number of illegal and/or aggressive behaviors. Some argue that these categories are different from the rest of the disorders in that they identify youths simply as "troublesome," without any underlying psychological theory to suggest that they are "troubled" in the way that is implied in other categories of disorder (Lambert, Wahler, Andrade, & Bickman, 2001; Richters, 1996). Some evidence in Chapter 2 will challenge that view. But as shown in later discussions in this chapter, recent studies estimating the proportion of juvenile justice youths with mental disorders render this a moot issue, because almost all delinquent youths diagnosed with disruptive behavior disorders *also* manifest disorders in one or more of the other categories in the list above. Setting aside the disruptive behavior disorders as "not really mental disorders" would barely change the picture of mental health needs in the juvenile justice system, because only a small proportion of youths manifest disruptive behavior disorders alone.

Prevalence of Psychiatric Diagnoses

To date, the three best studies of the prevalence of mental disorders among youths in the juvenile justice system were performed in juvenile detention and corrections facilities by three groups of researchers: Teplin and colleagues (2002; Abram, Teplin, & McClelland, 2003), Atkins, Pumariega, and Rogers (1999), and Wasserman and colleagues (2002). All studies used the Diagnostic Interview Schedule for Children (DISC; Shaffer et al., 1996; Shaffer, Fisher, Lucas, Dulcan, & Schwab-Stone, 2000) (although not all employed the same version), which identifies youths meeting various diagnostic conditions according to DSM-IV criteria (American Psychiatric Association, 1994). All studies also employed large samples, including both boys and girls, with adequate proportions of black, Hispanic, and white non-Hispanic youths.

These studies did not all find the same prevalence for specific types of disorders, probably because they sampled youths in different juvenile justice contexts (e.g., pretrial detention vs. postadjudication correctional programs). But all were in agreement at the broadest level of analysis, in that the prevalence of mental disorders among youths in their studies was between 60% and 70%. That is, *about two-thirds of youths in pretrial detention or juvenile corrections programs in these studies met criteria for one or more of the psychiatric disorders* within the mood, anxiety, substance use, disruptive behavior, and thought disorders categories. This prevalence is about two to three times higher than the prevalence of the same disorders among U.S. youths in general (Costello et al., 1996; Kazdin, 2000; Roberts, Attkinson, & Rosenblatt, 1998).

In addition to the overall prevalence of psychiatric diagnoses among youths in juvenile justice facilities, these studies provide three findings of primary importance. First, they report very high rates of youths with "comorbidity" (i.e., youths who met criteria for more than one mental disorder). (See Chapter 2 for a discussion of the importance and frequency of comorbidity of disorders during adolescence.) Abram and colleagues (2003), for example, found that about one-half of youths in pretrial detention met criteria for two or more mental disorders. Second, the studies report fairly consistent ethnic differences, with general prevalence of mental disorders being highest for white non-Hispanic youths and lowest (although still well over 50%) for black youths in juvenile justice settings. Finally, in almost all studies that included both boys and girls, the prevalence of mental disorders among girls in juvenile justice facilities was higher than for boys. (See Grisso, 2004, for a more detailed analysis of these studies.)

Three Caveats

These recent studies are of enormous benefit in defining the scope of the problem. Applying this information to decisions about policy and practice, however, requires certain cautions.

First, none of these primary studies of youths in juvenile justice programs included mental retardation or attention-deficit/hyperactivity disorder, both of which are found with significant frequency among delinquent youths (Mash & Barkley, 2003). Addition of these disorders would probably increase the proportion with psychiatric disorders reported in this population, although perhaps not substantially (since they are often comorbid with other disorders that have already been included in the studies).

Second, the fact that youths qualify for a psychiatric diagnosis does not necessarily define the proportion of youths in juvenile justice programs who need psychiatric care (Grisso, 2004). Youths who meet criteria for a particular mental disorder are not all alike. Some will be functioning fairly well in every day life despite their disorder, while others may be extremely impaired. Among the latter, many jurisdictions identify a class of youths—sometimes called "seriously emotionally disturbed" or "seriously mentally ill"—who have chronic, persistent, and multiple disorders (Davis & Vander Stoep, 1997). They constitute a small proportion of youths who meet psychiatric diagnostic criteria (about 9% to 13% of youths in the community: Friedman, Katz-Levy, Manderscheid, & Sondheimer, 1996), but their prevalence in juvenile justice programs is about twice as high as in the general community (Cocozza & Skowyra, 2000). They share some diagnoses with other youths who are less seriously or chronically disturbed. A psychiatric diagnosis alone does not allow us to distinguish the degree of need across youths who are given that particular diagnosis. Thus, in addition to diagnosis, some index of severity of disorder is needed when one is defining the meaning of diagnostic prevalence rates for the juvenile justice system's task of responding to youths' disorders.

Finally, psychiatric diagnoses are not the only way to describe the mental health needs of youths in juvenile justice programs. There are at least three other approaches (Chapter 2 describes these in more detail). Some studies examine symptom conditions (e.g., feeling depressed or anxious, experiencing suicidal ideation) and symptom severity, without identifying specific psychiatric diagnoses. Others have developed alternative dimensions of psychopathology that do not parallel DSM psychiatric diagnoses. Still others use a "problem-oriented" perspective, focusing less on diagnosis and more on youths' actual problem behaviors in school, family, or other social contexts. All of these approaches have a helpful role to play, along with psychiatric diagnosis, in addressing various policy questions and case-by-case decisions relevant for the juvenile justice system's response to youths' mental health needs. All of them have formed the basis for various instruments described later in this volume.

WHY IS THE JUVENILE JUSTICE SYSTEM OBLIGATED TO IDENTIFY YOUTHS' MENTAL DISORDERS?

Knowing that the majority of youths in juvenile justice programs have various mental disorders does not lead automatically to any particular conclusion about the system's obligations to respond to their needs. Few would doubt that there is such an obligation, but there is less agreement regarding its nature and extent. Juvenile justice settings were not designed as sites for comprehensive psychological and psychiatric treatment of adolescents' mental disorders. On the other hand, some level and some type of "essential" services seem necessary. What is the scope of the juvenile justice system's obligation to respond to youths' mental health needs?

To determine this requires considering the juvenile justice system's purposes as defined by its social and legal mandates. Such an analysis (Grisso, 2004) reveals three primary reasons why the juvenile justice system is obligated to respond to the mental health needs of youths in its custody: (1) a *custodial* obligation, (2) a *due process* obligation, and (3) a *public safety* obligation. Those response obligations provide the foundation for the general obligation to identify youths' mental health needs through screening and assessment.

Custodial Obligation

The first obligation to respond to youths' mental health needs resides in the condition of custody itself. Juvenile justice custody often restricts youths' access to public health services for which they have a pressing need and that they would otherwise be eligible to receive. Adolescents typically depend upon adults for access to most mental health services. While youths are in juvenile justice custody, those adults are the youths' juvenile justice custodians. Therefore, especially in circumstances of incarceration (e.g., pretrial detention, secure juvenile corrections), the juvenile justice system is obligated to provide access to emergency or other essential mental health services when youths are in significant distress or have acute disabilities that require immediate attention.

This obligation begins with awareness. Parents or other caregivers may be charged with abuse or neglect not only because of harmful acts, but also because they have failed to recognize physical and psychological conditions that are detrimental to their children. Similarly, ignorance of a youth's suicidal potential does not absolve a juvenile justice facility from its responsibility as custodian when a youth commits suicide. The facility must show that it took reasonable steps to identify whether the youth might have been at risk of suicide.

Identification of youths' mental conditions is therefore an obligation of the juvenile justice system as a part of its custodial role. Note that the custodial argument for the system's obligation to identify youths' mental health needs increases under two conditions: (1) when youths are incarcerated, which decreases their access to community services; and (2) with regard to acute mental conditions, which create the need for emergency services to avoid imminent distress, psychological deterioration, and harm to the youth.

Due Process Obligation

For youths who are charged with delinquencies, the juvenile justice system has a mandate to assure that the legal process judges their responsibility for their alleged delinquencies fairly, and that the system does not abuse its discretion in deciding on penalties and rehabilitative measures when youths are found delinquent. All states have identified due process requirements in the adjudication of youths; these follow from a series of important federal constitutional protections for youths charged with crimes or delinquencies that can result in loss of liberty (e.g., *Kent v. United States*, 1966; *In re Gault*, 1967; *Fare v. Michael C.*, 1979).

Among the due process rights of youths in juvenile court adjudication are the right to avoid self-incrimination, the right to waive or obtain representation by an attorney, and various rights associated with the process by which courts hear evidence and make determinations of guilt and disposition (sentencing). In addition, most states' legislatures or courts have determined in recent years that youths must be competent to stand trial in delinquency cases (Bonnie & Grisso, 2000; Redding & Frost, 2002). That is, they must be able to understand the trial process, assist counsel in developing a defense, and make important decisions about the waiver of their constitutional rights.

All of these legal protections are designed to assure fairness in police questioning of youths, youths' interactions with their attorneys, and youths' participation in their trials. In addition, they focus on the capacities of youths themselves to make decisions during the juvenile justice process that may have far-reaching implications for their lives. Youths with mental disorders and developmental disabilities are especially at risk of incapacities in the process of their trials that might jeopardize their fair defense (Grisso, 1997, 2000; Grisso et al., 2003). Thus the system's obligation to protect youths' due process rights includes identification of mental conditions that might impair their ability to make decisions during their adjudication.

This obligation has implications at several levels of juvenile justice protection: (1) promoting laws that recognize the relevance of mental disorders for youths' participation in their trials; (2) providing methods to identify youths with mental disorders for whom the question of mental incompetence should be raised, and to determine when this question should be raised; and (3) assuring the availability of adequate assessment services to determine whether a youth's mental disorder actually impairs the youth's functioning in a way that threatens due process in the youth's adjudication.

Public Safety Obligation

The juvenile justice system is charged with exercising reasonable efforts to protect the public from harm. This mandate drives two primary functions of the juvenile justice system. One function is to protect the public from the immediate risk of harm by youths who are imminently dangerous to others. This sometimes requires placement of youths in secure facilities at the pretrial stage of their adjudication and/or after they are found delinquent. The second way in which the mandate is expressed is in the juvenile justice system's responsibility to reduce recidivism by providing rehabilitative services intended to decrease the likelihood that youths will reoffend in the long run or pose a longer-term risk of harm to others.

Youths in the juvenile justice system who have mental disorders are not known to present a substantially greater risk of violence or harm to others than other youths in the juvenile justice system do (for a review, see Grisso, 2004). But when youths have mental disorders, their disorders do play a role in their aggression (Connor, 2002). Their mental disorders influence whether, how, and under what circumstances their aggression is likely to be expressed. Therefore, reducing their aggression requires a response to their mental disorders, which begins with the ability to identify these disorders and the level of risk that they present (Borum, 2000).

The mandate has implications for two kinds of identification: (1) assessing youths' level of risk of violence; and (2) if that risk is high, assessing youths' mental disorders as factors that may be related to that risk and therefore require intervention. Moreover, identification must focus on at least two kinds of risk of harm and their relation to mental disorders: (1) imminent risks requiring an immediate response to protect others; and (2) longer-range risks requiring appropriate treatment of youths' mental disorders as part of general rehabilitation efforts to reduce aggressive recidivism.

WHAT ARE MENTAL HEALTH SCREENING AND ASSESSMENT?

Given the evidence for high prevalence of youths with mental disorders, and in light of clear mandates to identify youths' mental disorders, juvenile justice programs throughout the nation are employing two broad ways to fulfill those mandates, typically called "screening" and "assessment." The field's choice of these terms is potentially confusing, because the term "assessment" is often used in the behavioral sciences to refer to *any* type of measurement of psychological characteristics. So the following discussions use the term "identification" or "measurement" for the broader concept, while referring to "screening" and "assessment" as two ways to measure and identify youths' mental health needs and behaviors.

A second source of potential confusion is the lack of consensual definitions of "screening" and "assessment" in the current juvenile justice literature (e.g., Grisso & Underwood, in press; Wasserman et al., 2003). Although there is considerable overlap, in specific instances one writer's "screening" may be another writer's "assessment." The definitions provided later in this section strive to incorporate what does seem to be consistent across earlier descriptions, with commentary where there may be divergence.

A final source of confusion is in authors' labeling of instruments as "screening tools" or "assessment tools." As will become evident, the present discussion does not use the terms to refer to names or types of instruments, but to two different identification processes. Some tools may work better for one process or the other. But the mere fact that an instrument's author has called it a "screening tool" does not guarantee that it will serve all juvenile justice programs' needs for a screening process. "Screening" and "assessment" provide the context within which we can decide what types of instruments can best accomplish the objectives of these two broad types of identification.

Defining Screening and Assessment

If you were developing a process to identify youths' mental health needs as they enter the juvenile justice system, what would it look like? In one ideal image of that process, all youths entering a detention center or an intake probation office would receive an extensive interview by a psychiatrist or clinical psychologist, several psychological tests to describe their personalities and diagnose their mental disorders, a detailed assessment of their risk of aggression and suicide, and an analysis of problem areas in their everyday lives. This information would be used to produce an individualized view of their immediate, emergency mental health needs, as well as longer-range plans for rehabilitation.

This objective is, of course, impossible. In a given year in the United States, about 1.7 million youths are arrested on delinquency charges, and about 320,000 youths are admitted to pretrial detention facilities (Snyder & Sickmund, 1999). Performing such comprehensive mental health inquiries with every youth referred to intake probation or pretrial detention would be far outside even the most generous definition of juvenile justice systems' resources, not to mention the availability of doctoral-level professionals to perform such services. Even if this ideal were possible, it would not be "ideal" at all. It would be wasteful of our resources for caring for youths, because for many youths we simply do not need this degree or depth of clinical scrutiny in order to meet their needs adequately. Providing it to all would inevitably mean that there would be fewer resources left for treatment services to those who genuinely need them. Moreover, there are good reasons to avoid any greater level of intrusion in youths' and families' lives than is clearly justified by the benefits to youths and society (Grisso, 2004).

The notions of "screening" and "assessment" are ways to deal with this problem. They are conceptualized as two levels of identification of youths' mental health needs. Screening provides a type of economical identification applied to all youths, whereas assessment, following after screening, provides more extensive and individualized identification of mental health needs to those youths whose screening results suggest that it is warranted.

Screening has two defining characteristics. First, it is applied with *every youth* at entry into some part of the juvenile justice system—for example, with every youth within the first day after his or her entrance to a pretrial detention center, or at the first interview contact by an intake probation department after every referral to the juvenile court. Second, screening tends to focus on identifying conditions that signal the potential need for some sort of *immediate response*—for example, the need to consider placing a youth on suicide watch, the need to consider transfer to an alcohol/drug detoxification unit, or the potential need to obtain additional clinical information on the youth's immediate need for psychoactive medication,

In contrast, assessment is performed *selectively* with some youths and not others, often in response to signals (e.g., indications during screening) that suggest the need for a more individualized and thorough identification of mental health needs than can be provided by screening. The timing of assessment methods is more variable. Assessment may occur soon after first contact in response to screening information, in which case it may be aimed at determining whether an emergency situation truly exists, what the specific nature of the emergency is in this particular youth's case, and how best to deal with it. Or it may be delayed if screening does not suggest an emergency situation, focusing instead on comprehensive collection of data aimed at developing longer-range treatment planning or meeting judicial needs for information related to a forensic question.

It is worth noting that screening and assessment do not necessarily differ in the mental health conditions they attempt to identify. Both may seek to learn about the presence and severity of symptoms often associated with mental disorders (e.g., depressed mood, anxiety), the potential for problem behaviors (e.g., suicide, aggression), specific psychiatric diagnoses (e.g., major depressive disorder), or problem areas in a youth's life (e.g., school difficulties, family problems). Yet, as explained later, screening typically identifies these conditions far more tentatively than assessment; its results are valid for a shorter period of time; and it provides a less individualized perspective on the nature of a youth's mental health needs. The reasons for this will become clear as we examine screening and assessment practices more closely.

The Nature of Screening

Screening involves every youth at high-volume points in juvenile justice processing. Its purpose is to do an initial "sorting" of youths into at least two groups: one group that is very unlikely to have the characteristics one wishes to identify (e.g., mental health needs, risk of harm to others), and another that is at least somewhat more likely to have those characteristics. The screening process is similar to triage in medical settings, where incoming patients are initially classified (in triage, into three categories) according to their level of urgency. Like triage, screening is useful in systems that have limited resources and therefore cannot respond comprehensively or immediately to every individual's particular needs. In these circumstances, identifying those who may be most greatly and most urgently in need is not just a defensible position, but the best one.

For reasons described in Chapter 3, tools that are likely to be favored for screening processes require no more than 10–30 minutes of administration time by persons who do not have advanced training in the provision of mental health evaluations or treatment. Those that work best for these purposes are standardized and highly structured, providing the same process (e.g., interview questions) for every youth. But as we will see in Parts II and III, they vary considerably in their specifics. Some focus on symptoms, others on social problem areas, still others on one dimension or several dimensions of psychopathology, and yet others on the risk of suicidal or aggressive behaviors.

The brevity of screening methods requires a tradeoff. Most screening methods sort youths into categories, but are not intended to provide sufficient detail about a youth's condition to allow for an individualized decision about the youth's need for specific services. For example, a brief 10-minute screen that focuses on symptoms of mental or emotional distress (e.g., the Massachusetts Youth Screening Instrument) will sort youths into those with no remarkable symptoms and those with significant symptoms, but it will not provide diagnoses for youths in the latter group. A lengthier, 1-hour screen that focuses on psychiatric diagnoses (e.g., the DISC) will sort youths into diagnostic categories and indicate degree of impairment, providing a better basis for deciding on certain types of responses (such as hospitalization). The cost, however, is greater in time and resources than many screening situations can afford.

The value of a screening method is its identification of a group of youths who are more greatly at risk of mental health problems than those in the group that is "screened out." Although only some of the "screened-in" youths may have the acute disorders that the screening targets, the proportion in that group will be much greater than the proportion among all youths admitted to a facility. Screening therefore allows a juvenile justice system to focus its efforts and its scarce resources on a group containing a higher proportion of higher-need youths.

The Nature of Assessment

In contrast to screening, assessment strives for a more comprehensive or individualized picture of a youth. The assessment tools described in Parts IV and V are chosen to verify the presence or absence of mental health needs among "screened-in" youths, determine how disorders are manifested in these specific youths, and focus on recommendations for some specific intervention. The instruments used in assessment often involve longer administration times (e.g., more than 30 minutes), and they are often supplemented with clinical interviews and with past records from other agencies. They may or may not be performed by mental health professionals (child-specialized psychiatrists, psychologists, or psychiatric social workers), depending on their nature and scope, but they all require considerable training and expertise. All of the costs of assessment are compensated for by greater depth, breadth, and clarity than usually can be offered by tools more suited for screening.

The comparative advantages and costs of screening and assessment methods have resulted in their symbiotic use in many juvenile justice programs. Screening is often used to determine which subset of youths is most likely to need the more comprehensive yet costly assessment methods.

A Note about Short-Range and Long-Range Objectives

Screening and assessment tend to address different types of questions about youths' mental health needs. In general, screening is more appropriate for addressing short-range questions about youths' needs and behaviors, while assessment, with its more comprehensive and individualized focus, is better for longer-range questions. There are several reasons why this is so.

Screening focuses to a large extent on the condition of youths as they are entering the system, often within a day or two after their arrest and at the very beginning of the adjudicative process. In addition, a significant part of the reason for screening is to identify conditions that may need a response within the very near future—that is, within hours or days. Because of both these factors, screening at intake may provide information that reflects not only a youth's enduring traits and characteristics, but also the youth's thoughts and feelings that are stimulated by immediate events—the offenses he or she has just committed, stresses at home that may have contributed to the delinquent behavior, or emotions (such as fear or anger) associated with arrest and placement in a secure facility. Were the youth to be given the instrument in a few weeks, after those circumstances had passed, it would not be surprising to find somewhat different results.

In contrast, assessment often occurs later in a youth's stay in a particular juvenile justice setting, after the youth has had some time to become accustomed to the setting and circumstances. In addition, the more comprehensive methods used in assessment allow a clinician to focus on the youth's general behavior in everyday life and on his or her psychological history. This allows the clinician to begin to identify which of the youth's thoughts, feelings, and problems are typical of him or her across time and which are primarily reactions to the current situation.

As a consequence, screening can be expected to reflect the youth's current condition and an estimate of the youth's circumstances for the immediate future. Will the youth need suicide precautions tonight? Should we expect a high risk of aggression during the next week or two while the youth is in detention? But screening results are typically less reliable for making longer-range judgments about a youth's treatment needs. In contrast, assessments are typically better suited to guide us in making disposition recommendations, long-term placements among various secure treatment programs, and plans for implementing various community resources to maximize rehabilitation efforts.

VARIATIONS IN SCREENING AND ASSESSMENT AT "DOORWAYS" IN THE JUVENILE JUSTICE SYSTEM

We have described screening as occurring at entry points in the juvenile justice process. By "entry points" we do not mean merely the point of arrest and the beginning of custody, but the many "doorways" through which youths pass as they move through the juvenile justice process. In addition, screening at these doorways may lead to assessment at several different points in juvenile justice processing. Although there are variations across jurisdictions, it is convenient and fairly common to identify at least five of these doorways as potential points for screening and/or assessment: (1) probation intake, (2) pretrial detention, (3) preadjudication and disposition, (4) juvenile corrections reception, and (5) community reentry. These five doorways are briefly described here, and the differing demands they place on tools used for screening and assessment are discussed in more detail in Chapter 3.

Probation Intake

Most youths referred to juvenile courts on delinquency charges have their first contact with the system at their first meeting with a probation intake officer (who may be part of either the community's probation department or the juvenile court itself). Some probation intake programs use a mental health screening instrument with every youth at the first intake interview. The volume of youths at this point is very high, so that individualized clinical assessments of every youth by mental health professionals are typically not possible.

The most common purpose of screening at this doorway is the identification of those youths who are most likely to have special mental health needs, requiring more detailed clinical assessment or emergency referral for community mental health services. Sometimes mental health screening (or assessment) at this point results in diversion from the juvenile justice process, with probation intake officers using their discretion to arrange for appropriate community services for youths instead of filing the cases for delinquency adjudication.

Pretrial Detention

Some youths referred to the juvenile court are immediately admitted to pretrial detention centers, which may be either secure or nonsecure. This admission (especially to a secure facility) is based on a judgment that they present a significant danger to themselves or to others if they are not detained, or that they themselves may be in danger if they are not in protective temporary custody. Mental health screening at the front door of a detention center—often between 1 and 12 hours after admission—has become routine in many jurisdictions nationwide. Detention centers typically have a high volume of admissions and high turnover of residents, calling for relatively inexpensive screening devices. Their purpose is to identify youths who need emergency services (e.g., referral to inpatient psychiatric facilities, suicide watches, referral for substance use detoxification), a more complex assessment, or consultation with a mental health professional. Some of the most frequent mental health concerns at this point include the immediate toxic effects of heavy substance use just prior to admission, suicide potential, significant depression or anxiety, and anger that might increase the risk of harm to staff or other residents.

Preadjudication and Disposition

Either through intake or detention screening, or by other means, some youths may be identified as having significant mental disorders that could impair their ability to participate in their defense (i.e., their competence to stand trial) (Barnum, 2000; Grisso, 1998). In other cases, a youth may be petitioned for a juvenile court hearing to determine whether he or she should be transferred (waived) to criminal court for trial as an adult—a decision that often requires consideration of the youth's mental status, treatment potential, and risk of harm to others (Fagan & Zimring, 2000). These forensic questions often require evaluations by mental health professionals. They are called "forensic" questions because answering them requires courts' decisions based on the application of legal criteria. Forensic evaluations typically do not involve screening methods, but rather full assessments by specially trained forensic mental health professionals. These examiners often use tools designed to provide comprehensive information about a youth's personality and psychopathology (Part IV), but in addition they may employ specialized tools to assess risk for violence (Part V) or to examine characteristics relevant for specific forensic questions (Part VI).

When youths are adjudicated delinquent, courts must then determine the proper disposition for each case. Most courts have a wide range of dispositions, which can be classified broadly as including community placements or out-of-community secure and nonsecure placements. Community placements can range from a youth's own home to staff-secure residential group homes, and community placement conditions often include referral to community mental health services or special treatment programs for delinquent youths with mental disorders. Out-of-community placements range from low-security to high-security juvenile facilities or programs, usually administered by a state's juvenile corrections department. States vary widely in the availability of mental health treatment for youths in juvenile corrections facilities.

Most large juvenile courts have the resources to order clinical assessments for youths with mental disorders, and the need for such assessments must be taken into account by the judges deciding on these youths' proper dispositions. The focus of these assessments is on necessary treatment for the mental disorders—for the youths' welfare and the reduction of delinquency recidivism—as well as on the degree of security required in each youth's immediate placement, in order to protect the public and the youth.

Juvenile Corrections Reception

When youths' dispositions include placement with the state's department of youth corrections, this is another doorway that often requires screening and assessment. Many juvenile corrections programs operate reception centers, where youths reside for a few weeks in order to ascertain their appropriate placement within corrections programs. Entrance to such a reception center frequently includes a mental health screen. The purpose is less often to determine the need for further assessment, since the purpose of reception centers is typically to provide assessment for all youths to determine their individual needs and appropriate placement. Therefore, screening in these settings serves as a "first look" to determine whether there are needs that require immediate attention, while the youth embarks on an assessment process that often will take several weeks. Screening is often needed as well when the youth finally arrives at the juvenile corrections placement that has been recommended, in order to determine the youth's immediate emotional response to incarceration.

Community Reentry

Youths who have been placed in secure corrections programs are eventually returned to their communities—either to their homes or to community-based residential programs. Assessment is sometimes necessary to identify a youth's readiness for community reentry, and to develop plans for obtaining necessary mental health services as part of the reentry plan. Arrival at a community residential program is often an appropriate point for screening to assess the youth's immediate emotional reactions to returning to the community, especially if he or she is returning to stressful circumstances.

CONCLUSION: PREPARING TO DESIGN SCREENING AND ASSESSMENT PROGRAMS

Parts II through VI of this book review a wide range of tools that are currently used in juvenile justice settings for screening and assessment of mental health needs and aggression risk. These tools are not interchangeable. Instruments in one category have very different purposes from those in another category, and even instruments within a category have their own unique features that may make them more or less suitable for specific settings and purposes.

Selecting among these instruments therefore requires an understanding of the reasons for wanting to evaluate youths' mental health needs. In addition, administrators and clinicians need to take into account a variety of factors with which to weigh the quality and feasibility of the available instruments. The three chapters in the remainder of Part I provide information to assist in the process of evaluating, choosing, and implementing tools for use in juvenile justice settings for screening and assessment of mental health needs and aggression risk.

Chapter 2 provides basic concepts in developmental psychopathology that are important to consider in weighing the value of screening and assessment. What makes a "child" screening or assessment tool different from an "adult" tool, and why are instruments designed for adults usually inappropriate in juvenile justice settings? What does one need to know about types of adolescent psychopathology in order to assure that an instrument is measuring the mental health concepts one wants to measure? What are the limits of screening and assessment, in light of the complex nature of adolescent psychopathology? And what (if anything) is different about adolescent psychopathology in delinquent populations, including its relation to aggression?

Chapter 3 focuses on the context for screening and assessment, especially the legal, policy, and practical demands encountered in developing screening and assessment methods and selecting appropriate instruments. From an administrator's perspective, any strategies for evaluating youths' mental health needs must be guided by law, policy, and agency objectives; constraints associated with staffing and budget resources; the specific population of youths within the facility or facilities; and the potential uses of information about youths' mental disorders. Screening and assessment occur in the context of a complex, practical set of circumstances, and this context places particular demands on instruments—demands that are somewhat different from those in other settings where psychological and psychiatric evaluations are performed. Some tools meet these pragmatic and legal demands better than others, and these matters play a significant role in one's decisions about their use.

Chapter 4 reviews the technical properties of screening and assessment tools, as well as important decisions about the screening and assessment process that must guide one's choice of instruments. In selecting methods, what does one need to know about how screening and assessment tools are developed? What are the important indicators of a method's dependability and accuracy, and how dependable and accurate does an instrument have to be in order to be useful for various specific purposes? Given that there are no perfect screening or assessment tools, how does one weigh the balance of their strengths and limitations when deciding among them?

The importance of being careful to choose the right tools and procedures for the job cannot be overemphasized. In these days when juvenile justice programs are urgently seeking assistance in dealing with the system's three most pressing issues—"mental health, mental health, and mental health"—there may be a tendency to reach for the first option that gets one's attention. Yet one can argue that ineffective measures can be worse than no measures at all, given the waste of resources that could be used to meet other important needs of youths. Proper identification of youths' mental health needs and risk of harm requires taking the time to make careful selections and to position the right tools within an effective screening and assessment process.

REFERENCES

Abram, K. M., Teplin, L., & McClelland, G. M. (2003). Comorbid psychiatric disorders in youth in juvenile detention. *Archives of General Psychiatry, 60,* 1097–1108.

American Psychiatric Association. (1994). *Diagnostic and statistical manual of mental disorders* (4th ed.). Washington, DC: Author.

American Psychiatric Association. (2000). *Diagnostic and statistical manual of mental disorders* (4th ed., text rev.). Washington, DC: Author.

Atkins, D., Pumariega, W., & Rogers, K. (1999). Mental health and incarcerated youth: I. Prevalence and nature of psychopathology. *Journal of Child and Family Studies, 8,* 193–204.

Barnum, R. (2000). Clinical and forensic evaluation of competence to stand trial in juvenile defendants. In T. Grisso & R. Schwartz (Eds.), *Youth on trial: A developmental perspective on juvenile justice* (pp. 193–224). Chicago: University of Chicago Press.

Blumstein, A. (1995). Youth violence, guns, and the illicit drug industry. *Journal of Criminal Law and Criminology, 86,* 10–36.

Blumstein, A., Rivara, F., & Rosenfeld, R. (2000). The rise and decline of homicide— and why. *Annual Review of Public Health, 21,* 505–541.

Bonnie, R., & Grisso, T. (2000). Adjudicative competence and youthful offenders. In T. Grisso & R. Schwartz (Eds.), *Youth on trial: A developmental perspective on juvenile justice* (pp. 73–103). Chicago: University of Chicago Press.

Borum, R. (2000). Assessing violence risk among youth. *Journal of Clinical Psychology, 56,* 1263–1288.

Burns, B., & Hoagwood, K. (Eds.). (2002). *Community treatment for youth: Evidence-based interventions for severe emotional and behavioral disorders.* New York: Oxford University Press.

Cocozza, J., & Skowyra, K. (2000). Youth with mental health disorders: Issues and emerging responses. *Juvenile Justice, 7*(1), 3–13.

Connor, D. (2002). *Aggression and antisocial behavior in children and adolescents: Research and treatment.* New York: Guilford Press.

Costello, E., Angold, A., Burns, H., Stangle, D., Tweed, D., Erkanli, A., et al. (1996). The Great Smoky Mountains Study of Youth: Goals, design, methods and the prevalence of DSM-III-R disorders. *Archives of General Psychiatry, 53,* 1129–1136.

Davis, M., & Vander Stoep, A. (1997). The transition to adulthood for youth who have serious emotional disturbance: Developmental transition and young adult outcomes. *Journal of Mental Health Administration, 24,* 400–427.

Fagan, J., & Zimring, F. (Eds.). (2000). *The changing borders of juvenile justice.* Chicago: University of Chicago Press.

Fare v. Michael C., 442 U.S. 707 (1979).

Friedman, R., Katz-Levy, J., Manderscheid, R., & Sondheimer, D. (1996). Prevalence of serious emotional disturbance in children and adolescents. In R. Manderscheid & M. Sonnenschein (Eds.), *Mental health in the United States, 1996* (pp. 71–89). Rockville, MD: U.S. Department of Health and Human Services.

Grisso, T. (1997). The competence of adolescents as trial defendants. *Psychology, Public Policy, and Law, 3,* 3–32.

Grisso, T. (1998). *Forensic evaluation of juveniles.* Sarasota, FL: Professional Resource Press.

Grisso, T. (2000). Forensic clinical evaluations related to waiver of jurisdiction. In J. Fagan & F. Zimring (Eds.), *The changing borders of juvenile justice* (pp. 321–352). Chicago: University of Chicago Press.

Grisso, T. (2004). *Double jeopardy: Adolescent offenders with mental disorders.* Chicago: University of Chicago Press.

Grisso, T., Steinberg, L., Woolard, J., Cauffman, E., Scott, E., Graham, S., et al. (2003). Juveniles' competence to stand trial: A comparison of adolescents' and adults' capacities as trial defendants. *Law and Human Behavior, 27,* 333–363.

Grisso, T., & Underwood, L. (in press). *Screening and assessing mental health and substance use disorders among youth in the juvenile justice system: A resource guide for practitioners*. Washington, DC: U.S. Department of Justice, Office of Juvenile Justice and Delinquency Prevention.

In re Gault, 387 U.S. 1 (1967).

Kazdin, A. (2000). Adolescent development, mental disorders, and decision making of delinquent youths. In T. Grisso & R. Schwartz (Eds.), *Youth on trial: A developmental perspective on juvenile justice* (pp. 33–65). Chicago: University of Chicago Press.

Kent v. United States, 383 U.S. 541 (1966).

Lambert, E., Wahler, R., Andrade, A., & Bickman, L. (2001). Looking for the disorder in conduct disorder. *Journal of Abnormal Psychology, 110*, 110–123.

Mash, E., & Barkley, R. (Eds.). (2003). *Childhood psychopathology* (2nd ed.). New York: Guilford Press.

Otto, R., Greenstein, J., Johnson, M., & Friedman, R. (1992). Prevalence of mental disorders among youth in the juvenile justice system. In J. Cocozza (Ed.), *Responding to the mental health needs of youth in the juvenile justice system* (pp. 7–48). Seattle, WA: National Coalition for the Mentally Ill in the Criminal Justice System.

Redding, R., & Frost, J. (2002). Adjudicative competence in the modern juvenile court. *Virginia Journal of Social Policy and Law, 9*, 353–410.

Richters, J. (1996). Disordered views of aggressive children: A late twentieth century perspective. In C. Ferris & T. Grisso (Eds.), *Understanding aggressive behavior in children* (pp. 208–223). New York: New York Academy of Sciences.

Roberts, R., Attkinson, C., & Rosenblatt, A. (1998). Prevalence of psychopathology among children and adolescents. *American Journal of Psychiatry, 155*, 715–725.

Shaffer, D., Fisher, P., Dulcan, M., Davies, M., Piacentini, J., Schwab-Stone, M., et al. (1996). The NIMH Diagnostic Interview Schedule for Children Version 2.3 (DISC-2.3): Description, acceptability, prevalence rates, and performance in the MECA study. *Journal of the American Academy of Child and Adolescent Psychiatry, 35*, 865–877.

Shaffer, D., Fisher, P., Lucas, C., Dulcan, M., & Schwab-Stone, M. (2000). The NIMH Diagnostic Interview Schedule for Children Version IV (DISC-IV): Description, differences from previous versions, and reliability of some common diagnoses. *Journal of the American Academy of Child and Adolescent Psychiatry, 39*, 28–37.

Snyder, H., & Sickmund, M. (1999). *Juvenile offenders and victims: 1999 national report*. Washington, DC: Office of Juvenile Justice and Delinquency Prevention.

Teplin, L., Abram, K., McClelland, G., Dulcan, M., & Mericle, A. (2002). Psychiatric disorders in youth in juvenile detention. *Archives of General Psychiatry, 59*, 1133–1143.

Wasserman, G. A., Jensen, P. S., & Ko, S. J. (2003). Mental health assessments in juvenile justice: Report on the Consensus Conference. *Journal of the American Academy of Child and Adolescent Psychiatry, 42*, 751–761.

Wasserman, G. A., McReynolds, L., Lucas, C., Fisher, P., & Santos, L. (2002). The Voice DISC-IV with incarcerated male youths: Prevalence of disorder. *Journal of the American Academy of Child and Adolescent Psychiatry, 41*, 314–321.

Zimring, F. (1998). *American youth violence*. New York: Oxford University Press.

CHAPTER 2

A Developmental Perspective on Adolescent Personality, Psychopathology, and Delinquency

Gina Vincent
Thomas Grisso

Identifying the mental health needs of youths in the juvenile justice system requires a basic understanding of the nature of mental disorders in adolescents, as well as the relation of such disorders to delinquency. This is not as simple a task as it might seem, because only in recent years have developmental psychologists and psychiatrists become fully aware of the ways in which adolescents' disorders are fundamentally different from those of adults. In this chapter, we briefly review some of those differences and examine the relation between mental disorders and delinquency. This background will be useful not only in deciding on the disorders for which one should screen and assess, but in understanding that screening and assessment can be very challenging, given the complex nature of youths' mental disorders.

WHAT IS DEVELOPMENTALLY DIFFERENT ABOUT MENTAL DISORDERS OF ADOLESCENCE?

Child clinical professionals have long been discontent with the mental health professions' way of defining mental disorders in adolescence. In fact, experts in the psychopathology of children and adolescents tell us that "there is little professional consensus on how to define psychopathology [in adolescence]" (Ingram & Price, 2001, p. 6). Thus far, the experts in child clinical psychopathology have not been able to find sets of symptoms that neatly go together and distinguish specific types of disorders.

Moreover, using adult diagnostic categories has been very unsatisfactory, for reasons that will become apparent later in this chapter. These discontents have led to a relatively new perspective called "developmental psychopathology" (Cicchetti, 1984, 1990; Cicchetti & Cohen, 1995; Cicchetti & Rogosch, 2002; Rutter & Garmezy, 1983; Sroufe & Rutter, 1984). Developmental psychopathology is not just the study of psychopathology in childhood and adolescence. It tries to describe how youths' mental disorders emerge and change in a developmental context—how it is guided by normal biological, cognitive, emotional, and social development during childhood, adolescence, and adulthood. In this perspective, adolescent disorders are not presumed to be simply "older" versions of childhood disorders; nor are they presumed to be "immature" versions of disorders of adulthood. They are examined in combination with the ways in which all adolescents grow and develop, and which make them different from adults (Steinberg, 2002).

Some of the concepts and findings that this perspective has produced are very helpful for grasping aspects of mental disorders in adolescence that complicate the screening and assessment of those disorders. These concepts include (1) age relativity, (2) discontinuity, (3) comorbidity, and (4) demographic differences.

Age Relativity

Age makes a difference in what kinds of behaviors or emotions we identify as "symptoms" of disorder. Many behaviors, emotions, or thoughts can be symptoms of disorders at one age, but not at another age. For example, a temper tantrum is not considered a sign of disorder for a preschooler, but it might be when seen in a 10th-grade classroom. Similarly, many behavioral, emotional, or cognitive characteristics of mental disorders in adults are relatively "normal" features among adolescents (Mash & Dozois, 2003). In other words, behaviors, emotions, or thoughts that are adaptive and "normal" at one age may be maladaptive and "abnormal" at another. As a consequence, developmental psychopathologists emphasize that characteristics can be considered symptoms of disorder only if they deviate from the "average" behavior of peers at a particular developmental stage, and if they result in life problems in the context of this developmental period (e.g., Cicchetti & Rogosch, 2002).

A good demonstration of the problem of age relativity is psychopathic personality disorder. This disorder is said to involve antisocial attitudes together with callousness and the absence of feelings of guilt, and it has been well defined in adults for many years (Hare, 2003). Recently the mental health field has used the concept to try to identify the disorder in children (e.g., Frick & Hare, 2001; Lynam, 1997; Murrie & Cornell, 2000) and adolescents (e.g., Andershed, Kerr, Stattin, & Levander, 2002; Forth, Kosson, & Hare, 2003).

But problems have arisen in these efforts, because several of the symptoms of psychopathy look like various attitudes and behaviors that are fairly common at various stages of child or adolescent development (Edens, Skeem, Cruise, & Cauffman, 2001; Hart, Watt, & Vincent, 2002; Seagrave & Grisso, 2002). For example, when youths are asked to respond to instruments said to measure psychopathic personality disorder, some degree of behavioral symptoms—impulsiveness, irresponsibility, stimulation seeking—is simply more common in adolescents than in adults (Vincent, 2002). Similarly, an egocentric (self-centered) attitude and an apparent lack of guilt feelings are fairly common among children or adolescents developing typically, but they are prominent symptoms of psychopathy in adulthood.

This problem of age relativity of symptoms somewhat complicates the identification of mental disorders in youths. One of the main lessons for screening and assessment is that adult measures of mental disorders are unlikely to be of much use with adolescents, whether they are evaluated in clinical settings or in juvenile justice programs. Screening and assessment tools must be developed specifically for adolescents, and often they must be concerned with whether so-called "symptoms" mean the same thing for younger adolescents as for older adolescents.

Discontinuity

If an individual has a mental disorder this week, or a level of symptoms that is very serious, what's the likelihood that this will continue to be the case for the next few weeks? Or the next few months? Or next year? When we obtain a diagnosis for a youth at a given time, there is a tendency for us to presume that the disorder is likely to continue into the future (especially if it is not treated), because this is what usually happens during adulthood. But with adolescents, the picture is a bit more complicated.

If untreated, some childhood disorders tend to continue into adulthood, whereas others tend not to (Mash & Dozois, 2003). Some mental disorders arise early in life and change greatly in nature or disappear altogether as a result of both biological and social developmental processes (Cicchetti & Cohen, 1995; Kazdin & Johnson, 1994; Pennington & Ozonoff, 1991). It is possible, then, for a child who appears to be prone to serious anxiety or depression to develop into an adult who does not meet criteria for anxiety or mood disorders (even without treatment). Alternatively, mental disorders may arise in adulthood without any obvious symptoms earlier in life. For instance, a person who appears relatively "normal" in adolescence could be diagnosed with bipolar disorder or schizophrenia in adulthood.

Two concepts are used to express the complex pathways to development and remission of disorders among children and adolescents (Cicchetti & Rogosch, 2002). "Equifinality" means that different pathways can lead to the same outcome. Thus, as a group, adolescents with serious depression will not always have had the same problems when they were younger, but might have had any of two or three different earlier disorders. "Multifinality" refers to the notion that similar starting points can lead to different disorders. For example, among youths with inhibited, introverted personality styles, some may progress to psychotic disorders in adulthood, while others will progress to anxiety disorders or avoidant personality disorder (Kagan, Resnick, Clark, Snidman, & Garcia-Coll, 1984).

Continuity is more likely for some childhood disorders than for others. For example, mental retardation or disorders with a basis in brain dysfunction are more likely to continue across the developmental life span, whereas mood disorders and anxiety disorders are less continuous (Albano, DiBartolo, Heimberg, & Barlow, 1995; Hammen & Rudolph, 2003).

Another kind of "discontinuity" in adolescence pertains not to the course of disorders, but to the instability of emotional states in youths. On average, adolescents' emotions tend to be more changeable from day to day; they react more readily to immediate situations that they are experiencing.

It is not difficult to imagine the problems these matters of discontinuity present for screening and assessment. With adults, if we identify a disorder at a particular time, we have good reason to believe that if they experience recurring symptoms in the future, these will be symptoms of a disorder much like the one they manifested earlier. With adolescents in juvenile justice settings, however, today's disorder is not necessarily the disorder we will see next year when some of these youths return to the detention center. We may be seeing the youths at a different stage in their development, and the way the disorder looks may have been transformed to some degree by that new stage. In addition, the greater instability in youths' emotions and behavior from week to week means that we must be careful not to presume that how the youths looked a few weeks ago at intake screening necessarily describes them well today. Because data on youths are likely to have a shorter "shelf life," periodic reevaluation is required if we are to have a current or up-to-date view of the youths' problems.

Comorbidity

As noted in Chapter 1, about one-half of youths in the juvenile justice system meet criteria for *two or more* mental disorders (Marsteller et al., 1997; Teplin, Abram, McClelland, Dulcan, & Mericle, 2002). Clinicians sometimes refer to this phenomenon as "comorbidity." They mean simply that a youth meets criteria for more than one disorder. Moreover, those who study youths' disorders find that some disorders tend to go together: When you see one of them, you often see the other (Achenbach, 1995; Caron & Rutter, 1991).

Comorbidity can occur at any point in the life span, but it is particularly evident during childhood and adolescence. One review found that the presence of depression among community youths increased the likelihood of receiving some additional diagnosis by 20 times (Angold & Costello, 1993). Depression and conduct disorder (CD) have high comorbidity among adolescents (see Hammen & Rudolph, 2003, for a review). About 30% to 50% of adolescents with attention-deficit/hyperactivity disorder (ADHD) meet criteria for oppositional defiant disorder (ODD) or CD in adolescence (Barkley, 1998). Substance use diagnoses occur at very high rates for youths with CD, anxiety disorders, and depression (Neighbors, Kempton, & Forehand, 1992; Richards, 1996; Teplin et al., 2002).

Why is comorbidity of disorders so common during childhood and adolescence? One possibility is that our categories for identifying youths' mental disorders simply do not work very well. But it's also possible that these frequent overlaps in symptoms and disorders are "real"—in other words, that adolescent disorders are just more "disorderly." Developmental psychology provides good reasons to believe that conditions such as depressed mood and anxiety may be almost the same thing in young children, then begin to separate during adolescence, and finally become more distinct symptoms in adulthood (Hinden, Compas, Achenbach, & Howell, 1997; Lilienfeld, Waldman, & Israel, 1994). Trying to find better ways to separate depressed mood and anxiety in adolescence may be an instance of searching for something that doesn't actually exist.

The implications of comorbidity for screening and assessment are fairly clear. Measures for adolescents need to be open to the possibility of multiple mental health problems, not aimed at locating "the" problem for a given youth. In addition, we cannot assume that youths scoring high on mental disorder X will all look alike. Those who score high on mental disorder X, but *also* on mental disorders Y or Z, will look somewhat different from those who score high on X alone.

Demographic Differences

The prevalence of mental disorders, and the ways they evolve and appear, sometimes vary according to race or ethnicity, gender, or environmental conditions. How mental health problems emerge and take shape seems to be influenced by the interaction of developmental processes with social factors (Mash & Dozois, 2003). For example, boys and girls develop in different social contexts that may contribute to gender-based differences in symptoms of a particular disorder. Similarly, during typical development, youths of different ethnicities may be inclined to develop somewhat different personality characteristics because of the different social contexts in which they grow up (Murray, Smith, & West, 1989).

Gender differences in the prevalence of psychiatric diagnoses are fairly well documented among youths. Especially in clinical populations, boys are more likely to be diagnosed with what are often called "externalizing" disorders (where mental health problems result in "external" actions, often aggressive), such as CD and ADHD (Szatmari, Boyle, & Offord, 1989); girls are more likely to be diagnosed with "internalizing" disorders, such as depression and anxiety disorders (e.g., Hartung & Widiger, 1998; Offord et al., 1987). Girls are also more likely to be diagnosed with comorbid disorders (Loeber &

Keenan, 1994). These differences seem to increase with age. Boys show more difficulties during childhood and early adolescence, while girls develop more problems in middle and later adolescence (Offord et al., 1987).

Recent studies in juvenile detention centers consistently report higher rates of almost all types of mental disorders and mental health problems, including anger, among girl offenders than boy offenders (e.g., Abram, Teplin, & McClelland, 2003; Grisso, Barnum, Fletcher, Cauffman, & Peuschold, 2001). However, since girls are still less likely than boys to be referred to detention facilities, detained girls' higher rate of mental health problems is probably caused by the fact that those girls who do get referred to detention are the most difficult or disturbed.

There is not a great deal of information about possible racial differences in mental health problems among youths (Cauffman & Grisso, in press; Isaacs, 1992). In the general population, a study that examined over 1,000 youths in rural North Carolina reported that about 20% of both white non-Hispanic and black youths met criteria for one or more disorders (Angold et al., 2002). White non-Hispanic youths had higher rates of depressive disorders, ODD, and anxiety disorders than did black youths. In general, few differences in rates of mental health referrals have been found between black and Hispanic youths after economic factors have been controlled for.

Concerning youths with mental disorders in juvenile justice samples, Teplin and colleagues' (2002) study of detained juveniles in Cook County, Illinois, reported higher rates of diagnoses among white non-Hispanic males than black males (for most disorders) and Hispanic males (for some disorders). Using samples of youths from several points of the juvenile justice systems in Massachusetts and California, Grisso and colleagues (2001) found that compared to black males, white non-Hispanic males were more likely to present with substance abuse and anger symptoms, and Hispanic males were more likely to exhibit depressed and anxious symptoms. Among girls, white non-Hispanic females presented with more substance abuse and trauma symptoms than black females did, and Hispanic females were more likely than black females to endorse somatic complaints and suicidal ideation.

Socioeconomic status is related, either directly or indirectly, to the prevalence of child and adolescent disorders. Mental health problems are overrepresented among the poor. Estimates indicate that 20% of inner-city youths have some form of impairment (Institute of Medicine, 1989; Schteingart, Molnar, Klein, Lowe, & Hartmann, 1995).

These demographic differences raise serious questions for administrators who are responsible for selecting and using screening and assessment tools. For example, are gender and ethnic differences due to actual tendencies for certain disorders to be more or less prevalent among certain groups? Or are they due to gender- or ethnic-based errors in the screening and assessment tools? It is possible that the higher rates of psychological disturbances among girls than boys in the community reflect girls' tendency on average to be more open in revealing their problems. Differences in rates for various ethnic groups might reflect "real" differences, or they might mean that something about an instrument's items has a biasing effect or lessens the instrument's ability to identify problems in the same way across ethnic groups. In the community, mental health problems do not appear to differ remarkably among youths from different racial groups. With respect to mental disorder in juvenile justice settings, however, large differences can arise as a product of differences in arrest patterns. Currently the field does not have sufficient information to sort out these possibilities for juvenile justice screening and assessment. But administrators should pay close attention to information that is (or is not) available in later chapters regarding the performance of specific instruments across gender and ethnic groups.

Summary of Developmental Differences

Many developmental factors complicate the identification of psychiatric disorders and mental health problems during childhood and adolescence. The concept of age relativity warns us that adolescent behaviors that appear to be "symptoms" of mental disorders can represent typical development at one stage and atypical conditions at another. Discontinuity in symptoms and disorders causes complications in making inferences about the cause or course of a youth's condition from diagnoses obtained at an earlier point during childhood or adolescence. There will also be greater variability among adolescents than adults in the projected meaning of the diagnosis. In some youths, the disorder will not persist; in others, it will; and in still others, initial disorders will develop into different disorders. This warns us that we can be less certain about the long-range consequences of many disorders in adolescents than in adults.

Comorbidity plays an important role in our definition of youths' mental disorders. The mere fact that a youth has received a particular diagnosis does not necessarily provide a meaningful guide to mental health needs, because youths with diagnoses tend to manifest any variety of other disorders. Moreover, considerable diagnostic "overlap" challenges our ability to define discrete treatment or rehabilitation needs according to particular diagnoses.

Finally, the higher rate of mental disorders among girls and white non-Hispanics in juvenile justice programs raises important questions. The literature warns us that in selecting screening and assessment tools for mental health problems in juvenile justice settings, we must consider the validity of their use across gender, racial, and age groups.

HOW CAN WE BEST DEFINE PSYCHOPATHOLOGY AMONG ADOLESCENTS?

Our predominant system for identifying and classifying mental disorders is the *Diagnostic and Statistical Manual of Mental Disorders* (DSM), the most recent versions of which are the DSM-IV and DSM-IV-TR (American Psychiatric Association, 1994, 2000). The DSM system deals with the classification of child and adolescent disorders in two broad ways. First, it offers a number of "disorders usually first diagnosed in infancy, childhood, or adolescence," organized into groups such as mental retardation, learning and communication disorders, pervasive developmental disorders, and attention-deficit and disruptive behavior disorders. Second, the system offers hundreds of categories for other conditions that have similar criteria for youth and adults, for the most part. Some examples of these diagnoses are substance-related, psychotic, mood, anxiety, and personality disorder categories. The most important of these categories, for purposes of youths' mental health needs in the juvenile justice system, have been outlined in Chapter 1. The DSM system relies on the presence or absence of specific criteria (behaviors, thoughts, or emotions) to satisfy the requirements for classifying a youth's symptoms as suggesting a particular disorder.

Although the DSM system is the best that we have for categorizing youths' disorders, it has some important limits for reasons noted earlier. Successive versions of the DSM system have sought to improve the applications of the criteria to children and adolescents. Nevertheless, mental health professionals and researchers who study, diagnose, and treat disorders of childhood and adolescence claim that the assumptions at the heart of the DSM classification system continue to result in difficulties when this system is applied to adolescents.

Despite these limits, there can be no doubt that DSM diagnoses play an exceptionally important role in the provision of mental health services to adolescents. For example, much research that tells us "what works" in treating adolescents' mental disorders has used DSM diagnoses in forming the research groups for whom better or poorer success is found. Therefore, such diagnoses become important in deciding which treatments to provide. Moreover, DSM diagnoses are the "gold standard" for organized mental health care; thus government programs that provide funding for mental health services will often require DSM diagnoses to identify cases eligible for reimbursement.

Yet there are reasons to examine additional ways of describing or identifying youths' mental health problems. Knowledge of a youth's DSM diagnosis does not necessarily capture some of what we need to know about the youth in order to meet his or her mental health needs. Therefore, other approaches have arisen for thinking about youths' psychopathology, and all of them can be used alongside DSM diagnoses to provide a more complete picture of youths' mental health problems. Developmental psychopathology offers us at least three of these additional approaches.

Symptom Condition Approach

One of these approaches is to describe youths according to "symptoms" (e.g., depressed mood, anxiety, suicide ideation) or "symptom severity," regardless of their specific psychiatric diagnoses. For example, depressed mood or angry thoughts can be examined as symptoms in and of themselves, without making assumptions about their relation to a DSM diagnosis. This is the focus of some screening instruments that do not attempt diagnosis, but simply try to identify whether a youth is manifesting troubling symptoms that increase the risk of poor functioning or an underlying disorder. The approach has value for those limited objectives. But it is not satisfactory as a sole way to describe and identify child psychopathology (Mash & Dozois, 2003).

Dimensional Approaches

A second alternative approach is to describe youths according to "conceptual dimensions" of psychopathology that comprise behaviors, feelings, or thoughts related to poor functioning, but are different from conventional psychiatric diagnostic categories. Generally, the use of this approach to develop an instrument begins with a number of items referring to various symptoms of behavioral, emotional, or mental disturbances. These symptoms are typically "clustered," via statistical techniques, into scales that define broad dimensions and narrow subdimensions of child psychopathology. Instruments using this approach provide overall ratings of an individual's level of severity within each dimension in the instrument, rather than supporting a conclusion that the youth has a particular DSM disorder.

    A good example of this is a system developed by Achenbach (1993; Achenbach & Edelbrock, 1984), represented by a family of measures called the Achenbach System of Empirically Based Assessment (see Chapter 11). The measures in this assessment system were formed by grouping problem behaviors and feelings, via statistical techniques, to determine the structures that best fit their appearance across large samples of youths. This resulted in eight dimensions (e.g., anxious–depressed, attention problems, aggressive behavior), further grouped into two more global dimensions called "externalizing" (undercontrolled, outer-directed) and "internalizing" (overcontrolled, inner-directed). Youths are not classified into categories in this system. Instead, psychopathology is identified according to the elevation of scores on the various dimensions or the two broader concepts. Dimensional systems like Achenbach's identify degrees and types of disturbance, as well as patterns of manifestation, without the use of discrete categories and presumptions regarding an underlying disease process.

Problem-Oriented Approaches

The third alternative is a "problem-oriented" approach, which identifies areas of strengths and impairments in practical, everyday functioning through behavioral observations and standardized tests. Often the information about a youth is organized according to common areas of activity for adolescents, such as family relations, peer relations, school functioning, work, leisure activities, and so forth. Level of functioning is typically expressed on scales that measure functioning according to the degree of impairment relative to same-age peers. This approach tends also to point out a youth's strengths, or areas in which the youth is functioning in a more satisfactory manner. Performance-based approaches provide information that can differentiate between youths with the same diagnoses or similar symptoms (Frick, 2000; Kazdin & Kagan, 1994). An interesting feature of this approach is that it allows youths' problems to be examined both individually and as a function of the environment's response to the youths.

In summary, the instruments encountered later, especially in Parts II through IV, tend to be organized around any of the four approaches we have just reviewed: They provide either (1) diagnoses, (2) symptom descriptions without diagnostic classifications, (3) a picture of youths' disorders based on dimensions that summarize symptom conditions, or (4) an analysis of youths' problems in functioning in various life areas. Each of these approaches has different advantages and disadvantages, depending largely on the nature of screening or assessment objectives in various parts of the juvenile justice system.

HOW CAN WE BEST IDENTIFY THE SERIOUSNESS OF YOUTHS' MENTAL HEALTH NEEDS?

A very large proportion of youths in juvenile justice programs meet criteria for mental disorders. But in order to know which ones are most in need of treatment, we need not only ways to identify them, but also ways to identify the degree of urgency associated with their conditions. A brief review of this topic here will be helpful, because instruments reviewed later in the volume have adopted various ways to identify the "seriousness" of disorders. They tend to be of two types: indexes of (1) the *severity* and (2) the *pervasiveness* of symptoms or disorders.

How Severe are the Youths' Symptoms?

Classification of symptom severity requires some definition of "high" scores needing special attention. Typically, this involves finding a group of youths whom we can all consider "seriously in need," then using that reference point when we evaluate future youths. But there are several ways in which this can be done.

First, we can use a "peer group comparison" approach. We can determine the average level of various behaviors, emotions, or disturbing thoughts for youths of various ages, then decide that youths of the same age who score well above that average are most in need of services. This has the advantage of allowing different actual levels of seriousness to be used for different ages. Recall from an earlier discussion that some behaviors and thoughts are relatively "normal" at one age but "abnormal" at others. Comparing youths to their same-age peers helps to deal with that problem.

A second approach can be called "clinical group comparison." Here we decide that youths' symptoms should be called "serious" when they are at a level that is found in youths who typically receive inpatient or outpatient mental health services in the community. Those are youths who have been judged by clinicians to be in need of psychiatric care. Thus, the average scores made by a group of youths in those settings help us to identify what we call "severe" levels of symptoms when we use the instruments with youths in juvenile justice settings.

A third approach is "outcome group comparison." For this approach, imagine a test that claims to measure anger, especially as it relates to future aggression. Professionals developing the test give it to a number of youths, then keep track of them to determine which youths subsequently engage in aggression. By looking at their anger scores, compared to those of youths who do not eventually engage in aggressive acts, they may find the appropriate level of the anger scale that best distinguishes one group from the other. This level on the scale becomes the indicator of severity that alerts us to consider the possibility that youths might engage in aggressive acts in the future.

How Pervasive Are the Youths' Symptoms?

All three of the approaches just described focus on severity in identifying the "seriousness" of symptoms or disorders. But "seriousness" can be defined in another way, according to the pervasiveness of youths' disorders.

Some youths' mental disorders occur during a particular period in their lives, whereas other youths experience mental health problems *persistently* across many years. Their mental health problems may wax and wane, and sometimes they may even seem to have different diagnostic conditions at different times. But their needs are relatively continuous across their childhood, adolescence, and sometimes adulthood as well. This creates another definition for "seriousness" that we want to take into account when we make treatment decisions. The symptoms that such youths experience may or may not be severe, but their persistence makes them especially troublesome.

Another type of pervasiveness arises when we encounter youths who have *multiple* disorders. We have noted earlier that many youths in juvenile justice settings meet criteria for two, three, and even four mental disorders. It is commonly observed that youths who require the greatest extent of mental health services across the longest period also have a large number of symptoms and multiple disorders (Davis & Vander Stoep, 1997). Thus there is some overlap between persistence and multiple disorders.

A final type of pervasiveness is the degree to which youths' symptoms or disorders have a detrimental *influence on everyday functioning*—their ability to manage what they have to do in their lives at home, at school, at work, and in relations with peers. In some cases, the effects of a youth's symptoms or disorder may pervade all of these areas of life and may be so serious that there is a major breakdown in the youth's ability to function. In other cases, these consequences may be less severe.

In summary, there is no formula for determining how serious youths' disorders must be in order to require immediate or long-term attention to their mental health needs. As we have seen, there are many ways to define what "seriousness" means, as well as a variety of ways to determine how "serious" conditions must be to warrant various types of intervention. Having some concepts like those we have described may help us to think through these issues during screening and assessment.

WHAT IS THE RELATION BETWEEN ADOLESCENTS' MENTAL DISORDERS AND VIOLENCE?

Chapter 1 has described the juvenile justice system's public safety obligation. In this context, it is important to consider what is known about the relation between adolescents' mental disorders and the aggressive and violent behaviors associated with delinquency. To the extent that such relations exist, then treating violent youths' mental disorders is part of the public safety mandate. Are youths with mental disorders any more violent than youths without them, and what is the actual connection between mental disorders and violence in adolescence? The answers to these questions clearly have implications for screening and assessment of mental disorders, because they will inform us about the need for special methods to assess risk of violence during evaluation of youths' mental disorders.

Research on the risk of violence among persons with mental disorders has progressed remarkably in the past decade with regard to adults (e.g., Link & Steuve, 1994; Monahan et al., 2001; Quinsey, Harris, Rice, & Cormier, 1998; Steadman et al., 1998). One of the things this research tells us is that in adults, there are different answers for different disorders. Some disorders, such as psychopathy (e.g., Hare, 1999), increase the risk; others do not; and still others, such as schizophrenia (e.g., Steadman et al., 1998), actually decrease the risk. However, all disorders present increased potential for violence in combination with substance abuse or dependence (e.g., Steadman et al., 1998; Swanson et al., 1997).

Unfortunately, research on the relation of violence and mental disorders among adolescent offenders lags far behind these advances with regard to adult patients and offenders. For reasons reviewed elsewhere (Grisso, 2004), evidence for the association between adolescents' mental disorders or mental health problems and risk of harm to others has been largely inconsistent. Nevertheless, a brief review will provide evidence that a connection between mental disorders in adolescence and risk of harm to others is emerging. The evidence does not at all suggest that most violence among youths is due to mental disorders. But it does suggest that when youths have certain mental disorders, there is reason to be more (or less) concerned that they may engage in violent behaviors.

Disruptive Behavior Disorders

ADHD, ODD, and CD form a cluster of disorders in DSM-IV and DSM-IV-TR (American Psychiatric Association, 1994, 2000) called "attention-deficit and disruptive behavior disorders." These disorders have some overlap, so it is not surprising that they frequently are found together. About 80% to 90% of youths with CD have been previously diagnosed as having ODD. But ODD does not predict CD well, because only about 25% of youths with ODD are later diagnosed with CD. About one-half of youths diagnosed with ADHD will eventually be diagnosed with CD, but more than two-thirds of youths with CD also carry a diagnosis of ADHD. (For reviews, see Barkley, 2003; Biederman, Newcorn, & Sprich, 1991; Connor, 2002; Frick, 1998; Loeber, Farrington, Stouthamer-Loeber, & Van Kammen, 1998).

Substantially higher rates of physically aggressive behavior are found for youths with any of these three disorders than for youths in general or youths with other mental disorders (Connor, 2002). Most importantly, youths who meet criteria for *both* ADHD and CD have substantially greater rates of delinquent acts during adolescence, harmful acts in later adolescence, and continued violence and offending into adulthood (e.g., Biederman, Mick, Faraone, & Burback, 2001; Fischer, Barkley, Fletcher, & Smallish, 1993; Frick, 1998; Mannuzza, Klein, Bessler, Mally, & LaPadula, 1993).

Children with hyperactivity–impulsivity–attention deficits and serious conduct problems may also be at risk for developing psychopathy (Lynam, 1997). Psychopathy is a personality disorder that, when found in adults, is the most powerful psychological predictor of long-term, severe, and violent criminal behaviors (Hare, 2003). Interpersonally, psychopathic individuals are arrogant and deceitful; emotionally, they are shallow and lacking in empathy; behaviorally, they are impulsive and stimulation-seeking (Hare, 1991, 2003).

Evidence that psychopathy begins to develop during childhood has generated a dramatic increase in research investigating whether we can identify this personality disorder in children and adolescents (e.g., Brandt, Kennedy, Patrick, & Curtin, 1997; Christian, Frick, Hill, Tyler, & Frazer, 1997; Forth et al., 2003; Frick, O'Brien, Wootton, & McBurnett, 1994; Lynam, 1998; Rogers, Johansen, Chang, & Salekin, 1997). Although research on the reliability and validity of measures of youth psychopathy is progressing, currently the research does not allow us to call this group "psychopathic" or even "prepsychopathic" (Edens et al., 2001; Hart et al., 2002; Salekin, Rogers, & Machin, 2001; Seagrave & Grisso, 2002). There is no evidence that psychopathic traits will be stable into adulthood for a substantial proportion of the adolescents who score high on youth psychopathy. The mere fact that adolescents manifest "psychopathic" characteristics, particularly behavioral characteristics (e.g., irresponsibility, impulsivity, stimulation seeking), does not mean that they have psychopathy. There is reason to believe that many youths manifest these tendencies as transient features of typical developmental stages, rather than as early signs of psychopathy (Edens et al., 2001; Seagrave & Grisso, 2002). Nonetheless, it seems that when adolescents have these features in combination with a general lack of empathy and remorse, they are more likely to remain violent and delinquent, at least into late adolescence and early adulthood (Vincent, Vitacco, Grisso, & Corrado, 2003).

Mood Disorders

Among the widely recognized characteristics of adolescents with various forms of depression are irritability, hostility, and anger (Biederman & Spencer, 1999; Goodyer & Cooper, 1993). Not all youths with depressive disorders are angry, but it is common. The significance of anger as a motivator for aggression is well known (Novaco, 1994). Youths who clearly manifest a sullen, angry, and belligerent attitude are more likely to get angry responses from other youths (and adults), thus increasing the risk of events that escalate into physical aggression. And an irritable youth is more likely to interpret ordinary annoyances by others as direct threats, increasing the risk that the youth will respond with defensive aggression.

Anxiety Disorders

Clinicians and researchers (Connor, 2002; Walker et al., 1991) find that youths with most types of anxiety disorders are shy and withdrawn, and tend to avoid fearful situations. Typically, therefore, they tend to be less aggressive than the average for youths of their age. Nonetheless, youths for whom anxiety is a long-term condition often have conduct problems (Frick, Lilienfeld, Ellis, Loney, & Silverthorn, 1999). The relation between posttraumatic stress disorder (PTSD) and youths' aggressive reactions is well known (for a review, see Connor, 2002). PTSD appears to be related to the conditioning of neurobiological fear responses that underlie the natural human tendencies to react aggressively and self-protectively when events occur that are reminders of an earlier trauma (Charney, Deutch, Krystal, Southwick, & Davis, 1993; Fletcher, 2003). Most youths with PTSD do not engage in serious harmful acts, but their risk is increased. For example, in juvenile justice samples, both boys (Steiner, Garcia, & Matthews, 1997) and girls (Cauffman, Feldman, Waterman, & Steiner, 1998) with CD and PTSD have been found to be more impulsive and aggressive than youths with CD alone.

Psychotic Disorders

Serious psychotic disorders such as schizophrenia are rare prior to early adulthood. The presence of delusional beliefs among persons with schizophrenia, often including paranoid notions about harm from others, might suggest an increased risk of aggression. Yet research on adults suggests that they present less risk of violence than persons with other serious mental illnesses (indeed, no greater risk than persons with no mental disorders; Monahan et al., 2001). The evidence for increased risk among adolescents with schizophrenia is weak (Connor, 2002).

Substance Use Disorders

A great deal of research tells us what is perhaps obvious: There is a strong relation between adolescents' substance use and aggression, as well as between substance use and the seriousness of delinquent behavior (for reviews, see Brady, Myrick, & McElroy, 1998; Huizinga & Jakob-Chien, 1998; Loeber & Dishion, 1983). For example, in one general community sample of adolescents, prevalence of problem alcohol use was 15% for nondelinquent youths, 38% for youths with minor delinquencies, and over 50% for youths with serious violent and nonviolent offenses (Loeber, Van Kammen, Krohn, & Huizinga, 1991). One comprehensive review of past studies found that substance use during middle childhood was one of the strongest predictors of serious delinquency, with substance users being 5 to 20 times more likely to exhibit later violence and delinquency (Lipsey & Derzon, 1998).

The relation of mental disorders to harmful behavior is addressed in greater detail in Part V of this volume. The introduction to Part V provides a review of factors that are known to increase the risk of future violence among adolescents. Assessment tools developed to estimate those risks use those factors as the bases for their test items. Interestingly, those instruments make little use of mental disorders as factors increasing the risk of violence. This is because the mental disorders we have reviewed above, though somewhat related to aggression, do not carry as much weight for predictive purposes as many other factors that will be reviewed in Part V.

But this brief review of the relationship between symptoms of mental disorders and violent behavior indicates that mental disorders cannot be overlooked in assessing potential harm to others. Some specific types of mental disorders do increase the risk of future violence. In addition, for those youths with mental disorders who do have a history of violence, typically their symptoms of mental disorder have contributed to their violent behavior. Thus reducing their future risk of violence will typically require identifying their disorders and, through comprehensive assessment, determining how they can be treated.

CONCLUSION: THE IMPORTANCE
OF A DEVELOPMENTAL PERSPECTIVE

The creation of instruments to assess youths' mental disorders has only recently begun to catch up to the mental health field's substantial earlier progress in the assessment of adults. Although the instruments in this book have predecessors, most of them have been developed only in the past 15 years.

One of the reasons for this recent progress is a change in the way child psychiatrists and child clinical psychologists think about youths' mental disorders. This change of perspective has focused primarily on the ways that typical child and adolescent development complicate the picture, including how we define symptoms and disorders, how they develop, what they mean for longer-range development, and why they are more difficult to identify and measure than in adults.

There are several important messages in this chapter's brief review for juvenile justice administrators and clinicians who are considering screening and assessment plans in juvenile justice contexts. We would summarize them this way:

- Identifying youths' mental disorders is greatly complicated by the normal developmental changes in youths across adolescence.
- Identifying youths' mental disorders requires methods that were developed for children and adolescents, not adults.
- Youths who have a mental disorder are quite likely to have more than one.
- Mental health information about youths is likely to have a shorter "shelf life" than such information about adults. Development and change are proceeding more rapidly for most youths than for most adults, so that what we see when we identify youths' mental disorders at a given time may change when we see them next year.
- Most youth violence is not "caused" by mental disorders. But many mental disorders increase the risk of delinquency and aggressive behavior.
- We need to think about the "seriousness" of youths' mental health needs in two ways. Some youths' disorders are serious because their symptoms are currently severe and require immediate attention. Other youths' disorders are serious because they are pervasive, involving chronic problems that have persisted since childhood and are likely to persist well into their adult years.

REFERENCES

Abram, K. M., Teplin, L., & McClelland, G. M. (2003). Comorbid psychiatric disorders in youth in juvenile detention. *Archives of General Psychiatry, 60,* 1097–1108.

Achenbach, T. (1993). *Empirically based taxonomy: How to use syndromes and profile types derived from the CHCL/4–18, TRF, and YSR.* Burlington: University of Vermont, Department of Psychiatry.

Achenbach, T. (1995). Diagnosis, assessment, and comorbidity in psychosocial treatment research. *Journal of Abnormal Psychology, 23,* 45–65.

Achenbach, T., & Edelbrock, C. (1984). Psychopathology of childhood. *Annual Review of Psychology, 35,* 227–256.

Albano, A., DiBartolo, P., Heimberg, R., & Barlow, D. (1995). Children and adolescents: Assessment and treatment. In R. Heimberg, M. Liebowitz, D. Hope, & F. Schneier (Eds.), *Social phobia: Diagnosis, assessment, and treatment* (pp. 387–425). New York: Guilford Press.

American Psychiatric Association. (1994). *Diagnostic and statistical manual of mental disorders* (4th ed.). Washington, DC: Author.

American Psychiatric Association. (2000). *Diagnostic and statistical manual of mental disorders* (4th ed., text rev.). Washington, DC: Author.

Andershed, H., Kerr, M., Stattin, H., & Levander, S. (2002). Psychopathic traits in non-referred youths: A new assessment tool. In E. Blaauw & L. Sheridan (Eds.), *Psychopaths: Current international perspectives* (pp. 131–158). Amsterdam, Netherlands: Elsevier.

Angold, A., & Costello, E. (1993). Depressive comorbidity in children and adolescents: Empirical, theoretical, and methodological issues. *American Journal of Psychiatry, 150,* 1779–1791.

Angold, A., Erkanli, A., Farmer, E., Fairbank, J., Burns, B., Keeler, G., & Costello, E. (2002). Psychiatric disorder, impairment, and service use in rural African American and white youth. *Archives of General Psychiatry, 59,* 893–901.

Barkley, R. (2003). Attention-deficit/hyperactivity disorder. In E. Mash & R. Barkley (Eds.), *Child psychopathology* (2nd ed., pp. 75–143). New York: Guilford Press.

Barkley, R. (1998). *Attention-deficit hyperactivity disorder: A handbook for diagnosis and treatment* (2nd ed.). New York: Guilford Press.

Biederman, J., Mick, E., Faraone, S., & Burback, M. (2001). Patterns of remission and symptom decline in conduct disorder: A four-year prospective study of an ADHD sample. *Journal of the American Academy of Child and Adolescent Psychiatry, 40,* 290–298.

Biederman, J., Newcorn, J., & Sprich, S. (1991). Comorbidity of attention deficit hyperactivity disorder with conduct, depressive, anxiety, and other disorders. *American Journal of Psychiatry, 148,* 564–577.

Biederman, J., & Spencer, T. (1999). Depressive disorders in childhood and adolescence: A clinical perspective. *Journal of Child and Adolescent Psychopharmacology, 9,* 233–237.

Brady, K., Myrick, H., & McElroy, S. (1998). The relationship between substance use disorders, impulse control disorders, and pathological aggression. *American Journal on Addictions, 7,* 221–230.

Brandt, J., Kennedy, W., Patrick, C., & Curtin, J. (1997). Assessment of psychopathy in a population of incarcerated adolescent offenders. *Psychological Assessment, 9,* 429–435.

Caron, C., & Rutter, M. (1991). Comorbidity in child psychopathology: Concepts, issues and research strategies. *Journal of Child Psychology and Psychiatry, 32,* 1063–1080.

Cauffman, E., Feldman, S., Waterman, J., & Steiner, H. (1998). Posttraumatic stress disorder among female juvenile offenders. *Journal of the American Academy of Child and Adolescent Psychiatry, 37,* 1209–1216.

Cauffman, E., & Grisso, T. (in press). Mental health issues among minority offenders in the juvenile justice system. In D. Hawkins & K. Leonard (Eds.), *Our children, their children: Confronting race and ethnic differences in American criminal justice.* Chicago: University of Chicago Press.

Charney, D., Deutch, A., Krystal, J., Southwick, S., & Davis, M. (1993). Psychobiological mechanisms of posttraumatic stress disorder. *Archives of General Psychiatry, 50*, 294–305.

Christian, R., Frick, P., Hill, N., Tyler, L., & Frazer, D. (1997). Psychopathy and conduct problems in children: II. Subtyping children with conduct problems based on their interpersonal and affective style. *Journal of the American Academy of Child and Adolescent Psychiatry, 36*, 233–241.

Cicchetti, D. (1984). The emergence of developmental psychopathology. *Child Development, 55*, 1–7.

Cicchetti, D. (1990). An historical perspective on the discipline of developmental psychopathology. In J. Rolf, A. Master, D. Cicchetti, K. Nuechterlien, & S. Weintraub (Eds.), *Risk and protective factors in the development of psychopathology* (pp. 2–28). New York: Cambridge University Press.

Cicchetti, D., & Cohen, D. (1995). *Developmental psychopathology* (2 vols.). New York: Wiley.

Cicchetti, D., & Rogosch, F. (2002). A developmental psychopathology perspective on adolescence. *Journal of Consulting and Clinical Psychology, 70*, 6–20.

Connor, D. (2002). *Aggression and antisocial behavior in children and adolescents: Research and treatment.* New York: Guilford Press.

Davis, M., & Vander Stoep, A. (1997). The transition to adulthood for youth who have serious emotional disturbance: Developmental transition and young adult outcomes. *Journal of Mental Health Administration, 24*, 400–427.

Edens, J., Skeem, J., Cruise, K., & Cauffman, E. (2001). Assessment of "juvenile psychopathy" and its association with violence: A critical review. *Behavioral Sciences and the Law, 19*, 53–80.

Fischer, M., Barkley, R., Fletcher, K., & Smallish, L. (1993). The stability of dimensions of behavior in ADHD and normal children over an 8-year follow-up. *Journal of Abnormal Child Psychology, 21*, 315–337.

Fletcher, K. (2003). Childhood posttraumatic stress disorder. In E. Mash & R. Barkley (Eds.), *Child psychopathology* (2nd ed., pp. 330–371). New York: Guilford Press.

Forth, A., Kosson, D., & Hare, R. (2003). *The Hare Psychopathy Checklist: Youth Version.* Toronto: Multi-Health Systems.

Frick, P. J. (1998). *Conduct disorders and severe antisocial behavior.* New York: Plenum Press.

Frick, P. J. (2000). Laboratory and performance-based measures of childhood disorders. *Journal of Clinical Child Psychology, 29*, 475–478.

Frick, P. J., & Hare, R. D. (2001). *The Antisocial Process Screening Device.* Toronto: Multi-Health Systems.

Frick, P. J., Lilienfeld, S. O., Ellis, M., Loney, B., & Silverthorn, P. (1999). The association between anxiety and psychopathy dimensions in children. *Journal of Abnormal Child Psychology, 27*, 383–392.

Frick, P. J., O'Brien, B., Wootton, J., & McBurnett, K. (1994). Psychopathy and conduct problems in children. *Journal of Abnormal Psychology, 103*, 700–707.

Goodyer, I., & Cooper, P. (1993). A community study of depression in adolescent girls: II. The clinical features of identified disorder. *British Journal of Psychiatry, 163*, 374–380.

Grisso, T. (2004). *Double jeopardy: Adolescent offenders with mental disorders.* Chicago: University of Chicago Press.

Grisso, T., Barnum, R., Fletcher, K., Cauffman, E., & Peuschold, D. (2001). Massachusetts Youth Screening Instrument for mental health needs of juvenile justice youths. *Journal of the American Academy of Child and Adolescent Psychiatry, 40,* 541–548.

Hammen, C., & Rudolph, K. (2003). Childhood depression. In E. Mash & R. Barkley (Eds.), *Child psychopathology* (2nd ed., pp. 233–278). New York: Guilford Press.

Hare, R. D. (1991). *The Hare Psychopathy Checklist—Revised.* Toronto: Multi-Health Systems.

Hare, R. D. (1999). Psychopathy as a risk factor for violence. *Psychiatric Quarterly, 70,* 181–197.

Hare, R. D. (2003). *The Hare Psychopathy Checklist—Revised* (2nd ed.). Toronto: Multi-Health Systems.

Hart, S., Watt, K., & Vincent, G. (2002). Commentary on Seagrave and Grisso: Impressions of the state of the art. *Law and Human Behavior, 26,* 241–245.

Hartung, C. M., & Widiger, T. A. (1998). Gender differences in the diagnosis of mental disorders: Conclusions and controversies of the DSM-IV. *Psychological Bulletin, 123,* 260–278.

Hinden, B. R., Compas, B. E., Achenbach, T. M., & Howell, D. (1997). Covariation of the anxious/depressed syndrome: Separating fact from artifact. *Journal of Consulting and Clinical Psychology, 65,* 6–14.

Huizinga, D., & Jakob-Chien, C. (1998). The contemporaneous co-occurrence of serious and violent juvenile offending and other problem behaviors. In R. Loeber & D. Farrington (Eds.), *Serious and violent juvenile offenders: Risk factors and successful interventions* (pp. 47–67). Thousand Oaks, CA: Sage.

Ingram, R., & Price, J. (Eds.). (2001). *Vulnerability to psychopathology: Risk across the lifespan.* New York: Guilford Press.

Institute of Medicine. (1989). *Research on children and adolescents with mental, behavioral, and developmental disorders: Mobilizing a national initiative* (Contract No. 278-88-0025). Washington, DC: U.S. Department of Health and Human Services, National Institute of Mental Health.

Isaacs, M. (1992). Assessing the mental health needs of children and adolescents of color in the juvenile justice system: Overcoming institutionalized perceptions and barriers. In J. Cocozza (Ed.), *Responding to the mental health needs of youth in the juvenile justice system* (pp. 143–163). Seattle, WA: National Coalition for the Mentally Ill in the Criminal Justice System.

Kagan, J., Resnick, J., Clark, C., Snidman, N., & Garcia-Coll, C. (1984). Behavioral inhibition to the unfamiliar. *Child Development, 55,* 2212–2225.

Kazdin, A., & Johnson, H. (1994). Advances in psychotherapy for children and adolescents: Interrelations of adjustment, development and intervention. *Journal of School Psychology, 32,* 217–246.

Kazdin, A., & Kagan, J. (1994). Models of dysfunction in developmental psychopathology. *Clinical Psychology: Science and Practice, 1,* 35–52.

Lilienfeld, S., Waldman, I., & Israel, A. (1994). A critical examination of the use of the term and concept of comorbidity in psychopathology research. *Clinical Psychology: Science and Practice, 1,* 71–83.

Link, B., & Steuve, A. (1994). Psychotic symptoms and the violent/illegal behavior of mental patients compared to community controls. In J. Monahan & H. Steadman

(Eds.), *Violence and mental disorder: Developments in risk assessment* (pp. 137–159). Chicago: University of Chicago Press.

Lipsey, M. W., & Derzon, J. H. (1998). Predictors of violence and serious delinquency in adolescence and early adulthood: A synthesis of longitudinal research. In R. Loeber & D. P. Farrington (Eds.), *Serious and violent juvenile offenders: Risk factors and successful interventions* (pp. 86–105). Thousand Oaks, CA: Sage.

Loeber, R., & Dishion, T. (1983). Early predictors of male delinquency: A review. *Psychological Bulletin, 94,* 68–99.

Loeber, R., Farrington, D., Stouthamer-Loeber, M., & Van Kammen, W. (1998). *Antisocial behavior and mental health problems: Explanatory factors in childhood and adolescence.* Mahwah, NJ: Erlbaum.

Loeber, R., & Keenan, K. (1994). Interaction between conduct disorder and its comorbid conditions: Effects of age and gender. *Clinical Psychology Review, 14,* 497–523.

Loeber, R., Van Kammen, W., Krohn, M., & Huizinga, D. (1991). The crime–substance use nexus in young people. In D. Huizinga, R. Loeber, & T. Thornberry (Eds.), *Urban delinquency and substance abuse* (pp. 488–515). Washington, DC: U.S. Department of Justice, Office of Juvenile Justice and Delinquency Prevention.

Lynam, D. (1997). Pursuing the psychopath: Capturing the fledgling psychopath in a nomological net. *Journal of Abnormal Psychology, 106,* 425–438.

Lynam, D. (1998). Early identification of the fledgling psychopath: Locating the psychopathic child in the current nomenclature. *Journal of Abnormal Psychology, 107,* 566–575.

Mannuzza, S., Klein, R., Bessler, A., Mally, P., & LaPadula, M. (1993). Adult outcome of hyperactive boys: Educational achievement, occupational rank, and psychiatric status. *Archives of General Psychiatry, 50,* 565–576.

Marsteller, F., Brogan, D., Smith, I., Ash, P., Daniels, D., Rolka, D., et al. (1997). *The prevalence of substance use disorders among juveniles admitted to regional youth detention centers operated by the Georgia Department of Children and Youth Services.* Rockville, MD: U.S. Department of Health and Human Services, Center for Substance Abuse Treatment.

Mash, E., & Dozois, D. (2003). Child psychopathology: A developmental–systems perspective. In E. Mash & R. Barkley (Eds.), *Child psychopathology* (2nd ed., pp. 3–71). New York: Guilford Press.

Monahan, J., Steadman, H., Silver, E., Appelbaum, P., Robbins, P., Mulvey, E., et al. (2001). *Rethinking risk assessment: The MacArthur study of mental disorder and violence.* New York: Oxford University Press.

Murray, C., Smith, S., & West, E. (1989). Comparative personality development in adolescence: A critique. In R. Jones (Ed.), *Black adolescents* (pp. 49–62). Berkeley, CA: Cobb & Henry.

Murrie, D. C., & Cornell, D. G. (2000). The Millon Adolescent Clinical Inventory and psychopathy. *Journal of Personality Assessment, 75,* 110–125.

Neighbors, H., Kempton, T., & Forehand, R. (1992). Co-occurrence of substance abuse with conduct, anxiety and depression disorders in juvenile delinquents. *Addictive Behaviors, 17,* 379–386.

Novaco, R. (1994). Anger as a risk factor for violence among the mentally disordered.

In J. Monahan & H. Steadman (Eds.), *Violence and mental disorder* (pp. 21–59). Chicago: University of Chicago Press.

Offord, D., Boyle, M., Szatmari, P., Rae-Grant, N., Links, P., Cadman, D., et al. (1987). Ontario Child Health Study, II: Six-month prevalence of disorder and rates of service utilization. *Archives of General Psychiatry, 44,* 832–836.

Pennington, B., & Ozonoff, S. (1991). A neuroscientific perspective on continuity and discontinuity in developmental psychopathology. In D. Cicchetti & S. Toth (Eds.), *Rochester Symposium on Developmental Psychopathology: Vol. 3. Models and integrations* (pp. 117–159). Rochester, NY: University of Rochester Press.

Quinsey, V., Harris, G., Rice, M., & Cormier, C. (1998). *Violent offenders: Appraising and managing risk.* Washington, DC: American Psychological Association.

Richards, I. (1996). Psychiatric disorder among adolescents in custody. *Australian and New Zealand Journal of Psychiatry, 30,* 788–793.

Rogers, R., Johansen, J., Chang, J., & Salekin, R. (1997). Predictors of adolescent psychopathy: Oppositional and conduct-disordered symptoms. *Journal of the American Academy of Psychiatry and the Law, 25,* 261–271.

Rutter, M., & Garmezy, H. (1983). Developmental psychopathology. In P. Mussen (Series Ed.) & E. Hetherington (Vol. Ed.), *Handbook of child psychology: Vol. 4. Socialization, personality, and social development* (pp. 775–911). New York: Wiley.

Salekin, R., Rogers, R., & Machin, D. (2001). Psychopathy in youth: Pursuing diagnostic clarity. *Journal of Youth and Adolescence, 30,* 173–194.

Schteingart, J. S., Molnar, J., Klein, T. P., Lowe, C. B., & Hartman, A. H. (1995). Homelessness and child functioning in the context of risk and protective factors moderating child outcomes. *Journal of Clinical Child Psychology, 24,* 320–331.

Seagrave, D., & Grisso, T. (2002). Adolescent development and the measurement of juvenile psychopathy. *Law and Human Behavior, 26,* 219–239.

Sroufe, L., & Rutter, M. (1984). The domain of developmental psychopathology. *Child Development, 55,* 17–29.

Steadman, H., Mulvey, E., Monahan, J., Robbins, P., Appelbaum, P., Grisso, T., et al. (1998). Violence by people discharged from acute psychiatric facilities and by others in the same neighborhoods. *Archives of General Psychiatry, 55,* 393–401.

Steinberg, L. (2002). Clinical adolescent psychology: What it is, and what it needs to be. *Journal of Consulting and Clinical Psychology, 70,* 124–128.

Steiner, H., Garcia, I., & Matthews, X. (1997). Posttraumatic stress disorder in incarcerated juvenile delinquents. *Journal of the American Academy of Child and Adolescent Psychiatry, 36,* 357–365.

Swanson, J., Estroff, S., Swartz, M., Borum, R., Lachicotte, W., Zimmer, C., et al. (1997). Violence and severe mental disorder in clinical and community populations: The effects of psychotic symptoms, comorbidity, and lack of treatment. *Psychiatry, 60,* 1–22.

Szatmari, P., Boyle, M., & Offord, D. (1989). ADHD and CD: Degree of diagnostic overlap and differences among correlates. *Journal of the American Academy of Child and Adolescent Psychiatry, 31,* 1036–1040.

Teplin, L., Abram, K., McClelland, G., Dulcan, M., & Mericle, A. (2002). Psychiatric disorders in youth in juvenile detention. *Archives of General Psychiatry, 59,* 1133–1143.

Vincent, G. (2002). *Investigating the legitimacy of adolescent psychopathy assessments: Contributions of item response theory.* Unpublished doctoral dissertation, Simon Fraser University, Burnaby, BC, Canada.

Vincent, G., Vitacco, M., Grisso, T., & Corrado, R. (2003). Subtypes of adolescent offenders: Affective traits and antisocial behavior patterns. *Behavioral Sciences and the Law, 21,* 695–712.

Walker, J., Lahey, B., Russo, M., Frick, P., Christ, M., McBurnett, K., et al. (1991). Anxiety, inhibition, and conduct disorder in children: I. Relations to social impairment. *Journal of the American Academy of Child and Adolescent Psychiatry, 30,* 187–191.

CHAPTER 3

The Context for Mental Health Screening and Assessment

Thomas Grisso
Gina Vincent

Effective screening and assessment require attention to the quality of the instruments themselves (see Chapter 4). But it is equally important to consider the degree to which an instrument can function *within the context* of juvenile justice settings. By "context," we mean the legal requirements, time pressures, limited resources, quality of personnel, potential for lawsuits, and a host of other practical considerations that form the "world" in which the instrument must work. Instruments vary in their capacities to withstand these circumstances. In addition, administrators can often do certain things to create circumstances in which screening and assessment tools will work better. This chapter reviews some of those circumstances, in order to prepare administrators and clinicians for the task of creating conditions that promote sound screening and assessment practices, and selecting instruments that best meet the contextual demands of juvenile justice programs. It begins by examining separately the contexts for screening and for assessment.

THE CONTEXT FOR SCREENING

As defined earlier, "screening" is a process for identifying the needs of all youths entering a particular doorway in the juvenile justice system—for example, a probation intake office, a pretrial detention center, or a secure juvenile corrections program. Determining how screening is to occur, what will facilitate its use, and what may frustrate its purposes requires considering a number of contextual factors, discussed below as related to (1) the objectives for screening within a particular setting, and (2) practical and financial feasibility.

Considering Objectives

The fundamental purpose for mental health screening of every youth entering a juvenile justice setting is to identify the likelihood that a youth will need immediate mental health or protective attention within a matter of days. Several additional motivations and reasons for screening, however, may have an impact on choices about how screening will be performed and what instruments will be used. Developing a screening process must begin with a clear view of those objectives, which are considered here in categories: (1) fulfilling regulatory requirements and professional standards, (2) improving staff members' decision making, and (3) managing resources.

Fulfilling Regulatory Requirements and Professional Standards

Some juvenile justice programs will develop mental health screening in part because they are required to do so by law, by state or county regulations, and/ or by professional standards to which they have committed themselves. Legal and regulatory directives focus on the identification not only of mental health and safety needs, but also of basic medical needs (e.g., acute or chronic medical conditions, allergies, current medications). In this context, mental health screening does not occur as a stand-alone activity. It is embedded in the necessity to collect a wider range of basic medical and behavioral information about youths, intended to assure that immediate, short-term needs are met and that emergencies are identified or averted. Therefore, in selecting screening tools, one must consider the degree to which each tool fits into the broader range of screening purposes required by law and regulations. For example, having to cover this wider range of purposes will have an influence on the length of screening tools that can be tolerated.

Most legal and regulatory directives do not specify precisely the types of mental health needs for which the system must screen. However, according to current authoritative sources (e.g., Boesky, 2003; Grisso, 2004; Grisso & Underwood, in press; Wasserman, Jensen, & Ko, 2003), fulfilling the intentions of laws and regulations for identification of youths' mental health needs will require screening tools that include the following at a minimum:

- One or more scales that focus on current affective (e.g., depression) and anxiety symptoms.
- An indicator of the short-range likelihood of aggression or of factors that might augment its likelihood (e.g., anger).
- An indicator of the likelihood that a youth is currently a significant risk for suicide or for physical self-harm in general.
- An indicator of recent or current serious alcohol or drug abuse or dependence.

Typically, the regulations that apply to juvenile justice programs regarding mental health screening do not specify any particular screening method. Unfortunately, some detention centers screen for mental health needs simply by asking a few questions with contents that seem to "make sense." In contrast, national standard-setting bodies (e.g., Council of Juvenile Correctional Administrators, 2001; Wasserman et al., 2003) emphasize that juvenile justice programs should employ "standardized" mental health screening tools (i.e., ones that are administered exactly the same way to all youths) with known "reliability" and "validity." Screening is likely to be a waste of time if there is no evidence that the method used for screening is a dependabe measure of the psychological conditions or psychiatric symptoms it is intended to identify. Therefore, selection of a screening method should take into consideration the degree to which research has demonstrated the reliability and validity of the instrument for purposes of meeting screening objectives. Chapter 4 provides more detail on the scientific criteria to apply in determining reliability and validity, and reviews of individual instruments later in this book evaluate each instrument according to these scientific criteria.

Improving Staff Decision Making

Another common purpose for developing standardized mental health screening is to assist staff members in the difficult process of making decisions about the management of youths in their custody. The personnel of juvenile justice programs have the daily responsibility to make decisions about youths' immediate mental health needs and their risk of harm to themselves or others. Many staff members of intake probation or detention centers do not have clinical expertise relevant to this task. Nevertheless, they are responsible for knowing when clinical attention may be necessary to avert an emergency, and which youths may need mental health consultations. Moreover, these nonclinical staff members must generally be responsible for screening, because the number of youths involved is usually too great to make it financially feasible to hire trained mental health professionals for this task.

Several features of screening tools require special scrutiny in order to fulfill this purpose. First, tools that have good structure and simplicity will better serve nonclinical staff members who perform screening duties. "Structure" refers to the clarity of a procedure. For example, a set of unvarying questions to ask youths in an unvarying sequence constitutes a high degree of structure, whereas procedures that call for staff members to decide whether to ask particular questions on a case-by-case basis are less structured. "Simplicity" refers to having a minimum number of steps in the process, as well as a minimum of complexity in the steps themselves. For example, a screening tool that requires simply counting the number of "yes" responses, or that is computerized so that scoring is automatic, is simpler than a tool that uses a 1-to-10 rating scale on each item or involves the application of scoring templates for each characteristic that the screening tool measures.

Second, screening tools can better meet the needs of nonclinical staff members when they have clear manuals and are accompanied by prepackaged training curricula. High structure and simplicity will minimize the amount of training time required to prepare staff for administering and using mental health screening tools. But at least some training (even if it is only a few hours of in-service orientation) is required for almost all such tools, in order to assure that staff members are comfortable with the tool and will implement it uniformly. This point cannot be overemphasized. The developers of screening tools may rightly claim good reliability and accuracy in their manuals, based on past research. But if a program's personnel do not administer an instrument as described in its manual, that same screening tool is likely to become unreliable and lose all credibility regarding the accuracy that it otherwise might have had. A tool with a good training curriculum helps to avoid this.

Third, screening tools that use cutoff scores will facilitate the consistency with which staff can make decisions based on the instrument's scores. A "cutoff score" is simply the point above which youths' scores are considered "high," "clinically significant," or "in need of a response." As described in more detail in Chapter 4, a cutoff score is typically determined in research on the instrument, showing that a particular point on a scale is the optimal score for separating youths into those who are more or less likely to actually have the characteristic being measured (i.e., the diagnosis or the symptom on which the scale focuses). Cutoff scores allow an institution to develop clear decision rules for personnel—for example, "Implement suicide precautions if score is above X"—rather than leaving personnel to their own unguided discretion regarding the use of scores to make intervention decisions.

Managing Resources

When selecting screening tools, administrators need to attend to the potential for instruments to contribute to broader program objectives. In addition to doing the day-to-day job of identifying youths' mental health needs, screening tools can improve administrators' abilities to manage practices and resources so as to meet responsibilities for fiscal and functional efficiency.

For example, administrators are responsible for assuring that necessary treatment is available to youths with serious mental health needs. Fulfilling this responsibility requires planning, which in turn requires data. For example, administrators may want to know what specific types of mental health needs arise with more or less frequency across time within their own juvenile justice facilities, and to have these data translated into the specific types of responses (e.g., hospitalization, psychiatric consultation) that are more or less often required. This information can be used to adjust budgets in order to place scarce resources where they are needed most, or to provide factual information when the administrators are lobbying for increases in financial resources to meet existing and future needs. Such information can also be used to adjust the functions of staff members or to identify the need for specialized staffing (e.g., a position for a specialized psychiatric social worker in a very high-need setting). A continuous flow of such information across time also permits the detection of changes that affect a facility's needs. For example, changes in police arrest and referral patterns, or changes in funding for child mental health agencies outside the juvenile justice system, may both influence the types of youths entering a justice facility. Such information allows for fine-tuning in the allocation of resources under changing conditions.

The key to identifying such matters in a particular program is the cumulative archiving of all screening cases. Each case needs to be entered into a data base that identifies the youth according to date of screening, some uniform demographic characteristics (such as identification number, age, gender, race, and offense charged), and scores on the screening instrument. (Ideally, such a system also records the facility's responses to cases in which youths meet screening criteria for some action by facility personnel.)

This record keeping can be accomplished in several ways. The least sophisticated method is to keep a file of the paper documentation for cases and tally them weekly or monthly. The most sophisticated method is to use screening tools that are administered by computer, automatically scored by computer, and automatically filed in an electronic data base that permits analyses and monthly comparisons of cases at any time. Screening tools differ with regard to the availability of software that can accomplish these purposes, as well as their compatibility with a facility's existing information systems. These electronic "packaging" features therefore become one of the characteristics of screening tools that should be considered in selecting among them.

In summary, administrators who are selecting mental health screening tools need to be clear about their objectives for implementing screening. Most good screening tools will serve the primary objective—to identify youths with mental health needs that may need immediate attention in order to prevent crises, and/or that may need further evaluation. But screening instruments may differ in their ability to meet the requirements associated with secondary objectives and motivations. Regulations may require that specific types of mental health needs receive special attention, and instruments differ somewhat in the needs that they assess. Instruments may be more or less useful in improving staff members' capacities to employ screening consistently. And instruments can differ in their ability to provide administrators with the record-keeping tools that they need for resource management and program planning.

Considering Practical and Financial Feasibility

Practical, everyday demands of juvenile justice programs and facilities raise a second set of institutional considerations in selecting mental health screening tools. Some of these factors have to do with increased time and effort, but all of them translate into financial costs in one way or another.

As a preface to this discussion, recall that "mental health screening" has been defined in Chapter 1 as a process that identifies mental health needs (1) for every youth at entry into some part of the juvenile justice system, in order to (2) signal the potential need for some sort of immediate response (often to avoid harm to a youth or to others as a consequence of an acute condition). Some tools described later in this book are labeled or self-defined as "screening instruments." In theory, however, every instrument described in later chapters could serve as a "screening" method, because in theory all of them could be used with every youth at entry to signal the need for emergency services. The reason why some are favored as screening tools and others are not is that the instruments differ enormously in the amount of resources that would be required to implement them with all youths and within the practical constraints of juvenile justice facilities and programs.

These demands will vary across different doorways in the juvenile justice system. In the following discussion, we consider three different doorways at which screening is often desirable or required. It is worthwhile to briefly consider the differences in circumstances across these settings before taking stock of their implications for selection of mental health screening methods.

One important doorway is the *intake interview*, which often begins with the arrival of a youth and a caretaker at the probation office on appointment a few days after the youth's arrest and referral to the juvenile court. Probation intake officers frequently have master's degrees in social work, and sometimes they have access to brief consultation from juvenile court clinicians with degrees in various mental health professions. Some youths appearing for intake interviews will already be known to the system through earlier contacts, and some information about their backgrounds and personal characteristics may already be on file for reference by the probation intake officer. For some other youths, however, this intake interview will be their first contact with the system, and virtually no background information will be available at the intake moment. A probation intake interview is typically not lengthy— perhaps 30–60 minutes at most. In this time, a probation intake officer must obtain enough information to make decisions about a youth's immediate safety needs, the potential need for further evaluation, and the safety of the community if the youth lives at home while awaiting further processing; the officer must also decide whether to try to work with the caretaker and youth informally, or to schedule the case for adjudication. Sometimes these decisions must be made "on the spot," as the officer moves literally from the interview to the court to register his or her recommendation.

A second important doorway is the *pretrial detention facility*. Often youths are brought to a detention center by law enforcement officers minutes or hours after being apprehended at home, on the street, or elsewhere in the community. Admissions to detention occur every day, often at any time of day or night. Some detention centers may have only 1 or 2 admissions a day, while others may have 40–50. Youths typically arrive without any accompanying information about them other than the law enforcement officers' report of the reasons for apprehension. Detention centers with computerized record systems may be able to obtain background records on youths who have been referred to the juvenile justice system before, but many will be first-time offenders or youths from outside the community who do not yet have a file in the juvenile court. Although the detention center may notify youths' parents or other caretakers very soon after the youths arrive, the vast majority of youths do not receive visits from caretakers for the first several days of their detention, and some youths never receive visits prior to their discharge. Some youths will remain in detention only a few days before they are released, while others will stay for many months while awaiting their trials.

Staff members are expected to obtain enough information early in each youth's stay to make decisions about the youth's safety, the safety of others in detention, and the youth's medical and mental health needs that may require immediate attention. Typically this must occur at least within the first 24 hours after the youth's admission, although delaying the collection of information beyond the first 6–12 hours increases the risk that emergency needs (e.g., suicide potential) will not be detected in time to prevent negative consequences. Screening in this context is often done by detention officers who are not clinically trained, but who have received in-service training on the screening process.

The third setting is intake into a *juvenile corrections program* after adjudication. Such programs range from secure facilities, usually outside the community, to nonsecure or staff-secure residential facilities within the community. Typically a range of information about each youth is available upon entry, in the form of probation intake records and evaluations that may have been done during the adjudication process in order to assist the court in making dispositional decisions. Nevertheless, correctional staff members are responsible for identifying the youth's *current* mental state upon admission, in order to determine whether any emotional conditions may require immediate caution or response. Current mental conditions may not be apparent from the general or even detailed personality descriptions that accompany the youth.

Given this general description of these three settings and their circumstances, let us examine some of the practical considerations regarding the feasibility of instruments as screening devices in each setting.

Informant Availability

The three settings differ considerably in the sources of information about youths' current and recent mental status that are available to staff members at entry. In some settings information can be obtained immediately from both youths and their parents or other caretakers, while in others the caretakers are not available. Research indicates that obtaining information from both sources is preferable, because they have differing limitations and strengths (Grills & Ollendick, 2002). Youths sometimes underreport their involvement in troubling *behaviors*, which are reported with somewhat more accuracy by caretakers. Yet youths are often better informants about their internal *emotions and thoughts* than are their caretakers. Moreover, caretakers' descriptions of their children at the time of intake interviews or detention admission may be influenced by the adults' own fear, anger at their children, or hostility toward juvenile authorities as a reaction to their children's arrest.

Probation intake officers typically will be able to address questions to caretakers and youths, both of whom typically attend intake interviews. But detention and youth corrections personnel typically have only the youths as direct sources of information for screening during the first 6–12 hours after entry. Some screening tools described in later chapters are designed specifically to obtain information from a youth alone, while others require information from both the youth and a caretaker. These differences need to be taken into account in selecting screening instruments that are best suited to the informant demands of a particular juvenile justice setting.

Expertise

Instruments differ in the degree of expertise required for their administration and the translation of scores into decisions about responding to youths' mental health needs. Some methods require doctoral- or master's-level training for their application, while others have been designed to be used by juvenile justice personnel without any advanced training in psychiatry, psychology, or social work. Most of the latter instruments require in-service training of personnel who will be administering the screening procedures and using their results. But they vary in the degree of training required.

Selecting a tool for screening therefore requires a commitment to the costs associated either with employing mental health professionals or with providing adequate training to non-mental-health juvenile justice staff. The volume of screening cases in many juvenile justice facilities or programs typically favors instruments that can be administered by sensitive non-mental-health staff members after they are provided brief in-service training. Training costs should thus be explored when potential tools for mental health screening are being considered. Some test developers have training teams or a network of consultants from whom administrators can purchase training workshops for staff members when a juvenile justice program is implementing the test developer's instrument.

Efficiency of Administration

The time and effort required for administration vary across instruments, because instruments differ in their ease of administration. Some instruments allow youths to respond to printed questions, while others require that staff members present the questions in interview form. Some can be administered to small groups of youths, while others must be individually administered. Some instruments may be administered by computer: A youth is able to answer questions in response to on-screen or computer-transmitted audible questions, without any staff involvement other than visual monitoring of the youth. Cost savings in staff time in the latter arrangements may be considerable, although equipment costs are greater for computer-assisted administration, of course. Tools to screen for youths' mental health needs vary in all these respects, requiring choices that fit a particular juvenile justice program's resources.

The time required to administer tools for mental health screening is important not only because of staff commitments, but also because of demands for case processing. Mental health screening often occurs in the context of gathering information about a wider range of data, including health information, family background, and developmental history. As noted earlier, some juvenile court intake procedures provide only an hour or so for this whole process. Tools that require longer time for gathering mental health information decrease the time for acquiring these other types of information.

This discussion may lead some to believe that the ideal screening choices are simply the tools requiring the least amount of time. But the matter is not that simple. There tends to be a relationship between the length of time tools require for administration and the breadth and quality of the information they provide. Designing a tool for 10-minute administration requires the test developer to sacrifice some of the advantages of lengthier instruments. Briefer tools typically obtain a more limited range of mental health information (e.g., number and types of symptoms or diagnoses), and the accuracy or dependability of the results is decreased. The choice therefore requires balancing the advantages of efficiency in obtaining information against the desire for maximum integrity of the information one acquires. But there is no formula for making this choice, and the "correct" choice will vary considerably across types of juvenile justice settings and doorways.

Financial Cost of Materials

Using instruments for mental health screening typically requires purchasing of materials of various kinds. Because instruments vary considerably in this respect, a system's resources will have some influence on which instruments are chosen.

Virtually all instruments require the purchase of manuals for use by the personnel who will perform screening procedures. In addition, some instruments require the use of individual, nonreusable answer forms and scoring forms. Some tests' publishers allow these to be photocopied without cost, while others require that forms be purchased in packages, creating a per-case cost.

As noted earlier, there is an increasing array of electronic services for mental health screening. For some instruments, youths' responses can be processed by computers, which use complex algorithms and item weightings to arrive at scores. These scoring systems sometimes are made available for downloading onto a juvenile justice program's personal computers. For some tests this is an optional arrangement, while for others it is the only way to score the test. For some tests these computer scoring programs can be used indefinitely, while others are programmed to score a specified number of cases, after which an additional purchase is necessary to "reload" the system for a new batch of cases. For a few assessment tools, users cannot purchase scoring programs at all, but instead must send youths' raw test data electronically to the test publishing company for scoring; the scores (and sometimes written interpretations) are communicated back within a few hours, and the user is billed a service fee per month or by the number of cases.

Finally, in recent years, a number of companies have begun to offer full online assessment services to juvenile justice programs. These companies typically pay a licensing fee to test publishers or authors in order to include their instruments among an array of online tools, from which a juvenile justice program may create its own screening package. When a facility has a youth who needs screening, the facility dials up the assessment service, which administers the package to the youth through the computer-based assessment process, provides the results to the facility, and bills the facility by case or by some other prior fee arrangement.

In summary, methods vary considerably in their practical and financial feasibility, both of which vary in turn across juvenile justice programs. Financial costs typically rise in relation to the practical efficiency of administration and scoring features. Similarly, administration time and effort rise in relation to the comprehensiveness of the instrument. Selecting a screening tool for use with every youth entering a juvenile justice facility requires weighing all these factors in light of the facility's objectives, fiscal responsibilities, program resources, and volume of cases.

THE CONTEXT FOR ASSESSMENT

As defined earlier, the term "assessment" pertains to mental health evaluations that are performed selectively (i.e., with some youths and not others). In contrast to screening, assessment usually seeks to obtain more comprehensive information about a youth than that provided by brief screening, as well as a more individualized picture of the youth's mental health needs.

Assessment of mental disorders is conducted for three purposes during juvenile justice processing of delinquency cases: (1) to follow up on screening results, (2) to address forensic questions in the adjudication process, and (3) to determine needs and construct plans for longer-term treatment. We examine each of these purposes, focusing on their implications for the selection and use of tools in assessment processes.

Assessments to Follow Up on Screening

Screening identifies potential high-need cases, but it is limited in its ability to provide all of the information facility personnel will want before authorizing emergency treatment procedures. This is largely because the relatively brief and simple formats of tools that are typically used in screening require some sacrifices in their accuracy and their ability to describe youths comprehensively. Therefore, screening is often followed by more careful and individualized assessments for those youths whose screening results place them in "at-risk" categories for various types of disorders or troubling conditions. These assessments are in part intended to determine more specifically the youths' current mental condition, and especially to clarify whether some intervention is needed immediately or relatively soon.

Assessment as a follow-up to screening occurs in different ways across juvenile justice programs. The following are two dimensions to consider, along with their implications for selecting assessment tools for this process.

Assessment Tools with or without Professional Consultation

Perhaps the most straightforward way to accomplish assessment after screening is to have a system that basically schedules all "screened-in" youths for a clinical interview by a psychiatrist (an MD), a doctoral-level clinical psychologist, or a master's-level psychologist or social worker shortly after the youths have been identified as "at risk" by the screening process. Many juvenile correctional intake programs will have these professionals on staff either full time or part time. Some pretrial detention centers are able to afford consultations with such professionals, while others will find these arrangements difficult, due to financial constraints or the lack of relevant mental health professionals in their community. When they are available, these professionals will sometimes use psychological assessment instruments selected from among those described in later chapters in this book (clinical psychologists will do this more often than psychiatrists). They will then combine data from these tests with the results of their own interviews of the youths, in order to arrive at clinical judgments about the nature and extent of the youths' immediate needs.

Some juvenile justice programs, however, choose to employ assessment tools as "second-screening" devices, thus reducing further the number of youths who will require referrals for professional consultation. In these arrangements, specially designated and trained staff members of the facility administer an assessment tool and use the results to decide on the best course of intervention, if any, in response to the data.

Assessment tools will differ in their suitability for these two arrangements. For example, some assessment instruments require doctoral-level training to administer and interpret. Others have been designed for administration and interpretation by master's-level counselors, psychologists, social workers, or other juvenile justice personnel who have been provided intensive training in the specific assessment method to be employed. Thus a wider range of assessment tools is available for the consultant-based model of screening follow-up than for the staff-based model. The question of who should or can administer and interpret a particular test may be answered by tests' publishers, who often restrict the sale of some instruments to doctoral-level professionals.

Focused versus Comprehensive Assessment

Screening follow-up assessments may be designed for two different objectives. One approach is to obtain more detailed and individualized information on specific conditions that have been identified as potential problems in screening. For example, youths who score high on measures of suicide potential or alcohol/drug use in screening may be provided with a follow-up assessment to define the degree and seriousness of the suicide risk or the substance use. The second approach is for youths who score high on any problem area in screening to be provided with a broader, more comprehensive assessment that does not focus exclusively on that specific problem area. For example, youths scoring high on any of several scales in a screening tool may be evaluated for the full range of basic psychiatric diagnoses, or may be given a battery of tests that generally assess personality traits and functioning pertaining to many different areas of youths' lives.

Some assessment instruments described later in this book focus on specific problem areas or disorders; for example, they provide a more detailed picture of a youth's substance use or risk of harmful behavior. Other assessment instruments have many scales that cover a wide range of personal characteristics and problem areas. A few instruments are versatile in this regard. The Diagnostic Interview Schedule for Children, for example, can be used to acquire information to determine whether a youth meets criteria for any of a wide range of psychiatric diagnoses, or it can be adapted so that the instrument's questions focus only on checking a specific diagnosis or a limited range of diagnoses. In any case, the selection of instruments for screening follow-up will be influenced by the focused or comprehensive approach employed in a particular juvenile justice setting.

Forensic Assessments

As noted in Chapter 1, one of the juvenile justice system's obligations is to assure due process in the adjudication of youths charged with delinquencies. Due process requirements assure that the jurisdiction will abide by various procedural and evidentiary rules in adjudicating delinquency. They are intended to protect against possible abuse of authority in proceedings that might restrict the liberties of the accused.

Several due process questions in juvenile courts raise the need for information about youths' mental disorders and developmental disabilities. Some pertain to the youths' capacities to make decisions that will influence their adjudication. For example, youths' confessions to police officers (usually made without the advice of an attorney) may be used as evidence in their trials only if their prior waivers of the rights to silence and to legal counsel were made "voluntarily, knowingly, and intelligently" after they were warned of their "*Miranda* rights" (Grisso, 1981, 2003). Attorneys and courts sometimes must consider whether mental illness or developmental disability might have influenced a youth's ability to understand the rights and the potential consequences of waiving them. Similarly, during the adjudication process (from arraignment through trial), defendants in criminal and in juvenile court delinquency trials must be competent to stand trial. That is, they must be able to grasp the nature of the trial process, work with their attorneys to construct a defense, and make important decisions about pleading and plea agreements (see generally Grisso & Schwartz, 2000). Mental disorders and developmental disabilities sometimes compromise youths' abilities to function within this legal context (Grisso et al., 2003).

Attention to mental disorders in the interest of due process arises also in cases in which the prosecution seeks to transfer (or waive) a youth from juvenile to criminal court, allowing the youth to be tried as an adult. In many states, transfer to criminal court occurs automatically for certain offenses. But most states also allow for transfer by judicial discretion. In states in which the latter option is possible, courts typically may decide to transfer only when there is substantial evidence that a youth (1) is not amenable to rehabilitation in the juvenile justice system and (2) presents a significant danger to the community if retained in the juvenile system. The evidence for these matters must be weighed in a formal "transfer hearing." Youths' mental disorders, and their possible relation to future aggression, are relevant to consider in the context of the two primary factors the court must address.

In cases in which these questions of youths' capacities and future prospects are raised, courts and attorneys often request that mental health professionals perform special evaluations to determine whether mental disorders or developmental disabilities (or sometimes even simple immaturity) may significantly impair the abilities relevant to these legal questions (e.g., Barnum, 2000; Oberlander, Goldstein, & Goldstein, 2003), or may influence the youths' rehabilitation prospects and degree of risk related to transfer criteria (Grisso, 1998, 2000). The fact that these evaluations are focused on the resolution of legal questions during the adjudicative process (e.g., competence to stand trial, transfer to criminal court), not primarily on the youths' actual clinical welfare, is what makes them "forensic" assessments rather than ordinary clinical assessments.

Evaluations to address forensic questions may call for the use of three different types of assessment tools: clinical instruments, risk-of-harm instruments, and what have been called "forensic assessment instruments" (Grisso, 1986, 2003). We discuss these with reference to evaluations for legal competencies in delinquency cases, especially competence to stand trial and the capacity to have made a valid waiver of *Miranda* rights at the time of police questioning.

Clinical Instruments

Forensic questions of youths' characteristics related to legal competencies and to transfer to criminal court usually require an evaluation of potential mental disorders and developmental disabilities (Grisso, 1998; Melton, Petrila, Poythress, & Slobogin, 1997). With regard to the transfer question, the presence of a mental disorder may indicate a need for treatment that has a good prospect of reducing future delinquency and that cannot be provided to an adolescent if the youth were transferred to the adult justice system. Regarding questions of competence to stand trial, most states' laws recognize mental illnesses and mental retardation as potential causes of defendants' inabilities to understand the trial process, to assist counsel in a defense, or to make important decisions about waiving rights (e.g., the decision whether to plead guilty). Thus diagnostic conditions are important to determine.

New laws in some states pertaining to juveniles' competencies present reasons for examiners to consider nondiagnostic conditions as well. That is, some courts have come to recognize developmental immaturity as a cause of incompetence to stand trial (Bonnie & Grisso, 2000; Redding & Frost, 2002). Emotional and psychosocial characteristics such as dependency, extreme impulsiveness, and poor perspective on the long-range consequences of decisions can be causes of the same inabilities described above. Some instruments in this book focus specifically on assessing these characteristics, while other tools focusing primarily on psychopathology may also be relevant. Yet not all of the psychopathology instruments assess personality dimensions that may vary as a consequence of immaturity. Clinicians will want to take this into consideration when selecting tools for use in forensic assessments related to youths' capacities in the delinquency adjudication process.

Instruments to Assess Risk of Harm to Others

Until recently, there have been no suitable tools for use with adolescents to assess specifically their "risk of harm to others" (or "violence risk"). Several such tools have been developed in recent years, however, and these are described in Part V of this book.

When selecting violence risk instruments, clinicians must carefully examine the evidence for each instrument's validity in predicting future violence, especially the type of violence that the instrument claims to predict and the time frame for that prediction (i.e., how far into the future it extends). Some research studies with youth violence instruments have defined "violence" broadly (e.g., any aggressive behavior) and others narrowly (e.g., injury to others). Some have examined instruments' abilities to predict violence within a month, and others within the coming year or two. Still others have examined whether a youth's current violence signifies a much longer-range chronic risk that will extend into adulthood. Clinicians must examine these research results to determine whether the type of violence risk that an instrument measures matches the future-harm questions posed by the court in a particular case.

Forensic Assessment Instruments

Forensic questions of youths' capacities related to legal competencies are not answered with determinations of their mental disorders alone, even if such disorders are relatively serious. (A defendant may have a mental illness yet be competent to stand trial.) A clinician must also discover specifically what a youth understands, believes, or can do that is necessary to function within the legal context in question (e.g., within the police interrogation where *Miranda* rights were waived, or within the trial process). If there are deficits in those functional abilities, then the clinician determines whether they are consequences of the youth's psychopathology.

The need to assess individuals' actual functional abilities associated with these legal contexts has resulted in the development of so-called "forensic assessment instruments" (Grisso, 1986, 2003). These tools provide a structured process wherein clinicians can assess specifically those characteristics of youths that have some essential connection to the legal definitions of the functional abilities relevant to the legal questions. Although many such instruments have been developed for use with adults (Grisso, 2003; Heilbrun, 2001; Melton et al., 1997), very few have yet been developed for use with adolescents. Part VI of this book describes three of these instruments.

Admissibility of Testimony Based on Instruments

Assessments for forensic mental health questions are unlike general clinical evaluations, in that they are intended primarily for use by judges and attorneys in their resolution of legal questions. Judges will often rely heavily on forensic clinicians' reports, and prosecutors as well as youths' defense attorneys often wish to challenge the results of such evaluations. This sometimes means that a clinician will be asked to testify during a hearing at which the clinician's results undergo close scrutiny, often involving cross-examination aimed at finding weaknesses in the clinician's methods or interpretations.

In this context, clinicians may encounter challenges to their use of certain psychological assessment tools. A clinician's opinions may be considered inadmissible as evidence if they are based on evaluation methods that do not meet certain standards that have been outlined for the courts in prior cases. This presents clinicians with an additional set of considerations when they are selecting instruments for use in their forensic evaluations, as opposed to their clinical evaluations. Specifically, to what extent will an instrument satisfy these legal standards if the question of admissibility of a clinician's testimony based on the instrument is raised?

Two types of standards are employed, depending on the state in which a clinician is practicing. Some states employ a criterion established in *Frye v. United States* (1923), which focuses on whether the method one uses (in this case, the instrument) has been generally accepted for use in one's field of practice. This older criterion, however, has given way in other states to a newer one established in *Daubert v. Merrell Dow Pharmaceuticals* (1993). When the question of the admissibility of testimony based on a specific instrument is raised in those states, *Daubert* standards direct judges to consider such matters as whether the validity of the method can be scientifically tested (and whether it has, and with what results); what is known about the degree of error in the method; whether the method has been peer-reviewed; and—as in the *Frye* standard—its degree of use or acceptance in the field (for discussions, see Heilbrun, 2001; Melton et al., 1997). Unfortunately, when one is choosing an instrument for use in forensic evaluation cases, there is no universal formula for evaluating whether the instrument will meet these legal criteria, because they are employed somewhat differently and often unevenly across cases and states.

Disposition Assessments

Perhaps the most frequent mental health assessments in juvenile courts are those that assist judicial decisions about the disposition of juvenile cases. "Disposition" is the juvenile court equivalent of "sentencing" in criminal courts; it involves a judgment regarding what will happen to a youth who is found delinquent. The juvenile court's rehabilitative mandate, however, directs the court to consider not only the appropriate punitive consequences, but also the course of commitment that has the best prospects for reducing the likelihood of future delinquency. Thus a clinician is often asked to perform an evaluation prior to the court's decision about a disposition for a delinquency case. The disposition hearing always occurs after the hearing at which the youth is found delinquent on the charges. The assessment itself is sometimes performed between those two events, but often it occurs prior to adjudication (while the youth is awaiting trial), in order to avoid a delay between the adjudication finding and the disposition hearing.

Disposition decisions often focus on two factors for which clinical assessments can be helpful (Grisso, 1998). One of these pertains to the youth's mental health needs: Does the youth have a mental disorder or other mental disability that requires treatment, and if so, what are the most appropriate community-based options or residential and correctional programs to meet that need? The second factor is risk of aggression: What does the court need to know about the youth in order to decide about the degree of security needed in the youth's placement to reduce the risk of harm to others?

The questions of youths' mental health needs and risk of violence are sometimes intertwined. Youths with mental disorders do not necessarily present a greater risk of harm to others than youths without mental disorders (see Chapter 2; for reviews, see Connor, 2002; Grisso, 2004). But when their aggression is in part stimulated by their mental disorders, then understanding their disorders and treating these appropriately are important parts of a rehabilitation plan that may reduce their future aggression and risk of harm to others.

Clinicians therefore have two needs for instruments in disposition assessments. They often use measures of child psychopathology to provide data that will be combined with their interviews and mental health record reviews to arrive at conclusions about youths' mental disorders and needs for treatment. In addition, they need special tools designed to assist them in estimating the future risk of violence and aggression. As noted earlier, the research behind violence risk instruments has sometimes focused on short-term predictions, sometimes on 1-year or 2-year predictions, and even sometimes on predictions about a youth's probable violence later in adulthood. Decisions about a youth's need for a secure placement during the next year will thus be assisted better by some instruments than by others, depending on the time frame for which they were validated.

POLICY CONSIDERATIONS
IN SCREENING AND ASSESSMENT

Implementing mental health screening and assessment requires more than choosing the right instrument for each job. One must also create the right circumstances for the use of the instrument. In many respects, the best instruments for screening and assessment are like any other well-made tools (be they computers, hammers, automobiles, laboratory instruments, or firearms): None have been made that can achieve their positive potential when they are used in the wrong situations, by the wrong people, or for the wrong purposes. In fact, no matter how skillfully tools are crafted and with whatever good intentions, the conditions under which they are used can render them useless at best and destructive at worst. In the case of screening and assessment in juvenile justice programs, it is in the *greater* interest of youths if program personnel do *not* employ the instruments in this book than if they use them thoughtlessly.

The burden of employing instruments for screening and assessment in ways that will maximize their potential and will not do damage lies squarely on the shoulders of (1) juvenile justice administrators who form, implement and maintain policies that regulate screening and assessment practices within their agencies; and (2) clinicians who perform assessments or consult to administrators on matters of clinical policy. Three areas of policy formation require careful consideration when these professionals are implementing mental health screening and assessment in juvenile justice programs: (1) decision rules, (2) personnel guidance, and (3) controlled use.

Policies about Decisions Based on Screening
and Assessment Results

The need for policy regarding decision rules begins with this recognition: No instrument ever provides results that literally tell anyone that a youth has a condition requiring a particular course of action. An examination of the instruments in this book will reveal no screening instrument that provides a "Get more comprehensive assessment" score. No mental health assessment instrument concludes with a "Psychoactive medication needed" score or a "Pursue inpatient commitment" score, and no violence risk instrument ends with a "Place in secure detention" score. They produce numbers that represent the presence or likelihood of symptoms, problems in functioning, psychiatric diagnoses, personality traits, probability of aggression, or degree of cognitive deficit. This is all they do.

Yet if screening and assessment lead only to obtaining those numbers, they have no compelling purpose in practice. The primary reason for using these instruments is to reach a decision about how to respond to a youth's mental condition—whether to implement a suicide watch, request a psychiatric consultation, pursue more comprehensive assessment, seek a more secure placement, or recommend a future mental health treatment plan as part of the youth's disposition.

It follows that a system's commitment to use instruments in mental health screening and assessment entails a commitment on the part of administrators and clinicians to construct "decision rules" that translate instruments' scores into systematic responses to youths' mental health needs. These rules then provide guidance and structure at every level of the agency. Facility staff members know exactly what response to make when particular screening scores are obtained. Supervisors know what mechanisms need to be in place for staff members to implement those responses. And juvenile justice administrators will be able to respond confidently when asked by the public specifically how they deal with youths with mental health needs. But they will not know these things simply because the system is collecting scores. They will know them because administrators and clinicians have established rules about how the scores are to be used to make decisions.

Recent years have brought increased pressure on juvenile justice administrators to implement mental health screening and assessment, as well as increased guidance in the choice of screening and assessment methods (Cocozza & Skowyra, 2000, in press). By contrast, administrators find little in the literature to guide policy formation regarding the decision rules to apply to results of the screening and assessment methods they choose. How serious does a mental disorder have to be, or how high a symptom score is required, to signal that a particular mental health response should be made? Do all types of mental disorders necessarily require an immediate response while youths are in detention, or can some of them wait until a stable placement is found? What cutoff score on a screening tool measuring degrees of depression should be used to signal a call to the consulting psychiatrist to examine a youth more closely, or to hospitalize the youth? Almost no literature answers these questions for administrators. But a structure that may help them in their formation of policies about these decisions revolves around four considerations, which we call the "four R's": *responses, research, resources,* and *risk*.

Responses

A first step in arriving at decision rules based on mental health screening or assessment results is to take stock of the possible responses to various types of juvenile mental health needs. Some of these responses are in effect additional assessment, as when the results of a screening tool are used to decide on a "second screening" to further determine the seriousness of the first screening's results (Grisso & Barnum, 2003), or when the results are used to decide to ask for consultation or more comprehensive assessment by a clinician. Other potential responses include immediate interventions (e.g., instigating a suicide watch or applying for psychiatric hospitalization), whereas still others involve setting up a longer-term treatment plan. Taking stock of all possible responses will not translate directly into decision rules for the use of assessment data, but it is a necessary first step.

Research

Although instruments' scores do not indicate specifically how to respond, sometimes the research involved in the instruments' development provides information that can help in making policy decisions about appropriate responses. For example, validity studies for some instruments have examined the scores of youths who were or were not considered appropriate for inpatient clinical services. Sometimes this has been translated to provide meaning for the scores—for example, "Among youths requiring inpatient psychiatric care, 75% scored above [X, the cutoff score], while only 20% of youths in the general community exceeded this score." This research-based cutoff score thus begins to provide a basis for forming policy about how particular scores might appropriately lead to particular responses. But it still does not tell the policymakers whether X should be used to trigger a particular intervention, because there are other matters to consider.

Resources

Decision rules about a system's response to youths' mental health needs will be determined in part by the resources available to the system for implementing various potential responses. Sometimes the type of responses that can be implemented are limited by circumstances—for example, the lack of any child psychiatric facilities or child psychiatrists in a rural area. At other times they are limited by scarce financial resources.

In the latter case, developing decision rules about how to respond to youths' mental health needs requires policymakers to deal with the question of resources in either of two ways. One approach is to adjust decision rules (e.g., how high a score has to be in order to trigger a particular response) so that they do not identify a greater proportion of youths than the system's financial resources can bear. For example, when the costs of a particular type of intervention challenge the system's financial capacity, cutoff scores for triggering that intervention can be set higher, thus reducing the number of youths whose scores would call for that intervention. Alternatively, the cutoff score can be set at a level that is driven by some index of need rather than financial considerations. For example, policymakers may create a decision rule that all youths scoring in the "clinically significant" range on an instrument must receive treatment, and then argue for procurement of the financial resources to meet this need if it triggers a greater number of positive cases than the system can currently afford.

Many child advocates would argue that the latter approach is preferable. Yet a knee-jerk presumption that "more treatment is better" is not responsible management. Resources are always limited, and money spent in one part of a system may often mean that needs in another part of the system go unmet (Grisso, 2004). For example, might additional funding to support more frequent psychiatric hospitalization have a negative effect on a request at another time to fund an important community-based treatment for adolescents' substance use?

Managing this aspect of decision rules for responding to screening and assessment scores is complex and difficult. The answers cannot be reduced to simple arguments for either "cost reduction" or "treatment for kids at any cost." The ultimate answers often require much soul searching regarding basic priorities and values, and implementing screening or assessment often requires laying these values on the table for close and painful scrutiny.

Risk

In the formation of decision rules about responses to screening and assessment results, lowering or raising the standard (i.e., the cutoff score) does more than merely increase or decrease the number of youths that will receive a particular intervention. It also increases or decreases the number of times that staff members will make wrong decisions about youths. Moreover, these adjustments to standards create more than one way to be wrong, so that policymakers must decide what kinds of risks of wrong decisions are more bearable. Chapter 4 will describe why this is so in some detail, but the following is a preview of that discussion.

Forming policies about cutoff scores requires consideration of the consequences of setting higher or lower cutoffs. One of the consequences of using a higher cutoff score is that most of the youths who score above it actually need services. This is because fewer youths who do *not* really need services will score that high, so it reduces the number of youths to whom further services will be provided unnecessarily. However, raising the cutoff score also means that more youths who actually *do* need services will be missed, whereas a slightly lower cutoff score could have allowed more of them to be identified.

In other words, policymakers will be wrong in either instance, but in different ways. If they lower the cutoff, they will more often be wrong by providing services for some youths who are *not* greatly in need. They are increasing the risk of ineffective use of the system's financial resources, which could be employed in other ways to benefit youths and society. Yet if they raise the cutoff score, they will more often be wrong by missing youths who *are* truly in need. Being wrong in this instance sometimes means dealing with a youth's successful suicide, learning about a murder by a youth with a mental disorder who did not receive services at the appropriate time, or presiding over a juvenile justice system with an extraordinarily high recidivism rate that might have been lower if more youths had received necessary mental health services. Setting decision rules for use of screening and assessment results therefore requires policymakers to analyze the types of risks they believe are more necessary to take.

Working with the "Four R's"

Although there is no formula for their use, the "four R's"—responses, research, resources, and risk—can be used creatively to arrive at decision rules. For example, policymakers can work within limited *resources* by using a higher cutoff score (reducing the number of youths who will receive services) and bearing the *risk* of neglecting some who are in need, or by maintaining a lower cutoff score suggested by *research* but mandating a type of *response* that is of lower cost than the intervention they might prefer if they had unlimited funds. Whatever the strategy, there must be one. Failure to attend to policy regarding the translation of instruments' scores into intervention decisions nullifies the value of any screening and assessment program.

Policies about Screening and Assessment Personnel

The value of screening and assessment is also nullified by failure to establish policies about the personnel on whom these processes depend. Haphazard administration of the best screening instruments can render them invalid, and improper administration and use of assessment tools by clinicians can produce misleading information. Administrators must have policies that minimize these negative potentials and maximize the usefulness of mental health screening and assessment.

Some juvenile detention centers are operated by personnel who are flexible to new demands, are concerned about youths' mental health problems, and look for ways to improve their impact on youths. Other detention centers are staffed by workers who resist any new demands, are concerned primarily about the problems that youths create for them, and look for ways to do the job with the least effort possible. Many detention centers fall between these two extremes.

Staff members at these two types of detention centers will react differently to a system's intention to put into place a new mental health screening procedure, for example. Those in the first type of setting cautiously welcome it as something that they might adopt as daily practice, that they might learn from, and that might increase their effectiveness. Staff members at the second type of detention center regard the plan grudgingly, resist until they are forced to adopt it, and then learn ways to comply with orders for screening while minimizing any additional effort beyond that to which they have been accustomed. Personnel at many detention centers manifest some of both attitudes.

In order for screening and assessment instruments to have value, they must be used by personnel who at least are open to their potential values, and therefore are motivated to employ them in as effective a manner as possible. Administrators are responsible for creating those conditions. This is often done by careful selection of the personnel who will actually be involved in screening or assessment processes. Creating the proper conditions also requires appropriate in-service education for all staff members who will be responsible for administration of screening instruments and who will be using the results to make decisions about interventions. These educational preparations should focus not only on the mechanics of the process, but also on its potential value. Screening and assessment can be shown to be of value not only to youths, but also to youth workers who need a way to think about the difficult behaviors of delinquent youths with mental disorders, and who need ways to respond that reduce their own frustrations.

Such efforts to promote positive staff attitudes toward mental health screening and assessment can be facilitated if the instruments chosen are straightforward in meaning and capable of being administered efficiently. In addition, as noted earlier, staff members are likely to appreciate the structure provided by clear administrative polices that translate scores on these instruments into decisions about responding to youths.

Policies Controlling the Use of Screening and Assessment Data

Chapter 1 has discussed three obligations of the juvenile justice system in responding to youths' mental health needs: a custodial obligation to attend to youths' welfare and treatment, a due process obligation to protect their legal interests, and a public safety obligation to reduce the risk of harm to others. The need to attend to all three of these obligations sometimes produces conflicts when administrators are developing policies and practices for appropriate mental health screening and assessment. These conflicts tend to focus on the ways in which mental health information about youths might be used or misused, or on various purposes related to these obligations.

Avoiding Therapeutically Inappropriate Use of Screening Data

The purpose of mental health screening is to determine whether youths have immediate mental health needs that require a therapeutic response, and whether they present a risk of harm to themselves or others within the relatively short-range future. There is the danger, however, that the system will attempt to use the results of mental health screening tools for purposes that exceed these intentions and the capacities of the tools themselves.

One of these dangers lies in the use of screening tool results for disposition hearings. As noted earlier, a disposition hearing follows adjudication and involves judicial decisions about a youth's longer-term placement, rehabilitation, and treatment. The types of information about a youth with mental disorders that a disposition hearing requires include diagnoses, a knowledge of the youth's personality traits, and a relatively individualized clinical picture of the youth's psychopathology. Most tools used for initial screening have not been designed to provide those types of information. Their structure and purposes allow them to separate youths into a few broad categories, but not to produce the finer-grained descriptions on which disposition decisions should be based. Moreover, they are administered at a time and place—admission to some part of the justice system—when youths' screening results may reflect a mix of temporary and enduring characteristics, so that within a week or two youths may look somewhat different from what their screening results would suggest.

Despite these limitations on the value of screening data for longer-range treatment planning, some juvenile justice systems are tempted to use screening data for those purposes. This can happen because the screening data are the only information they have, or because they wish to avoid the expense of more comprehensive assessments that would provide the type of data disposition decisions really require. Yet this is one of those situations in which *some* data are *not* better than no data at all. Making long-range treatment plans solely on the basis of tools that were not designed for that purpose can result in misguided treatment that is not only damaging to youths' longer-range welfare, but also wasteful of resources.

Administrators must avoid this misuse by developing policies that limit the use of screening data to short-range mental health decisions—for example, to decisions about responses to youths' current and immediate mental health needs within a few days or weeks of screening. Such policies may have to be implemented across various parts of a juvenile justice program, rather than merely within the facility where screening occurs. For example, screening results in detention centers are often communicated to nondetention personnel, such as the probation officers who are assigned to youths to work with them as they move through the pretrial process. These probation officers are often responsible for making disposition recommendations to courts after the youths' adjudication. Therefore, the need for a policy to avoid the use of screening data alone for longer-range treatment planning sometimes must originate from detention administrators, but must be developed in collaboration with the court's probation department.

Avoiding Prejudicial Use of Screening Data

By "prejudicial use," we mean the use of screening results in ways that might jeopardize the legal interests of youths as defendants. The risks of prejudicial use of screening are greatest when screening occurs prior to adjudication on current charges—for example, during pretrial first contact with a probation intake officer or at a pretrial detention center. We are aware of several instances in which prosecutors, learning that their local detention center was going to begin systematic mental health screening, issued a memo to detention center administrators that all screening results should routinely be sent to the prosecutors' office. Considering the content of some screening instruments, this would make available to prosecutors such information as youths' admissions to drug and alcohol use, tendencies toward anger and revenge, harm to others, and poor attitudes toward school. This information could potentially be used against the youths in plea bargaining, at trial, or after adjudication (to argue for more restrictive dispositions). In other instances, defense attorneys have objected to the implementation of routine screening tools in detention centers, anticipating that their young clients may be providing "self-incriminating" or at least defense-jeopardizing information to probation officers and prosecutors.

These legal implications of screening present juvenile justice administrators with conflicting demands. On the one hand, they are often required by law or juvenile justice policy to perform health and mental health screening. On the other hand, they are obligated by law to protect the due process rights of youths. Often it seems that the obligation to care for youths' psychological welfare when they are in custody is in conflict with the obligation to protect their right to a defense that seeks to resist custody. The conflict, however, may not be difficult to resolve. There are at least two ways to reduce the risk that screening instruments will be prejudicially used.

One way is to select screening tools in part on the basis of the degree of jeopardy associated with their content. A screening tool that asks, "Have you recently physically injured someone on purpose?" has a more potentially prejudicial effect than one that asks, "Do you sometimes get into fights?" Selection of tools therefore might involve careful attention to each item's potential prejudicial content, weighed against the necessity for the item's wording. The objective is to minimize the potential for prejudice as much as possible, while still meeting mental health objectives. Note, however, that this must be done at the level of *tool* selection, not *item* selection. One should not simply remove or reword offending items in an existing screening instrument. In addition to violating copyright laws, removing or rewriting test items means that whatever is known about the instrument's validity will no longer apply.

Another way to reduce the danger is to develop policies that restrict the use of pretrial mental health screening information to the primary use for which it is intended. We are aware of a number of ways that juvenile justice programs have restricted the use of screening results. In one instance, a prohibition of the use of mental health screening information in any legal proceeding against youths was inserted into a state's juvenile justice legislation. More often the matter is settled locally through an agreement between the prosecutor's office and the juvenile defense bar, to the effect that screening results will not be communicated to prosecutors or will not be used in any legal proceeding related to a youth's adjudication. The agreement can be translated into a "rule of the court" by the local chief juvenile court judge, thus establishing it as formal policy with legal authority.

Arriving at this agreement will certainly involve debate within the court and the detention system, in which all parties will raise issues. The judge may contend, "We must screen youths for mental health needs; to do otherwise fails to meet our legal and moral obligations while they are minors in our custody." The defense may argue, "A defendant should not be required to provide information that assists the court in restricting the defendant's liberty." The prosecution may insist, "Some information related to screening must be released to persons outside the probation or detention setting. For example, we are all required by law to identify youths who are themselves in danger of being abused so that we can protect them, or who might endanger others so that we can protect the public."

Almost all such conflicts can be resolved with proper attention, because the parties themselves have a variety of reasons to work collaboratively to seek mutually beneficial ends. But it is the role of the probation supervisor or the detention administrator to anticipate and raise these issues for policy resolution before selecting and implementing mental health screening procedures.

CONCLUSION: FINDING THE FIT
BETWEEN INSTRUMENTS AND SETTINGS

This chapter has focused on the importance of context in choosing instruments for screening and assessment, and in implementing them within juvenile justice programs. The discussion has identified two broad ways in which context matters: Context makes demands on instruments, and instruments make demands on the context.

Concerning the first context–instrument consideration, the selection of tools from among those that appear later in this book must take into account the purposes, demands, and constraints of the situations in which they will be used. They must be chosen for their feasibility with regard to administration and use. And they must be able to tell us what users want to know, when they want to know it, within the context in which they need to apply them. In short, the tools must fit the context.

Juvenile justice contexts are often quite different from the clinical contexts of hospitals and community mental health centers. Moreover, there are many contexts within juvenile justice systems—the probation intake interview, the admission to pretrial detention, and the front door of the secure juvenile corrections facility. Each of these contexts may require somewhat different kinds of information about youths' mental health conditions, and each provides somewhat different conditions in which the information can be obtained. The instruments in this book are not "interchangeable" in this regard; some will fit certain settings better than others.

Second, finding the "fit" often requires modifying the setting to accommodate the instrument. This requires managing the context itself, and sometimes altering it, in order to maximize the value of the instruments chosen for screening and assessment. No instrument can simply be inserted into an existing context and be expected to fulfill its mission. The setting itself must be prepared for its use: Legal issues must be resolved, staff members trained, clinicians contracted and briefed, and policies established for how the system will respond to the results of screening and assessment.

Thus context is extraordinarily important as a factor in selecting instruments for mental health screening and assessment. The other part of the selection process, however, consists of examining and evaluating the properties of the screening and assessment instruments themselves. Chapter 4 therefore discusses "looking inside" these instruments to determine their potential and to compare their relative values.

REFERENCES

Barnum, R. (2000). Clinical and forensic evaluation of competence to stand trial in juvenile defendants. In T. Grisso & R. Schwartz (Eds.), *Youth on trial: A developmental perspective on juvenile justice* (pp. 193–224). Chicago: University of Chicago Press.

Boesky, L. (2002). *Juvenile offenders with mental health disorders*. Lanham, MD: American Correctional Association.

Bonnie, R., & Grisso, T. (2000). Adjudicative competence and youthful offenders. In T. Grisso & R. Schwartz (Eds.), *Youth on trial: A developmental perspective on juvenile justice* (pp. 73–103). Chicago: University of Chicago Press.

Cocozza, J., & Skowyra, K. (2000). Youth with mental health disorders: Issues and emerging responses. *Juvenile Justice, 7*(1), 3–13.

Cocozza, J., & Skowyra, K. (Eds.). (in press). *Mental health needs of juvenile offenders: A comprehensive review*. Washington, DC: U.S. Department of Justice, Office of Juvenile Justice and Delinquency Prevention.

Connor, D. (2002). *Aggression and antisocial behavior in children and adolescents: Research and treatment*. New York: Guilford Press.

Council of Juvenile Correctional Administrators. (2001). *Performance-based standards for juvenile correction and detention facilities*. Retrieved from *http://www.performance.standards.org*

Daubert v. Merrell Dow Pharmaceuticals, 113 S.Ct. 2786 (1993).

Frye v. United States, 293 F. 1013 (D.C. Circuit 1923).

Grills, A., & Ollendick, T. (2002). Issues in parent–child agreement: The case of structured diagnostic interviews. *Clinical Child and Family Psychology Review, 5*, 57–83.

Grisso, T. (1981). *Juveniles' waiver of rights: legal and psychological competence*. New York: Plenum Press.

Grisso, T. (1986). *Evaluating competencies: Forensic assessments and instruments*. New York: Plenum Press.

Grisso, T. (1998). *Forensic evaluation of juveniles*. Sarasota, FL: Professional Resource Press.

Grisso, T. (2003). *Evaluating competencies: Forensic assessments and instruments* (2nd ed.). New York: Kluwer Academic/Plenum.

Grisso, T. (2004). *Double jeopardy: Adolescent offenders with mental disorders*. Chicago: University of Chicago Press.

Grisso, T., & Barnum, R. (2003). *Massachusetts Youth Screening Instrument—Version 2: User's manual and technical report*. Sarasota, FL: Professional Resource Press.

Grisso, T., & Schwartz, R. (Eds.). (2000). *Youth on trial: A developmental perspective on juvenile justice*. Chicago: University of Chicago Press.

Grisso, T., Steinberg, L., Woolard, J., Cauffman, E., Scott, E., Graham, S., et al. (2003). Juveniles' competence to stand trial: A comparison of adolescents' and adults' capacities as trial defendants. *Law and Human Behavior, 27*, 333–363.

Grisso, T., & Underwood, L. (in press). *Screening and assessing mental health and substance use disorders among youth in the juvenile justice system: A resource guide for practitioners*. Washington, DC: U.S. Department of Justice, Office of Juvenile Justice and Delinquency Prevention.

Heilbrun, K. (2001). *Principles of forensic mental health assessment*. New York: Kluwer Academic/Plenum.

Melton, G., Petrila, J., Poythress, N., & Slobogin, C. (1997). *Psychological evaluations for the courts* (2nd ed.). New York: Guilford Press.

Oberlander, L., Goldstein, N., & Goldstein, A. (2003). Competence to confess. In I. B. Weiner (Series Ed.) & A. Goldstein (Vol. Ed.), *Handbook of psychology: Vol. 11. Forensic psychology* (pp. 335–357). New York: Wiley.

Redding, R., & Frost, J. (2002). Adjudicative competence in the modern juvenile court. *Virginia Journal of Social Policy and Law, 9*, 353–410.

Wasserman, G. A., Jensen, P. S., & Ko, S. J. (2003). Mental health assessments in juvenile justice: Report on the Consensus Conference. *Journal of the American Academy of Child and Adolescent Psychiatry, 42*, 751–761.

CHAPTER 4

Evaluating the Properties
of Instruments
for Screening and Assessment

Thomas Grisso

Chapter 3 has described many of the practical considerations that one should have in mind when reviewing the appropriateness of various tools and instruments for the juvenile justice purposes and settings in which they might be used. The present chapter turns to the internal properties of the instruments themselves. Do they focus on the mental health characteristics that one wants to measure? What formats do they use to do this? How well do they do it? How does one know whether they measure anything dependably, and if they do, do they actually measure the thing they say they intend to measure?

The manner in which this chapter describes these internal properties of screening and assessment tools is aimed primarily at enhancing the understanding of administrators, judges, lawyers, and counselors in juvenile justice settings. It focuses on selecting existing tools, not constructing new ones. Therefore, the chapter omits a number of concepts and discussions that would be found in textbooks for psychometricians and clinical psychologists who develop such instruments or are professionally trained to use them. These professionals will find the present chapter helpful as a perspective on the psychometric relevance of their work for test consumers, but they will find neither the depth nor the specificity that characterizes their own literature.

Because of the special focus of this chapter on the consumer's selection of tests, we have written it in the second person. We feel this is a somewhat more friendly and consultative way to try to communicate what otherwise may seem to be a morass of impossibly technical concepts and considerations. The chapter covers the following topics and questions:

- Constructs (What does the tool claim to measure?)
- Content (How have the tool's intentions been translated into item content?)
- Procedure (How is it administered and scored?)
- Norm sample (What types of youths have been involved in the tool's development?)
- Internal integrity (Do the content and structure of the tool make sense?)
- Dependability of measurement, usually called "reliability" (Does the tool measure something consistently?)
- Confidence about meaning, usually called "validity" (Does the tool measure what it claims to measure?)

EXAMINING CONSTRUCTS

All tools begin with a set of concepts that identify what the test developer wants to measure. Some tools are designed to measure just one concept (e.g., "depression"), while others are designed to measure several mental health concepts. A few measure several concepts and then combine them to form a larger concept (e.g., several specific concepts such as "depression," "anxiety," and "anger" may then be combined to form a more general concept like "emotional distress"). These concepts are represented in the tool by labels for scales. There are several things to keep in mind as you review these labels in the process of determining whether this tool will tell you what you want to know about youths in your own screening or assessment situation.

Constructs and Their Text Definitions

When you look at the labels for what the tool says it measures, the thing to which each label refers is a "construct.". This is the same thing as a "concept," "notion," or "idea." But calling it a "construct" helps you remember that the "thing" the tool intends to measure—for example, depression—has been "constructed" by the test developer or someone else. In the world of test development, there is nothing comparable to a government's Bureau of Weights and Measures; there is no place to go to find the universally acceptable definition of any psychological concept. There are many different definitions of almost all labels for psychological conditions.

For instance, two tools may both have scales labeled "Depression," but their test developers may have constructed somewhat different notions of "depression." One test developer's construction of depression may focus primarily on "moodiness," while another's may emphasize self-defeating thoughts and a belief that one is of little worth. Neither developer is wrong in calling this construct "depression," but they do not necessarily intend to measure the same thing; one is focusing on feelings and the other on thoughts.

Therefore, you should not simply read the labels and conclude that you know what they intend to measure. You will also need to read the definition of each construct that the test developer has provided.

Types of Constructs

Different tools measure fundamentally different types of constructs. This is another way in which one tool's "depression" is not necessarily like another's. Here is a list covering most of the types of constructs that tools in this book seek to measure.

- *Behaviors*: Things that youths do and that you can see them doing. Some tests attempt to measure the likelihood that youths will do specific things in the future (e.g., violent behaviors, suicide attempts).
- *States*: Conditions (usually emotional) that vary across time, usually in response to situations that youths are currently in or have recently encountered.
- *Traits*: Psychological characteristics that are more enduring—characteristics you would use to describe what the youth is "typically" like, across time or across situations.
- *Psychiatric diagnosis*: Formally, a label given to a disorder defined in the *Diagnostic and Statistical Manual of Mental Disorders* (the most recent editions are DSM-IV and DSM-IV-TR; American Psychiatric Association, 1994, 2000). Each disorder is identified as the presence of a specific set of symptoms.
- *Symptom*: A behavior, state, or trait-like condition that has often been identified as being one of the criteria for a diagnostic disorder (although a symptom often occurs without fitting into a set of symptoms that would define a diagnostic condition).
- *Psychosocial problem*: An area of poor functioning in a youth's everyday life in relations with others (e.g., at school, at home, in relations with peers). Typically a consequence of maladaptive behaviors or troubling states, traits, symptoms or diagnostic conditions

Note that a notion of "depression" can arise in all of these types of constructs. One tool might seek to measure *behaviors* that are theoretically related to depression (e.g., suicidal behavior), while others will seek to measure current depressed mood *states*, depression as a *trait*-like characteristic that is relatively typical for a particular person across time and circumstances, depression as a cluster of *symptoms* that define a formal psychiatric *diagnosis* called "depression," or *problems* that arise within the context of interpersonal relationships because of a youth's withdrawn behavior or depressed mood.

Even two tools that claim to measure a behavior—such as "aggressive behavior"—may not be measuring the same construct. Given two tools that claim to predict "aggressive behavior," one may be aimed at predicting behaviors that do physical damage to others (often labeled "violence"), while another may be designed to predict a range of "aggressive" behaviors from assault to verbal insult to property damage. Other constructs that have widely varying meanings are "anger," "hostility," "impulsiveness," "anxiety," and "delinquent behavior."

This problem of varying definitions for similar labels is not really a problem, as long as you avoid simply assuming that you can tell from its name what a scale measures. You must look beyond the label to the actual text definition that the test developer will have provided.

The Selection of Constructs

Test developers have an enormous range of constructs from which they can choose when they set out to develop "a tool to measure mental disorders in adolescents." How do they decide which ones to include?

The process typically combines many different concerns. As noted in Chapter 2, although there are hundreds of diagnostic conditions in DSM-IV, only a much smaller number are found with sufficient frequency to warrant adoption as constructs within tools for arriving at diagnoses. Some symptoms are so frequently found across so many different diagnostic conditions that they are essential to include in a symptom checklist, while other symptoms are too rare to warrant their use. Concerns related specifically to juvenile justice objectives sometimes influence the inclusion of certain constructs, especially those pertaining to harm to self or others.

Chapters 2 and 3 have discussed some of the mental health constructs that are most often of interest for screening and assessment in juvenile justice settings. Comparing the constructs reviewed there to the tools that are available, you will find that most of the instruments reviewed later in this book provide measures of these constructs. But few will provide measures of the constructs that are important for *all* juvenile justice circumstances. You will be looking for tests with constructs that best match the specific questions raised in your juvenile justice setting.

EVALUATING CONTENT

By "content," we mean the words and phrases in an instrument's items that youths or other test takers must answer, or the questions that interviewers must ask. The constructs that test developers intend to measure are used to create the content of these items. This step in test development is exceptionally important. Up to this point, the test developer has only been working with an "idea"—the construct and the developer's verbal definition of it. In contrast, the items that the developer generates constitute the test developer's "real" definition of the construct. They do more than represent the construct; one could say that the construct does not even exist in any practical or observable sense without them.

Test content can be developed in many ways. A detailed knowledge of how this is done is not necessary to evaluate the quality of a tool, but a few comments about the process may be helpful.

As you read descriptions of screening and assessment tools in later chapters, test developers will sometimes speak of using "theory" regarding a construct to guide the content of their instruments' items. This typically means that the construct is part of a larger view of how the construct works in accounting for human behavior. For example, the construct "depression" may reside within a theory that assumes certain causes of depression, as well as certain ways that depression manifests itself in real human experience. It influences a person's thoughts (self-deprecating), emotions (sad), and behaviors (slowed down, effortful). This theory, then, produces a guide suggesting the content of potential test items that will represent this range of expressions of depression. Other ways to generate item content is to draw statements from clinical records of youths who are known to have particular types of mental disorders, or to review items developed for other tests that are intended to measure the same thing.

What should you be looking for when you read the items in a tool? Here are some things to consider.

Content Validity

Imagine that you are reading five items that make up a "Fighting" scale, focused on the construct "tendency to get into physical fights." As you look across the items, are they worded in a way that would seem to cover an adequate *range of content* to get at the construct? For example, if all of the items are worded in ways that refer to gang fights, isn't it possible that the scale is viewing the construct too narrowly? If this is supposed to be a "Fighting" scale (not a "Gang Fighting" scale), wouldn't it be better if some items pertained to fights with school acquaintances and other items to fights with brothers and sisters, as well as items involving gang encounters? Content validity simply focuses on whether the items in a scale are varied enough to capture the various ways in which the construct may operate in everyday life.

Face Validity

The term "face validity" refers simply to whether the item, "on its face," seems to be related to the scale to which it contributes (or the construct that it is said to represent). If you were to read the item "When you have been mad, have you stayed mad for a long time?", you would not be surprised if a "yes" on this item contributed to a "Fighting" or "Anger" scale. The content seems consistent with the construct as you understand it. But if the item appeared in a test's "Suicide" scale, you would probably question its relevance at face value. (Note, however, that our intuitions about these matters are not always clear-cut. For some adolescents, intense anger *does* accompany suicidal thoughts.)

Reading and Vocabulary Level

Item construction includes attention not only to representing the construct, but also to wording the item in a way that will be understood by the youths to whom the instrument will be administered. Do the items seem understandable and likely to have about the same meaning to a wide variety of youths? Part of this question is answered by the school-grade reading difficulty of the items; this will often be described by test developers, who have calculated it with "reading-ease" formulas. The reading abilities of youths in the juvenile justice system vary extremely, but the average is about a fifth- to sixth-grade reading level. Tests requiring more than a seventh-grade reading level will be outside the ability range of a significant proportion of these youths.

Reading difficulty, however, is not the only factor to consider; you must also think about reading comprehension. Reading-ease formulas only take into account such factors as sentence lengths, number of sentences in paragraphs, or number of syllables within a fixed number of words. Yet reading ease and comprehension are somewhat different matters. Many easy-to-read two-syllable words are incomprehensible to many youths (e.g., "entail"). Certain reference books will tell you whether the meanings of specific words are more or less difficult to comprehend. But perhaps the most straightforward way is to enlist the aid of a few teenagers who will read the items for you and identify words that they do not understand.

Policy Concerns

As discussed in Chapter 3, sometimes tools contain items that raise concerns from a legal or policy perspective. For example, some test items ask youths to indicate whether they have engaged in various illegal or dangerous behaviors. Answering them raises the risk that the information could jeopardize the youths' defense. The presence of such items should not rule out the instrument's use. But you will want to acknowledge that they exist, in order to determine what issues will need to be resolved if the instrument is selected for use.

CONSIDERING THE INSTRUMENT'S PROCEDURE

Every screening or assessment instrument requires that the person administering the tool (1) gets information from someone (the "source") (2) according to some procedure for obtaining and scoring the information (the "format"), and then (3) employs the tool's method for determining the importance of the scores (the "norms"). How this is done varies across tools, and some source, format, and norms procedures may work better than others for the demands of your own particular screening and assessment situation.

When reviewing these procedural features of a tool, you should recognize that if you select the tool, its procedures must be used just as they are described. You cannot choose the tool with the intention of somewhat altering its procedure to fit your needs. This point is related to the testing concept of "standardization." This simply means that a given tool must include a description of the "standard" way to administer and score it, and that anyone who uses the tool must employ this "standard" process consistently across all youths and across all settings in which the tool is used. *To do otherwise invalidates the results of the tool.* All that is known about the meaning of the scores (e.g., whether the tool actually measures what it intends to measure) has been discovered through studies that administered the tool in this standardized way. If your examiners administer it in a different way, you have no idea whether the scores they obtain can lay claim to the validity that was demonstrated in those past studies.

Data Source

Most screening and assessment tools require that examiners get information from one or more of four sources: self-report by the person being evaluated; the reports of other persons, such as family members or teachers; review of past records and documents; and/or the examiner's observations of the person's behavior. Test developers and clinicians who perform comprehensive assessments are aware that some sources are better than others for certain types of information. For example, self-reports and information from family members are better than past records for obtaining information about a youth's current mental state, but records often provide information (e.g., about past mental health treatment) that youths and caretakers have forgotten. Youths have some information that their caretakers often do not have (e.g., about their own thoughts and feelings), while caretakers will sometimes report information about their children's disruptive behaviors that youths choose not to share.

As you consider the sources of information used by various tools, your main concerns will be about feasibility. Is the source of information that this tool requires actually available at the time and place that you plan to use screening or assessment procedures? (For example, family members are typically not available to provide information at the time that a youth is admitted to a pretrial detention center.) Does the tool require special interviewing or observational skills, which must be considered when you are deciding what types of personnel are needed to use the tool?

Format for Administration and Scoring

Administration

Some tools require interviews and review of records, but most require youths to respond to questions (test items) that are posed to them. Three aspects of format require attention: the stimulus format, the response format, and design features.

The most common stimulus format is a paper questionnaire form listing the items and requiring the youth to read them. But there are many variations. Some tools allow an examiner to read the items to a youth one by one if the youth cannot read. Other tools come with software that permits items to be presented on a computer screen, and some even use the computer's audio system so that the youth can not only read but also hear the items presented. The most common response format is for the youth to use a pencil to answer each question by circling "yes" or "no" for the item, marking a number from 1 to 3 or from 1 to 5 indicating the degree to which the item is true for him- or herself, or making the computerized versions of these responses (touching the appropriate keys). All of these stimulus and response formats "look" somewhat different across tools because they have various design features involving the physical layout of the items and response options. What is the size of the type? Is the layout clear and simple, or does the page look complex and initially intimidating? Does responding require filling in "bubbles," circling, checking, or writing numbers? Does the tool seem "user-friendly" for your youths? There is more involved here than simple consumer sensitivity. How youths feel when visually confronted with a task may influence their motivation to do it and the quality of the information they provide your examiners.

Scoring

Most tools require the examiner to convert item scores to a total score for a scale. This is done separately for several scales on tools that measure more than one construct, and sometimes the scores for each of these scales are combined to form a total score for the whole test if the test measures some general construct like "emotional distress." Tools vary in their design features for accomplishing this scoring process. Some require counting; others use a plastic template; and computer versions often automatically calculate the scale scores without any manual effort.

A few of the tools you will read about in later chapters do not require scoring. For example, the Voice DISC combines the pattern of a youth's answers to questions to arrive at a psychiatric diagnosis. Some other tools require the examiner to use interview data and record reviews to rate the youth on a construct.

Test Norms

After the scale scores have been obtained, most tools call for them to be transferred to a form that offers a visual summary of all the scale scores. Often this is a diagram or table, and it is here that you discover the importance or significance of a youth's scores—basically, whether they are high or low. This diagram or table was put together by the test developer to show how the youth's score compares to the scores of other youths. Whether they are considered high or low depends on where they fall in comparison to "norms." A tool's norms are based on the test developer's administration of the tool to a large number of youths (the "norm sample"), whose scores become the foundation for interpreting the significance of any youth's score on the tool.

How the data from these norm samples have been analyzed in order to create the comparative table or diagram is a complex topic. There are various ways in which test developers turn raw scale scores into special psychometric scales that improve their utility. One of these conversions from raw scale scores to scale scores—called "*T*-scores"—is discussed below. If you need a more complete understanding of those concepts, you should consult a psychologist who understands the psychometric properties of tests. Basically, however, you do need to be aware of three features of norms as you inspect a tool for possible selection.

Score Distributions

If scores for a large sample of youths are arranged in order of their frequency, they will be "distributed" from highest to lowest in different ways, depending on the construct that the tool measures. There are two main types of score distributions for the tools with which we are concerned: "normal" and "skewed." Normal distributions are the well-known "bell-shaped curves." They are found with certain types of human characteristics (e.g., intelligence, assertiveness, and perhaps anger), for which most people score in the middle of the scale, with smaller and smaller numbers of people scoring higher or lower than the middle. In contrast, skewed distributions occur when you are measuring something that most people do not manifest (e.g., suicidal thoughts) or that most people do manifest (e.g., the ability to read). Most people score at the bottom of scales for the former, or at the top of scales for the latter types of abilities. Therefore, a youth is scoring like "average youths" if his or her score is in the middle of a normally distributed scale, or if it is near the top or bottom on a skewed scale.

Ways to Identify Significant Scores

Most tools then provide a way to determine whether a youth's score is "significantly different" from the average (i.e., different enough to warrant special attention). This may be expressed in a number of ways.

Some tests use "percentiles." That is, they have translated raw scores into a percentage figure showing where the youth falls in comparison to other youths (so that a youth above the 80th percentile has a score that is in the top 20% for youths on this scale). Other tests have translated their raw scores into "*T*-scores." Basically, they have found the average raw score for the group of youths and have assigned this average a *T*-score of 50. If scores on the test are normally distributed, the 50 is the middle of the bell-shaped curve, with the curve tailing off for lower and higher scores. This is useful, because it can tell you approximately what percentage of youths score above or below various

T-scores. On a scale using *T*-scores, about 15% of youths score below a *T*-score of 40, and only about 3% below a *T*-score of 30. Similarly, only about 15% of youths score higher than a *T*-score of 60, and only about 3% above a *T*-score of 70.

Quite often a tool will provide a "cutoff score," indicating that scores at or above that point place the youth at a "significant" level. On a scale using *T*-scores, often the cutoff (signaling clinical significance or importance) is 60, 65, or 70, depending on the choices made by the test developer. As noted in Chapter 3, this does not tell you what to do in response to the youth. It merely tells you that the youth is scoring at a substantially higher level than most youths—one that requires "attention."

Most test manuals provide information about the accuracy of the cutoff score. For example, for a tool that claims to measure suicidal intentions, the manual for a screening tool might tell you that in research to develop the tool, 75% of youths who scored above the cutoff actually turned out to be suicide risks, according to subsequent interviews by expert clinicians. Some of the things to consider when you are reading about the accuracy of cutoff scores will be described later in this chapter when we discuss test validity.

Characteristics of the Norm Sample

Almost everything about the use of norms depends on the norm sample—those hundreds or thousands of youths to whom the test developer gave the tool in order to establish what is "average" and what is "significantly different" from the average. It is the comparison of your youth's score to the scores in this norm group that makes your youth's score "significantly" high or low. If your daughter's gymnastic coach says that she has "way above average talent," it makes a difference whether the coach is comparing her to other gymnasts on her high school team, or to gymnasts her age who have moved on to work with coaches in the national network that feeds the Olympics. Similarly, when you learn that a tool indicates that a youth is "significantly more aggressive" than the average youths in the norm sample, there are very good reasons to want to know who those youths were. For example, were they a random sample of high school students, or were they youths in correctional programs? This issue is so important that it requires its own section to discuss the implications.

EXAMINING THE NORM SAMPLE

The sample of youths that was tested in order to establish the tool's norms represents the population of youths for which the tool was devised. By "population," we mean that *portion* of the general population of children for which the test developers intended the tool to be used. Often this is restricted to a certain age range, includes either one or both genders, and has other characteristics that we will discuss below.

In most cases, you should avoid using a tool designed for very different populations from the ones with which you intend to use the tool. The constructs and items were not developed with your youths in mind, and comparing your youths' scores to those of a different population may produce misleading conclusions.

But there are exceptions. Researchers sometimes find that a tool designed for a particular population (e.g., adolescent psychiatric inpatients) works well with other populations that the developer did not have in mind (e.g., adolescents in juvenile justice custody). If this evidence is substantial and consistent, then you could consider the instrument's use despite its original intentions for use in a different population. However, without that evidence, you should not use a tool to assess adolescent offenders when it was originally developed to assess other groups of youths (e.g., college students).

What population characteristics are important to consider when you are judging this "similarity" between your youths and the instrument's norm sample? Chapter 2 has discussed the nature of child psychopathology, both generally and as it is manifested specifically among delinquent youths. Those principles will now be helpful in identifying what population characteristics are more or less important. Because those characteristics have already been explained in Chapter 2, we use them here without extensive explanation regarding their relevance.

Adults, Adolescents, and the Adolescent Age Range

Most of the instruments encountered later in this book have been developed specifically for use with adolescents. Instruments that were designed originally for use in identifying mental health needs and characteristics of adults typically will not be suitable for use with adolescents. For example, recall that some diagnostic forms of mental disorder among adults occur only rarely in adolescence (e.g., schizophrenia), and some forms of disorder in adolescence are not assessed in most adult measures (e.g., attention-deficit/hyperactivity disorder). Moreover, some disorders are manifested very differently in adolescence versus adulthood (e.g., adolescents' tendencies toward anger when depressed). Thus the constructs chosen for adult measurement may be inappropriate or inadequate for describing youths. Later we will also discuss the significance of norms for identifying youths who are particularly "high" in certain characteristics. Instruments that only permit adolescents to be compared to adult-based norms are usually unusable in juvenile justice settings. What may be considered a "high" level of a particular symptom for adults may be relatively typical among adolescents.

Age range is also important to consider. Tools designed for use with adolescents typically cover ages ranging from 12 or 13 through 17 or 18. Occasionally, however, the samples on which they have been tested have relatively low numbers of youths in the younger adolescent range, largely because youths of that age were more difficult to obtain in the types of juvenile justice settings in which the instrument was developed. Chapter 2 has noted some differences in certain mental health problems between younger and older adolescents. Therefore, tools that have examined scores with adequate numbers of both younger and older youths offer more confidence for their use across the relevant age range for most juvenile justice programs.

Boys and Girls

Tools designed for juvenile justice settings have often been developed with delinquent boys in mind, largely because boys have always constituted a substantial majority of youths in the juvenile justice system. This may influence the content of instruments to some extent, and it creates a tendency to focus on boys when test developers are doing initial studies to develop instruments. However, recent years have seen the proportion of girls in juvenile justice custody nearly double, so that they now account for closer to 20% of the juvenile justice population. Moreover, we know that girls in juvenile justice programs on average have greater mental health needs than boys (see Chapters 1 and 2).

The development of some instruments has included a sufficient number of girls in juvenile justice programs that these tools will be useful for both boys and girls. Others have not, and one cannot automatically presume that the screening or assessment data obtained with these instruments will have the same meaning for girls as for boys unless subsequent research demonstrates it. This will be of greater or lesser importance to you, depending on whether the setting or settings in which you will apply the instrument serve boys, girls, or both.

Ethnicity

As noted in earlier chapters, ethnic minority youths are overrepresented in the juvenile justice system, in comparison to their proportions in the U.S. general population. Yet some tools were initially developed with samples in which the majority of youths were white non-Hispanic. This is not a fatal flaw, as long as there were sufficient numbers of youths from ethnic minority groups to determine that the test does not operate in a very different manner across various ethnic groups.

This problem of "equivalence" across ethnic groups, however, is fraught with problems that the field simply has not yet solved. For example, what if a mental health screening tool consistently finds a greater proportion of white non-Hispanic youths than black youths with higher levels of mental health needs? Is the tool operating differently in some way for the two ethnic groups, thus underidentifying mental disorders in the black youths? Or is it representing true differences between the two groups? The current research on ethnic differences in adolescent psychopathology does not provide a sufficient baseline with which to answer these questions.

Although you should be concerned about this issue, the current state of the art provides almost no guidance regarding what you should look for in a tool when considering its use with youths from various ethnic groups. You should certainly consider at least three things, however. First, substantial proportions of ethnic minority youths should at least have been included in the samples that were used to test the value of the tool. Second, you should note whether the test developer has provided data on the average scores of different ethnic groups on the instrument's scales. Third, if your population of youths includes many for whom English is a second language, you should note whether the items on the instrument have been translated into the languages that are relevant for your youths.

Clinical and Justice System Populations

A number of instruments that you will encounter later in this book were originally developed and normed for use with adolescents in clinical care settings, especially inpatient psychiatric facilities and community mental health centers. Can you trust such an instrument to produce meaningful descriptions of mental health needs among delinquent youths in a detention center? In many instances you can, but with certain cautions.

Researchers have discovered a significant overlap between the population of youths served by community public health programs and youths in contact with a community's juvenile court (see Chapter 1). Many youths are served by both the clinical and juvenile justice systems, and it is almost certain that the "clinical" samples of youths on which some instruments are based included many youths—perhaps a majority of them—who had juvenile justice contact at one time or another.

Less certain, however, is the effect of "setting" on the development of a tool. If a tool's initial development was based on its administration to youths in clinical surroundings, can you trust the tool to operate in the same way when it is administered to youths who are not experiencing clinical care, but rather the privations and tensions of incarceration in a secure facility while they await trial? You will find that few instrument descriptions answer this question for you. But you can at least examine whether the tool, despite its origins in a clinical system, has subsequently been examined for its value with samples of delinquent youths in custody.

Finally, you will find that some tools have been normed on *general* adolescent populations, not populations of youths obtained specifically in either clinical or juvenile justice settings. Comparison of youths in juvenile justice programs to norms for youths in the general community is not inappropriate. When doing this, however, you must remember to translate the results correctly. On a test based on a general sample of youths, if a youth scores high on an "Aggression" scale, the youth is scoring high in relation to the average high school student, not the average youth within the juvenile justice system. A youth who scores above the cutoff on such a scale may be no more aggressive than the average for youths with whom you work in a juvenile detention center.

We turn now to three final categories of information that represent different ways of addressing the true value of an instrument: its (1) internal integrity, (2) dependability (i.e., reliability), and (3) value in terms of meaning (i.e., validity).

CONSIDERING INTERNAL INTEGRITY

By "internal integrity," we mean the degree to which the items within an instrument go together, relate to each other, or are arranged in ways that are meaningful and logical. Of all the properties of instruments that we discuss in this chapter, this is probably the least likely to need your attention, because it is primarily a concern for test developers. If they do not handle this aspect of test construction well, later research will probably find weaknesses in the instrument's overall performance, or validity. If you use those later validity studies as the basis of your selection process, then looking at their internal integrity is less critical from a consumer's perspective. Nevertheless, we will cover just enough of this topic to provide a grasp of the essentials.

Internal Integrity of a Scale

Imagine a "Hostility" scale that has 10 items. The sum of the "yes" responses on those items is the instrument's Hostility score. If we give these 10 items to a large number of youths, and if each of those items is homing in on a single construct, then there should be a tendency for them to be related. That is, youths who answer "yes" to any one of them will often answer "yes" to others, and youths who answer "no" to any one of them will often answer "no" to others. Rarely are items in a scale perfectly related (so that youths who answer "yes" to one *always* answer "yes" to the others), but the *tendency* should be there if all of the items are really focusing in common on the single construct of "hostility."

Test developers use statistical procedures called "correlations" to determine these relations between items in a scale. Correlations range from 0.00 (no relation at all) to 1.00 (a "perfect" relation—you can always predict the response to one item by knowing the response to the other). If an item is correlating poorly with other items in the scale, it is often removed during test construction, on the presumption that it is not tapping into the construct that the other items seem to be sharing. Test developers often describe these item-to-item relations by using another statistic called an "alpha coefficient" (also ranging from 0.00 to 1.00), which is simply a way of using a single correlation to sum up the relations of all items within the scale. Test developers are usually satisfied when the alpha coefficient for items in a scale is above .60. Finally, they may also describe the "item–total correlation" for each item—the degree to which responses on the item relate to the total scale score.

Interscale Integrity

When an instrument has more than one scale, test developers usually examine the degree to which the scales relate to each other. For example, imagine that scores on an instrument's "Depression" scale and its "Anxiety" scale correlate

.90. This means that a youth's position on one of these scales will almost always identify the youth's position on the other scale (i.e., if the youth scores high on one, then he or she will almost always score high on the other). When this happens, the test developer steps back and ponders two questions. First, are both of these scales really needed, given that they seem to be saying the same thing? Second, if they are supposed to be measuring two *different* things ("Depression" and "Anxiety"), why are they producing the same scores? They don't seem to be measuring two different constructs, or if they are, then they are measuring two constructs that always rise and fall together. In either case, the test developer is likely to make some adjustments before proceeding further with the construction of the instrument.

You might think that the relation between scales within an instrument should be very low, in order to assure that they are all measuring some distinctly different symptoms, traits, or aspects of mental disorder. But a moment's reflection on the discussion of comorbidity within adolescent psychopathology (Chapter 2) indicates why this is not a reasonable assumption. When youths manifest mental disorders, they are more likely than adults to manifest more than one disorder. Moreover, many symptoms cut across mental disorders. Given that this is the true nature of adolescent psychopathology, we would expect many scales (or constructs) for adolescents' disorders and symptoms to have at least moderate interscale correlations.

Factor Analysis

A few of the instruments encountered in later chapters have been developed by using a statistical method called "factor analysis." Whereas many tests begin with constructs and with items written to represent each of them, factor analysis begins simply with a large set of items. Factor analysis is a statistical way to allow those items to group themselves into "factors," or potential scales. If you imagine a computer process that finds all possible item-to-item correlations, then sorts them into groups of items with correlations suggesting that they tend to go together, this is approximately what factor analysis does. Then the test developer reviews the content of all items within a factor, attempting to learn what symptom, trait, or behavior the factor and its items seem to represent. If the meaning of the factor is fairly clear, it may become a scale in the instrument.

EXAMINING DEPENDABILITY
OF MEASUREMENT (RELIABILITY)

Two of the most common terms that one hears when referring to the quality of screening and assessment instruments are "reliability" and "validity." Their difference is important and can be explained with an example.

Measuring a distance by taking long paces, you begin at one end of a hallway and stop at the 10th pace. Then you go back to the starting point and do this several more times. If your 10th pace always puts you at exactly the same spot, we can conclude that your method of measuring distance is "reliable," or highly dependable. There is little or no error in your measurement; every time you do it, you get the same result. Now let us imagine this: You claim that your paces are 3 feet in length, and therefore you believe that the spot where you took your 10th pace is 30 feet from your starting point. If we use a tape measure to verify this and find that you are right, we can conclude that your method of measuring distance is "valid." That is, we can be confident that your paces *actually* measure what you claim to measure.

Notice that your way of measuring distance may be highly reliable, but that we may discover that it isn't valid—for example, that it is always 2 feet short of 30 feet, so that it is consistent but wrong. Tests need both reliability and validity. They must measure dependably, and there must be some evidence that they measure what we expect them to measure. The following are two types of reliability (dependability) most commonly found in descriptions of instruments. (We will examine validity later.)

Test–Retest Reliability

One way to determine the dependability of a test is to give it to a group of youths, then give it to them again at a later time (often a few days or a week later) and compare their scores. The degree of similarity between the two administrations is typically expressed as a correlation. High correlations (e.g., over .70) are desirable, but there are a few cautions to keep in mind when you are inspecting a scale's "test–retest" figure.

First, the correlation does not always have to be high. This depends on the type of construct the instrument claims to measure. If the construct is a "trait"—some characteristic that is expected to be part of a youth's basic personality and therefore enduring across time—then the measure should produce a high test–retest correlation. Similarly, if an "Alcohol Use" scale has items that ask a youth to report on drinking behavior over the past year, we would hope that if we asked the youth those questions twice within the same month, we would get approximately the same answers. But some scales are intended to measure a symptom or an emotional state that is ordinarily expected to fluctuate across time. Thus we should not be too concerned if their test–retest correlations are not so high.

Second, the fact that test–retest reliability is good does not necessarily mean that youths' scores do not change across the time between test and retest. For example, from the first to the second testing, the highest scorers may continue to be the highest scorers on retest, and the lowest scorers may continue to be the lowest scorers on retest, yet almost everyone's score is lower on retest than their first score. This will produce a high correlation, even though almost everyone's scores have gone down.

Interscorer or Interrater Reliability

People who use an instrument sometimes make errors in their scoring. Similarly, when instruments require examiners to assign ratings based on their judgments (e.g., "Rate the youth's degree of distress from 1 to 10"), different raters may have somewhat different notions of the thing they are asked to rate, producing somewhat different results. Obviously, these "interscorer" or "interrater" sources of error are not desirable, because they impair the dependability of the instrument's results. Some instruments are more resistant to scoring error than others. To discover the degree of error, test developers frequently do studies that require several trained persons to score or rate the same set of cases. Then they examine the correlations between these scores or ratings. Instruments that require only counting should produce very high interscorer correlations (at least above .90). Tools that require examiners to use their judgment in making ratings will typically contain greater error, but still should produce interrater correlations above .70.

When test manuals provide these results, they do not necessarily indicate the level of scoring or rating reliability that you will find when the instrument is used in your juvenile justice program. This will depend in part on whether your own examiners have had the same degree of training and experience with the instrument as the test developer's scorers at the time that their reliability was established.

CONSIDERING CONFIDENCE
ABOUT MEANING (VALIDITY)

Is an instrument valid? That is, how confident can you be that the instrument measures what it says it measures, and that youths scoring above the cutoff score on a scale really will have the characteristic that the scale was designed to identify? Do the scores mean what the test developer wanted them to mean?

Descriptions of instruments in later chapters will provide much evidence about validity, based on research studies. Three types of information will assist you in sorting through the evidence for an instrument's validity. First, we take stock of several different types of validity that are mentioned in these descriptions of screening and assessment instruments. Second, we define some terms that test developers use to express how well an instrument performs. Finally, we offer some guidance for drawing conclusions about an instrument's validity and utility from its research evidence.

Types of Validity

An earlier section ("Evaluating Content") has described the "face validity" (whether the item appears "on its face" to be relevant for the thing that is being measured) and "content validity" (whether the items in a scale seem to cover a sufficient range to fully represent the construct that the scale is measuring). Research studies are typically not needed to examine these types of validity. They are merely discerned on the basis of a notion of what is or is not relevant to the construct the instrument is intended to measure. The remaining types of validity, however, require controlled research studies to provide the necessary information. They are "construct validity," "concurrent or criterion validity," and "predictive validity."

Construct Validity

Confidence in the meaning of a mental health screening or assessment measure is increased when its results are helpful in advancing our knowledge about the disorders or symptoms that it measures. For example, imagine a biological or psychological theory of depression suggesting that youths with parents who have been seriously depressed are at greater risk of experiencing serious depression themselves. To examine this notion, a study selects two groups of parents who did or did not receive clinical treatment for depression in their own adolescent years, then tests all of their children with a tool that claims to measure depression. The study finds much higher scores, on average, among the children of the parents with a history of depression than among those of nondepressed parents. In addition to providing support for the theory, the measure of depression that the study has used gains construct validity. We do not know from this study whether the tool actually measures depression or not. But the fact that it has found results consistent with a logical theory gives us some degree of confidence that it does. It is successful in representing a construct—that is, depression—in a way that has advanced our knowledge.

Test theorists consider this one of the most important and elegant forms of test validity. Yet you will not encounter it as often in the descriptions of screening and assessment tools in later chapters as the other forms of validity discussed next.

Concurrent or Criterion Validity

Perhaps the most common test of the validity of an instrument is to compare its scores to something else that claims to be an indicator of the same construct that the instrument was designed to measure. Do the instrument and the other indicator agree?

When the other indicator is another instrument, this is often called a test of "concurrent validity" (examining whether the two tests "concur"). Sometimes a new instrument will be examined for its relation to another instrument that has been around longer and has established a track record in clinical use. When the comparison indicator is some other external method, such as expert clinicians' diagnoses, the comparison is often called a test of "criterion validity" (examining how closely the instrument parallels this other "criterion" or "gold standard").

Either concurrent or criterion validity can be helpful in contributing to your confidence in the meaning of an instrument, but both have some drawbacks. These are important to remember when research results suggest that the instrument is not agreeing very well with the other indicator to which it is being compared. In those circumstances, you should consider two possibilities (in addition to the possible poor validity of the instrument).

First, consider what evidence exists for the reliability and validity of the measure or criterion to which the instrument is being compared. The mere fact that the criterion is an expert clinician panel does not guarantee that those clinicians' diagnoses were either reliable or valid. (In fact, studies of psychiatrists' and psychologists' diagnostic opinions offer reasons to question their reliability.) Similarly, instruments with longer track records do not always have excellent evidence for their reliability and validity. Even if they do, often this evidence was established primarily with other studies that compared *those* instruments to yet *other* instruments (about which the same question of *their* validity could be raised).

Second, when an instrument is being compared to another instrument, examine closely the comparison instrument's definition for the construct and the content of the items that represent the construct. As discussed at the start of this chapter, when it comes to mental health constructs, "a rose is *not* a rose is *not* a rose." There is no single definition for "depression," "hostility," "thought disorder," or any other symptom or psychological condition. The "Depression" instrument in question may not be agreeing with the comparison "Depression" instrument because they are not measuring the same thing—or they are measuring different aspects of "depression" that can only be expected to overlap to some degree, rather than to concur closely.

Therefore, when an instrument does not agree with other criteria for the same thing that it claims to measure, you should not automatically presume that it has "failed." It may have failed, or it just may not have been given a fair test.

Predictive Validity

Some instruments are designed to predict future behaviors, such as future delinquent acts, violent acts, or suicidal behavior. Some research studies obtain scores for youths on such a measure, identify those who are predicted to engage in the behavior in the future, and then follow them to see how accurately the instrument has identified those who do manifest the behavior and those who do not.

When the results are good, the instrument gains "predictive validity." As in the case of concurrent validity, poor results in predictive validity studies are not always the fault of the instrument. For example, imagine that "future delinquent behavior," the thing to be predicted, is determined by keeping track of youths' future arrests. Some youths may engage in much delinquent behavior for which they are never arrested. If so, it is possible that the instrument has "failed" in predicting "future delinquent behavior" because the indicator of future delinquent behavior is a poor definition of the thing the instrument was designed to predict.

One word of caution about terminology is in order. Some researchers use the term "predict" in a broader sense than we have defined it. For example, if a measure of adolescent psychopathy (delinquency-prone personality characteristics) successfully distinguishes youths who have been more versus less delinquent *in the past*, some researchers will report that the instrument has successfully "predicted" seriousness of delinquency. In our opinion, it would be more consistent to refer to that result as an instance of either criterion or construct validity, and to reserve the term "predictive" for the identification of *future* behaviors. But researchers are not in agreement about this. Therefore, in reading about a tool's evidence for validity, you may encounter the term "predictive" in circumstances that do not involve the prediction of future behavior.

Ways to Describe Accuracy

Test developers and researchers have several ways of describing how accurately an instrument's cutoff scores separate youths into those who do and those who do not manifest a particular characteristic. These ways of expressing accuracy arise in studies involving all of the types of validity described earlier. For example, how well does the instrument's cutoff score identify youths who score above the cutoff on another instrument (concurrent validity)? How well does it identify youths who have or have not engaged in suicidal behavior in the past (criterion validity), or who do and don't engage in it in the future (predictive validity)? Throughout this section, however, we use examples that refer to predictive validity, simply because it creates the clearest communication.

The key to understanding the terms we describe is to recognize that in all predictive cases we are working with a "yes" or "no" on the instrument (youths score above or below the cutoff) and a "yes" or "no" on the thing to which it is being compared (the behavior does or does not occur). This results in four possibilities for any case, two of which are correct predictions and two of which are not:

- "Yes–yes": Predicted to occur, and it does (correct).
- "No–no": Not predicted to occur, and it does not (correct).
- "Yes–no": Predicted to occur, and it does not (incorrect).
- "No–yes": Not predicted to occur, and it does (incorrect).

The simplest way to express the accuracy of the measure is to indicate the percentage of cases in which the instrument is correct, or the "hit rate." Yet there are several reasons why this is not sufficient information for determining your confidence in the instrument. For example, Figure 4.1 shows the results of a "Suicide" scale and whether or not the youths actually engage in suicide behavior in the next several months. The hit rate is 82% (only 18% of the pre-

Score is above cutoff?

		Yes	No	
Makes suicide attempt?	Yes	2	8	= 10
	No	10	80	= 90

FIGURE 4.1. Results of a "Suicide" scale versus actaul suicide behavior in subsequent months.

dictions are incorrect). But youths in the correct "no–no" category are 80% of the total cases, and those in the correct "yes–yes" category are only 2% of the cases. Moreover, imagine that those 2% are 2 youths out of 10 who *do* make suicide attempts. Thus, although the hit rate is 82% (which sounds good), the instrument has identified only 1 in 5 youths who eventually engage in suicide behavior. Thus a high "hit rate" alone is not a final basis for deciding your level of confidence in an instrument.

Because hit rates do not provide the information you need for policy decisions about the use of predictors, several other ways to express the accuracy of an instrument's cutoff scores have been developed. Table 4.1 provides their names and definitions, all of which you will encounter in later descriptions of screening and assessment tools. For each term, the table includes (1) a formal definition, (2) an example of a general question that each measure of accuracy answers, and (3) an example of a policy or practice question that the measure addresses. All these ways of describing accuracy are typically expressed as percentages.

Drawing Conclusions about Validity

How you judge the evidence for an instrument's validity will have a significant impact on your decision to use it or to look elsewhere. But as this discussion has shown, there are many ways to express the validity of an instrument, and reaching a conclusion about its validity is not an easy matter. How much evidence of validity is needed to conclude that an instrument is "valid"? There are several reasons why this question cannot be answered in a straightforward way (and, indeed, may not be the right question).

The field of psychological assessment does not have any standard that declares an instrument "valid" or "invalid." As research studies arise that examine an instrument's validity, our confidence in the instrument either accumulates or deteriorates. But there is no exact number of encouraging studies that we need in order to reach a reasonable level of confidence in it. Moreover, saying that an instrument is "valid" is somewhat misleading without also indicating the *use* for which it is valid. For example, certain studies might increase our confidence in a "Suicide Risk" scale for identifying youths who have suicidal *thoughts*, while other studies might find that it does not do

TABLE 4.1. Ways of Expressing the Accuracy of an Instrument and Its Cutoff Score

Among youths scoring *above* the cutoff

Positive predictive value	The proportion who *do* engage in the criterion behavior.
	When the tool identifies a youth as suicidal, what is the probability that it is *right* about that youth?
False-positive rate	The proportion who *do not* engage in the criterion behavior.
	When the tool identifies a youth as suicidal, what is the probability that it is *wrong* about that youth?
Policy-relevant question	If I place on suicide watch all youths scoring above the cutoff, what proportion will actually need it, and what proportion will be placed on suicide watch unnecessarily?

Among youths scoring *below* the cutoff

Negative predictive value	The proportion who *do not* engage in the criterion behavior.
	When the tool identifies a youth as nonsuicidal, what is the probability that it is *right* about that youth?
False-negative rate	The proportion who *do* engage in the criterion behavior.
	When the tool identifies a youth as nonsuicidal, what is the probability that it is *wrong* about that youth?
Policy-relevant question	If I do not place on suicide watch any youths scoring below the cutoff, what proportion of them will be treated correctly, and what proportion will not?

Among youths who *do* engage in the behavior

Sensitivity	The proportion who *do* score above the cutoff.
	What proportion of all suicidal youths does the cutoff score identify as suicidal?
Policy-relevant question	Does this instrument correctly identify enough of the suicidal youths to meet my objectives?

Among youths who *do not* engage in the behavior

Specificity	The proportion who *do not* score above the cutoff.
	What proportion of all nonsuicidal youths does the cutoff score identify as nonsuicidal?
Policy-relevant question	Does this instrument correctly identify enough of the nonsuicidal youths to meet my objectives?

Note. All values and rates are typically expressed as percentages—as proportions of a group.

as well as we would wish in predicting suicide *attempts*. If someone tells you that a scale is valid, you might logically reply, "For what?" No instrument is valid for all the possible uses that we might wish.

The mere quantity of studies that suggest an instrument's validity is therefore not a good basis for determining your confidence in it. Instead, you might approach a report of research on an instrument's validity with several other factors in mind.

First, the *quality* of the research matters. One excellent, comprehensive study of validity may be worth far more than 20 studies of questionable quality. The quality of research is often difficult for a nonresearcher to judge; determining this sometimes requires consultation from a professional trained in clinical research methods.

Second, the *type* of validity also matters. For example, a test that claims to predict some future behavior may have a considerable amount of research evidence for various types of validity. But if there are no studies of its *predictive* validity, you really do not have the data that you need in order to determine the confidence you can place in the instrument to make actual predictions.

Finally, the *research sample* matters a great deal. A dozen good studies demonstrating the validity of an instrument for some purpose are worth little to you if the research samples consisted of boys and you are looking for an instrument to use with girls. An instrument's successful prediction of aggression in a sample of white non-Hispanic youths in psychiatric inpatient facilities will not necessarily give you confidence in its validity for use in your detention center if two-thirds of the detention center's population is not white non-Hispanic.

CONCLUSION: THE STATE OF THE ART

The instruments described in Parts II through VI are among the best currently available to your field. Yet, as you begin to review them, you may find less evidence than you had expected—or less than you would wish—for some of the instruments' reliability, validity, or use with specific types of youths in juvenile justice settings. Our decision to include those instruments in this volume was based on their current use in juvenile justice settings or their promise for filling a gap in juvenile justice mental health screening and assessment needs. Explaining our judgment about those matters may help you to avoid overlooking some instruments simply because they seem to provide less research evidence for their utility than others.

Most of the instruments in this volume are new. Many basic psychological tools—for example, the Wechsler intelligence tests—have been around for over 60 years. In contrast, only a few of the manuals for the instruments in this volume have publication dates prior to 1990; most of them were first published in the past 15 years, and some only after 2000. It takes a long time for research to accumulate on an instrument after it has been published. Therefore, it is not at all surprising to find that some of the instruments are supported by only a few studies beyond the original validation research performed by the instruments' authors. When instruments are in this stage of development, we can be a bit forgiving if the strength of evidence for their use is not yet available, provided that the initial research with which the authors developed the instrument inspires confidence in the instrument's potential.

In addition, we must remember that tools developed to assess adolescent psychopathology are faced with substantial challenges that are less often encountered in the assessment of mental disorders in adults. As Chapter 2 has explained, the fact that adolescents are continuously developing into the adults they will become means that they are "moving targets," and the accuracy of assessment becomes much more difficult. Youths' disorders often manifest discontinuity, so that a youth's disorder today might not be the disorder we identify for the same youth next year. Behaviors that are "symptoms" of disorders at one stage of development are virtually "average behaviors" for youths at another stage. And youths' emotional conditions are simply less stable across time.

Given this developmental chaos, it is not surprising that instruments designed to assess youths' mental and emotional conditions often do not reach the levels of reliability, or achieve the impressive evidence for validity, that are seen in many tools developed to assess adult psychopathology. If our instruments for mental health screening and assessment in juvenile justice sometimes do not meet our expectations, developmental psychopathologists who understand the complicated world of youths' disorders may tell us that our expectations are too high. No instrument can produce a high degree of order when the thing it is measuring is as disorderly as adolescent psychopathology appears to be.

Viewed in this light, the instruments described in the following chapters are remarkable in a number of ways. As a group, they have not been reviewed before now, because until recently there would not have been enough of them to review. As a class of instruments, they demonstrate an extraordinary diversity for such a young field, covering a wide range of purposes. Given the inherent difficulties associated with measuring youths' developing characteristics, the instruments are testaments to the dedication and ingenuity of those who are seeking to improve our ability to identify mental disorders among youths in the juvenile justice system.

REFERENCES

American Psychiatric Association. (1994). *Diagnostic and statistical manual of mental disorders* (4th ed.). Washington, DC: Author.

American Psychiatric Association. (2000). *Diagnostic and statistical manual of mental disorders* (4th ed., text rev.). Washington, DC: Author.

Multidimensional Brief Screening Tools

Part II reviews brief (i.e., requiring less than 30 minutes) multidimensional instruments designed to identify several different characteristics of youths at intake screening—the first step in the juvenile justice process for addressing mental health needs. Recall from Chapter 1 that screening tools should be used with every youth at entry points to the juvenile justice process, to identify those most likely in need of emergency mental health services or immediate attention for further assessment. As such, screening tools should be efficient and cost-effective; mainly, they should be relatively quick to administer, should require little data collection, and should be usable by examiners with little or no specialized training. Screening tools are not intended to acquire sufficient detail for permitting decision making about long-range treatment. Rather, developers of these tools generally expect that test scores falling within a specific range will be followed with more detailed assessments or emergency care.

Few instruments have been designed or validated specifically for mental health screening in juvenile justice settings, and the three tools included in Part II appear to be the most common. Each tool is multidimensional, tapping into several types of mental health needs. But they are not interchangeable; they vary in their approaches and the constructs that they address. Juvenile justice professionals interested in adopting mental health screening procedures should consider the constructs measured in light of their agencies' purposes and objectives, as well as the feasibility of each of the instruments reviewed in this section.

In Chapter 5, Grisso and Quinlan describe the Massachusetts Youth Screening Instrument—Version 2 (MAYSI-2). The MAYSI-2 measures symptoms on seven scales pertaining to areas of emotional, behavioral, or psychological disturbance. This screening tool was designed specifically for use in juvenile justice settings. The MAYSI-2 targets youths in need of emergency care and/or more comprehensive assessment upon entry into probation intake, pretrial detention, or corrections reception juvenile justice settings. It is a self-report inventory that can be administered by nonprofessional staff members and completed by youths within 10–15 minutes. The sole uses of the MAYSI-2 are to identify possible emergency conditions and to indicate the need for further assessment. The MAYSI-2 is not intended for longer-term treatment planning or psychiatric diagnoses.

In contrast, the instrument described by Dembo and Anderson in Chapter 6—the Problem-Oriented Screening Instrument for Teenagers (POSIT)—has been used for both emergency screening and treatment planning, depending on the context in which it is used. The POSIT measures 10 areas of psychosocial functioning to target those youths likely in need of further assessment and/or intervention. Typically, as a screening tool, the POSIT is used with every youth at intake in juvenile assessment centers or pretrial detention facilities. However, professionals can also use the POSIT in residential or community treatment settings to guide intervention plans. The POSIT is a self-report inventory that youths can complete within 20–30 minutes when it is administered by nonprofessional staff members.

Finally, in Chapter 7, Hodges describes the Child and Adolescent Functional Assessment Scale (CAFAS). The CAFAS uses behavioral indicators to measure impairments in several areas of psychosocial functioning to identify youths who may be at risk for developing psychiatric, emotional, behavioral, or substance use problems. Unlike the other tools in this section, the CAFAS was originally designed for use in child mental health settings to identify youths eligible for "serious emotional disturbance" services or to assess treatment outcomes. In juvenile justice settings, the CAFAS is particularly suited for probation intake settings to generate treatment and intervention plans for youths who have been court-ordered to receive community services. The CAFAS offers several different methods for obtaining the behavioral data required to rate these youths. Some of these methods require more time than may be feasible for screening in intake settings, but "screener" forms have been developed that shorten the process and are adequate for some screening purposes. Thus, like the POSIT and the MAYSI-2, the CAFAS can be used as a screening tool that can be employed with every youth and requires a reasonably short administration time. And like the POSIT (but unlike the MAYSI-2), it can also be used as an assessment instrument in some settings—that is, as the agency's treatment planning tool—although it requires somewhat more collateral information when used as an assessment tool. As such, it lies on the boundary between screening (initial identification of need) and assessment (individualized information obtained by trained mental health personnel to guide longer-term treatment).

In addition to these three tools, readers looking for a brief intake screening method should consider two other instruments described in Part IV, which discusses comprehensive assessment instruments. In Chapter 11, Achenbach describes a family of tools (the Achenbach System of Empirically Based Assessment) for assessing a wide range of youth mental health problems. The system requires obtaining information from a range of informants, which makes it less than "brief." But one of the tools in that family, the Youth Self-Report, obtains the youth's own perspective, and it requires about the same time to administer (15–20 minutes) as the multidimensional brief screening tools reviewed in Part II. The other instrument in Part IV that can sometimes serve as a brief screening tool is the Present State Voice version of the Diagnostic Interview Schedule for Children (Chapter 13). The instrument requires about 50–60 minutes when administered in its usual form. However, the number of diagnostic categories employed may be decreased to suit the user's needs, which will reduce the procedure to a brief version of the tool.

CHAPTER 5

Massachusetts Youth Screening Instrument—Version 2

Thomas Grisso
Judith C. Quinlan

PURPOSE

The Massachusetts Youth Screening Instrument—Version 2 (MAYSI-2; Grisso & Barnum, 2003) was developed as a brief, self-report tool that can be administered by persons without clinical training to youths at any entry or transitional placement point in the juvenile justice system (e.g., probation intake, pretrial detention, or correctional programs). It was designed to identify youths experiencing thoughts, feelings, or behaviors that may be indicative of mental disorders and/or acute emotional crises requiring immediate attention. As of 2004, 36 states had adopted the MAYSI-2 for statewide use within at least one branch of their juvenile justice systems (e.g., all juvenile probation offices, or all of a state's detention centers).

The prevalence of mental disorders is high among youths in juvenile justice settings—about 60–70% of youths in detention centers (Teplin, Abram, McClelland, Dulcan, & Mericle, 2002) and in juvenile corrections (Wasserman, McReynolds, Lucas, Fisher, & Santos, 2002)—as is the presence of youths with serious and chronic mental disorders (about 20%; Cocozza & Skowyra, 2000). Not all such youths present with emergency treatment needs at intake probation contacts or at admission to detention centers. However, some do need immediate attention, especially for serious depression, suicide risk, aggression that might harm others in detention, and potential consequences of substance use withdrawal. Accurate identification of mental, behavioral, and emotional disturbances is essential as youths enter the juvenile justice system, since many state juvenile justice facilities have a legal responsibility to respond to the mental health needs of adolescents in their custody, and all such facilities can be argued to have a moral responsibility (Grisso, 2004).

The identification of youths in need of immediate attention upon intake into juvenile justice programs is often difficult for two reasons. First, parents or other caregivers are typically not available to provide information for at least several days or weeks. Second, these circumstances require evaluation of every youth entering the system, so assessing all such youths with comprehensive psychometric instruments would require more time and a higher level of clinical expertise than most juvenile justice programs can afford. The MAYSI-2 was designed to meet the specific needs of juvenile justice intake personnel for a standardized, reliable, and valid screening instrument that is feasible (brief, simple, requiring no clinical expertise) for use with every youth entering juvenile facilities.

BASIC DESCRIPTION

The MAYSI-2 screens for symptoms of mental and emotional disturbance, as well as potential crisis problems, in the context of youths seen for their first intake probation interview or in the first 24 hours of admission to pretrial detention and juvenile correctional facilities. It is appropriate for use with boys and girls ages 12–17, and administration and scoring require about 10–15 minutes.

The instrument consists of a Questionnaire, a Scoring Key, and a Scoring Summary form. The MAYSI-2 Questionnaire is a paper-and-pencil, self-report inventory of 52 questions, contained on two sides of a single piece of paper. Youths circle "yes" or "no" concerning whether each item has been true for them "within the past few months" on six of the scales, and "ever in your whole life" for one scale. The six primary scales are Alcohol/Drug Use, Angry–Irritable, Depressed–Anxious, Somatic Complaints, Suicide Ideation, and Thought Disturbance (for boys, as explained later). The seventh scale, Traumatic Experiences, provides information about potential recent traumas. Table 5.1 defines the scales and provides sample items.

The instrument can be administered in three ways: (1) Youths can read the items themselves (the MAYSI-2 has a fifth-grade level of readability) and circle their answers; (2) the items can be read to youths by juvenile justice staff members if youths cannot read the form, while youths circle their answers; or (3) facilities that have personal computers with audio capacity can use the MAYSI-2 CD-ROM, a computer application that administers the test via audio presentation simultaneous with items' appearance on the screen, while youths respond by using the keyboard or mouse. The paper-and-pencil instrument is available in Spanish (a CD-ROM Spanish version is in production). Users have produced MAYSI-2 translations in Korean, Flemish, Greek, Norwegian, Swedish, and Vietnamese.

TABLE 5.1. MAYSI-2 Scale Definitions

Scales	Sample items and definitions
Alcohol/Drug Use	"Have you used alcohol or drugs to make you feel better?" Frequent use of alcohol/drugs; risk of substance dependence and/or abuse, and psychological reaction to lack of access to substances.
Angry–Irritable	"When you have been mad, have you stayed mad for a long time?" Experiences of frustration, lasting anger, moodiness; risk of angry reaction, fighting, aggressive behavior.
Depressed–Anxious	"Have nervous or worried feelings kept you from doing things you want to do?" Experiences of depressed and anxious feelings; risk of depression or anxiety disorders.
Somatic Complaints	"Have you had bad headaches?" Experiences of bodily aches/pains associated with distress; risk of psychological distress not otherwise evident.
Suicide Ideation	"Have you felt like hurting yourself?" Thoughts and intentions to harm oneself; risk of suicide attempts or gestures.
Thought Disturbance (boys only)	"Have you heard voices other people can't hear?" Unusual beliefs/perceptions; risk of thought disturbance.
Traumatic Experiences	"Have you ever seen someone severely injured or killed (in person—not in movies or on TV)?" Lifetime exposure to traumatic events (e.g., abuse, rape, observed murder). Questions refer a youth to "ever in the past"; risk of trauma-related stress disorder.

Youths' "yes" answers are summed for each scale; this is done either with the paper-and-pencil scoring key (requiring about 3 minutes), or automatically if the CD-ROM version is used. The scale scores are recorded on the Scoring Summary form. Youths' answers contribute to six clinical scales for boys and five for girls (see scale labels and descriptions in Table 5.1), in addition to a "nonclinical" scale for both genders that screens for potentially traumatizing experiences in a youth's past. Each scale consists of five to nine items, with some items contributing to more than one scale. A few items contribute to none of the scales; they were retained from an earlier prototype for research purposes, despite their deletion from the scales for clinical purposes during scale development. Because the scales are independent, they are not added together; there is no MAYSI-2 "total score."

Scores on each scale are compared to cutoff scores suggested in the manual. Scores above the "Caution" cutoff signify a "clinical level of signifi-cance," while scores above the "Warning" cutoff indicate that a youth has scored higher than 90% of the Massachusetts normative sample at juvenile justice intake. The procedure does not require specific staff responses to scores on specific scales over the cutoffs. How a program responds to scores at or above the two cutoff levels, as manifested on particular scales or combinations of scales, is determined by policy specific to the agency that is using the instru-ment. Recommendations for establishing policy and procedure in response to high scores are discussed in the manual.

HISTORY OF THE METHOD'S DEVELOPMENT

Development of the MAYSI-2 has proceeded through five phases, involving both research and action designed to augment its use in juvenile justice pro-grams nationally:

- *1994–1996*: Initial drafting and pilot-testing of the MAYSI prototype.
- *1996–1998*: A study funded by the William T. Grant Foundation to identify the scales, develop norms and cutoff scores, and determine psychometric properties.
- *1998–1999*: Additional analyses of the Massachusetts data, leading to a second version (the MAYSI-2) and a new manual (Grisso & Barnum, 2000).
- *2000–2002*: With support from the John D. and Catherine T. MacAr-thur Foundation, development and implementation of a technical assis-tance center (National Youth Screening Assistance Project, or NYSAP), to assist juvenile justice programs with their implementation of the instrument and to stimulate research.
- *2003–2005*: Continued technical assistance (MacArthur Foundation); an updated user's manual (Grisso & Barnum, 2003); and two studies (in progress) designed to (1) develop national norms for the MAYSI-2 and identify any consistent differences in MAYSI-2 scores based on gender, age, and ethnicity (William T. Grant Foundation), and (2) examine how the MAYSI-2 is used nationally and with what outcomes for youths' mental health services (MacArthur Foundation).

Item development began in 1994 with a review of symptoms associated with the more prevalent mental disorders, emotional disturbances, and behav-ioral problems (e.g., suicidal behavior) among adolescents. Pools of potential items were developed for each of the problem areas, guided by consultation with national assessment experts. The initial item pool was administered to a small sample of youths in Massachusetts Department of Youth Services facili-ties. Those youths were also consulted as a "youth panel," discussing with the authors any difficulties in understanding the words and phrases, and brainstorming alternatives that they believed would be more understandable. Further revisions resulted in the final 52-item form.

For purposes of initial exploration, the items were assigned to eight scales, with some items included in more than one scale. This version was the original MAYSI. The instrument was pilot-tested with 176 male and female youths in Massachusetts Department of Youth Services pretrial and correctional facilities. Data were analyzed for the initial (pilot) scales to examine item–scale correlations and other indexes of internal consistency. Given these preparations, 1,279 Massachusetts youths between the ages of 12 and 17 received the prototype items for the MAYSI (Grisso, Barnum, Fletcher, Cauffman, & Peuschold, 2001). A subsample ($n = 749$) also received the Millon Adolescent Clinical Inventory (MACI; Millon, 1993) and the Youth Self-Report (YSR; Achenbach, 1991). Youths in this study were assessed in three settings: 227 at their first interview with intake probation officers soon after arrest, 819 at the time of admission to pretrial detention centers, and 233 at admission to youth correctional assessment centers soon after their delinquency adjudications. Girls constituted about one-third of the sample (by way of oversampling), and ethnic groups were represented in proportions found in the programs and facilities where they were assessed (44% white non-Hispanic, 23% black, 22% Hispanic, and 11% Asian and other). A second sample was obtained independently by Elizabeth Cauffman; this sample was composed of 3,766 boys and 238 girls, ages 13–17, at entry to assessment centers after commitment to the California Youth Authority. The ethnic distribution of the sample differed substantially from that of the Massachusetts sample (14% white non-Hispanic, 28% black, 59% Hispanic, and 6% Asian).

Factor analyses performed on the Massachusetts sample led to decisions about final scales and their items (Grisso et al., 2001). These analyses produced seven interpretable scales for boys and six for girls (see Table 5.1), and resulted in the MAYSI-2. The Thought Disturbance scale is for use with boys only, as the factor analysis for girls did not produce a coherent factor of items that could be interpreted as indicators of "thought disturbance." Internal consistency of the scales was examined in several ways with the Massachusetts sample, and factor analyses and internal-consistency indexes were subsequently performed on the California sample to confirm the Massachusetts results (see "Research Evidence," below). Finally, analyses were performed to determine "Caution" cutoff scores on the six clinical MAYSI-2 scales that produced optimal balances of sensitivity and specificity in identifying youths scoring in the clinically significant range on conceptually similar MACI or YSR scales.

RESEARCH EVIDENCE

The studies reported here were performed with youths in juvenile justice intake probation, pretrial detention facilities, and youth correctional facilities.

Internal Consistency and Reliability

As reported in the primary study (Grisso et al., 2001), factor analyses of the California youth corrections sample produced the same factors for boys and girls as in the Massachusetts sample, although item loadings on two factors (Somatic Complaints and Depressed–Anxious) manifested modest differences for girls. Measures of internal consistency (alpha coefficients) of items within scales ranged from .61 to .86 in both samples, and differences in alpha coefficients between ethnic groups were few (for boys, Asians had less consistency on the Suicide Ideation scale than others; for girls, blacks and Hispanics had less consistency on the Somatic Complaints scale than white non-Hispanics). Median item–total correlations ranged from .35 to .62 for the various scales.

Additional research has affirmed the instrument's initial reliability and internal consistency. A replication of the primary study with male and female youths in detention in Virginia produced practically equivalent alpha coefficients and an almost identical factor structure (Archer, Stredny, & Mason, 2004). A recent confirmatory factor analysis, using males with conduct disorder, also resulted in a factor structure similar to the norm data (Fisher, 2002). Moreover, the reliability of the MAYSI-2 was supported in a sample of 1,587 youths (Cruise, Dandreaux, & Marsee, 2004), with alpha coefficients ranging from .65 to .84 and average item–total correlations ranging from .40 to .56, exhibiting better internal consistency for the MAYSI-2 than in the primary study.

Concerning test–retest results, the primary study revealed changes in a few MAYSI-2 scale scores for boys with an interval of about 1 week between admistrations (Grisso et al., 2001). Nonetheless, intraclass correlations were significant for most scales across genders—a finding that was replicated by Archer and colleagues (2004). In addition, Cauffman (2004) found that test–retest MAYSI-2 scores were strongly correlated even with 3 months between administrations. Cauffman (2004) also found that among youths taking the MAYSI-2 for the first time, those receiving it in the first few hours after admission achieved somewhat lower scores on the Alcohol Drug/Use, Angry–Irritable, Depressed–Anxious, Somatic Complaints, and Suicide Ideation scales than did youths taking the MAYSI-2 a day or more after admission.

Validity

In the primary study (Grisso et al., 2001), four scales on the MACI and four scales on the CBCL-YSR were designated as conceptually parallel to various MAYSI-2 scales, based on examination of the constructs that they intended to measure. Comparison of youths' scores on those scales with their scores on the parallel MAYSI-2 scales indicated that in all but one instance, they correlated better with their parallel MAYSI-2 scales than with nonparallel MAYSI-2 scales. In other comparisons of the MAYSI-2 to personality measures, Rasmussen, Watt, and Diener (2004a) found associations between the MACI Expressed Concerns scales and certain MAYSI-2 scales (e.g., the MACI Childhood Abuse scale was related to six clinical MAYSI-2 scales). Espelage and colleagues (2003) used the MAYSI-2 to measure mental health symptoms in their study of young offenders' profiles on the Minnesota Multiphasic Personality Inventory (MMPI; Hathaway & McKinley, 1967). Cluster analysis revealed meaningful relationships between MAYSI-2 scores and distinct MMPI profiles. Finally, the MAYSI-2 scales were found to correspond meaningfully to various scales on the Brief Symptom Inventory (Land, 1998; Reppucci & Redding, 2000).

Examining the relation of MAYSI-2 scales to *Diagnostic and Statistical Manual of Mental Disorders*, fourth edition (DSM-IV) diagnostic criteria as measured by the Diagnostic Interview Schedule for Children—Version IV (DISC-IV), Wasserman and colleagues (2004) found that most of the scales—especially Alcohol/Drug Use and Depressed–Anxious—correlated best with DSM-IV diagnostic clusters with which they would have been expected to relate theoretically. The Suicide Ideation scale was especially effective in identifying youths who reported recent or lifetime suicide attempts on the DISC-IV. In contrast, the Angry–Irritable scale was no more closely associated with conduct disorder than it was with many other diagnoses, possibly because anger is manifested across various disorders in adolescence.

Several studies found that MAYSI-2 scores predicted future behaviors or conditions, including institutional maladjustment (e.g., isolation for inappropriate behavior); service provision by mental health and juvenile justice professionals (Rasmussen, Watt, & Diener, 2004b); lengthier sentences for higher scorers (Stewart & Trupin, 2003); and staff intervention for suicide risk, sexual misconduct, and assaults on staff members (Cauffman, 2004).

Separating groups of youths into clusters of generally high and generally low scorers on the MAYSI-2, Stewart and Trupin (2003) found that high scorers had substantially more past involvement with mental health systems, according to official records, than did low scorers. In contrast, Svoboda (2001) reported no differences in MAYSI-2 scores corresponding to youths' own reported past mental health treatment. The discrepancy between these findings might suggest that youths were reluctant to report a history of involvement with mental health systems. In other studies of postdictive relations, Steele (2000) found that youths who scored high on the Alcohol/Drug Use scale, while concurrently scoring high on other MAYSI-2 scales, were more likely to have been victims of sexual and physical abuse. Archer and colleagues (2004) found that youths with higher scores on the Suicide Ideation scale had a greater frequency of past suicide ideation and attempts.

Studies have examined MAYSI-2 mean scores for demographic groups, as well as the proportion of youths meeting or exceeding the "Caution" and "Warning" cutoff scores. Concerning age differences, younger adolescents generally score the same or higher on most scales than do older adolescents (but lower on Alcohol/Drug Use) (Cauffman, 2004; Grisso et al., 2001; Warren, Aaron, Ryan, Chauhan, & DuVal, 2003). On average, girls score higher on most scales (Cauffman, 2004; Espelage et al., 2003; Goldstein et al., 2003; Grisso et al., 2001; Nordness et al., 2002; Rasmussen et al., 2004a; Stewart & Trupin, 2003; Wasserman et al., 2004); this is consistent with findings regarding psychopathology in delinquent girls (Chesney-Lind & Sheldon, 1992; Teplin et al., 2002). In a sample of 18,607 detained youths, Cauffman (2004) found that the proportion of youths above the "Caution" cutoff ranged from 18% to 59% on various scales, with 70% of males and 81% of females scoring over the "Caution" cutoff on one or more scales.

Results for various ethnic groups on the MAYSI-2 scales vary across existing studies, showing few differences in some and significant differences in others. When differences were reported, MAYSI-2 scores tended to be higher for white non-Hispanic youths than for youths of ethnic minority backgrounds (Cauffman, 2001, 2004; Grisso et al., 2001; Stewart & Trupin, 2003; Wasserman et al., 2004). No studies have examined the meaning of these differences, but they are consistent with reports of prevalence of mental disorders among youthful offenders (Grisso, 2004; Teplin et al., 2002).

In 2005, results will be reported for the MAYSI-2 National Norms Study (conducted by the developers of the MAYSI-2). This project is using over 70,000 MAYSI-2 cases, contributed by juvenile justice programs in 18 states, to develop national norms for the instrument and to determine what differences (if any) arise consistently as a function of age, gender, and race differences across a wide range of juvenile justice programs.

APPLICATION

The *MAYSI-2: User's Manual and Technical Report* (Grisso & Barnum, 2003) is available from a commercial publisher (Professional Resource Press). The test's authors operate a technical assistance service for MAYSI-2 users, the NYSAP (*http://www.umassmed.edu/nysap*), with support from the Mac-Arthur Foundation. Public sector juvenile justice programs that purchase the manual may use the MAYSI-2 without per-case cost. However, the MAYSI-2 is copyrighted, and users must register with the NYSAP in order to be authorized to use the instrument. Registration involves signing an agreement that the user will not alter the items or format of the instrument and will not sell or distribute it for financial profit.

The MAYSI-2 can be administered and scored by front-line juvenile justice staffers without specialized clinical training or experience, although brief in-service training is strongly recommended. Typically, the MAYSI-2 is administered during the first intake interview in juvenile probation intake offices, or during the first day following admission to pretrial detention centers or postadjudication facilities. It can be administered to individuals or in small groups, although the former is necessary if a youth must have the items read to him or her. To minimize socially desirable responding when items are read to them, youths should be asked to circle their responses rather than responding aloud. Likewise, youths should be afforded sufficient privacy while taking the MAYSI-2, without staff members "looking over their shoulders" at paper-and-pencil responses or at the computer screen when the test is administered by CD-ROM.

The MAYSI-2 manual recommends that facilities use a "secondary-screening" process when youths score above the "Caution" cutoff on any of the scales. This process involves asking examinees a few questions (provided in the manual) that allow staff members to judge whether responses may have been due to factors that would reduce or augment concern about high scores. (For instance, see "Case Example," below.)

It is necessary for facilities or agencies that use the MAYSI-2 to devise their own decision rules about how the scales and their cutoff scores will be used by staff members to trigger certain actions or services. (Again, see the "Case Example" for a description.) What services will be triggered vary from one agency to another, but may range from "closer monitoring" to making a request for a psychological or psychiatric consultation (or, in serious cases, referral to outpatient or inpatient psychiatric services).

Benefits frequently mentioned in surveys of users by the NYSAP include ease of administration, relevance of the scale content, perceived meaningfulness of the results, and the instrument's low cost. Three limitations are mentioned most often. First, like most self-report brief screening instruments, the MAYSI-2 has no built-in mechanism for judging when youths may be underreporting or overreporting in describing their thoughts and feelings. Second is the absence of a Thought Disturbance scale for girls. Factor analysis simply did not identify a set of items with content that could be interpreted as suggesting "thought disturbance" in girls, whereas a set of such items did appear in the factor analysis of boys' responses. Third, users are aware of the potential for instruments to perform differently with youths of various ethnic groups, and they are in need of more information about this possibility. Research by the MAYSI-2 developers is underway to address this important question—one that is not unique to the MAYSI-2.

Implementation of the MAYSI-2 (and many other brief mental health screening instruments) requires careful attention to avoid three potential misuses of the instrument. First, no brief screening instrument for symptoms of mental disturbance should be interpreted as providing psychiatric diagnoses or as providing sufficient information with which to make long-term treatment plans. The MAYSI-2 identifies *current* mental and emotional states. In some cases, these will be enduring characteristics of youths; in others, they will be transient emotional reactions to changing circumstances.

Second, some agencies that use the MAYSI-2 have attempted to modify it in order to make it even shorter (e.g., reducing the number of items per scale, or changing the response format). This invalidates the screen, because scores will no longer have any known relation to the supporting norms and psychometric properties.

Third, juvenile defense attorneys in some jurisdictions have initially objected to MAYSI-2 screening (or to the use of any brief mental health screening instrument) with youths entering detention centers, out of concern that the information (e.g., admitting to the use of substances) might be used against their defendants at delinquency hearings. Similarly, prosecutors have sometimes asked that MAYSI-2 data be sent routinely to their offices. These problems can be avoided if agencies establish legal protections (e.g., a judge's general rule for the court) prohibiting the use of MAYSI-2 information for purposes other than screening in order to respond to youths' mental health needs at the pretrial stage.

CASE EXAMPLE

Police officers brought Carlos, a 14-year-old Hispanic male, to the admitting door of Carver Juvenile Detention Center at 3:00 P.M. on a Thursday. An officer led him to the admitting office, where he was given a chair, had his shackles removed, and was met by a staff member responsible for intake. The officer reported that Carlos had been apprehended at about 8:00 A.M. at the home of a friend, where police were led in their investigation of a group assault, which had taken place the previous evening and involved the stabbing of a homeless man. Officers had been unable to contact Carlos's parents, but they had questioned him and had charged him with participation in the stabbing. They learned that he had been suspended from school the previous Friday, and that he had been "on the street" since that time; he had been using the friend's residence where he was apprehended as his home base. The friend's parents had been out of town for 2 days.

When the officer left, the staff member asked Carlos questions that were needed in order to complete a detention intake form. A call to the home phone number Carlos gave did not produce a response, and Carlos said he did not know where his mother might be. The staff member noted that Carlos looked very tired, was slumped in his chair, and stared vacantly out a window across the room. His eyes became teary when she asked questions about his family members and why they would not have reported him missing since last week. Carlos was then introduced to another detention staff member, who got him some clean clothes and assigned him a bed in one of the four-person rooms in the 40-bed detention center.

The detention center's policies included health and mental health screening of all youths within 3–12 hours after admission. This was the responsibility of two intake workers, one for the day shift and one for the evening shift. Screening typically took place between 10:00 and 11:00 A.M. and 8:00 and 9:00 P.M. The evening shift intake worker (who had not done the daytime intakes) had Carlos and two other boys to screen this evening. After looking over their paperwork, he took them to a room and explained that he would be asking them some questions to see whether they needed special attention for medical or emotional reasons. Seating them at separate tables, he gave each youth a MAYSI-2 Questionnaire and explained how to complete it. He then went to each boy individually to have him read one of the questions aloud, in order to determine whether any of the boys might need to have the items read to them. All of the boys were able to read the questionnaire. After completing the MAYSI-2 Questionnaire, the boys were escorted to the day room while the intake worker scored each boy's responses and transferred the scores onto the instrument's Scoring Summary form.

The intake worker then called for Carlos and began by asking him a standard set of health questions (e.g., history of important illnesses, injuries, medical services received, current medications). Turning to the MAYSI-2, the intake worker found that Carlos had scored in the "Caution" zone on the Angry–Irritable scale and in the "Warning" zone on the Depressed–Anxious and Suicide Ideation scales. Following detention center policy, the intake worker asked several "second-screening" questions from the MAYSI-2 manual's page on Suicide Ideation: "On the questionnaire, you circled 'yes' to some questions about feeling like hurting yourself and wishing you were dead. Is that the way you are feeling right now—today—or something you were feeling in the past but not now?" Carlos answered, "Both," explaining that he had felt that way in the past but also was feeling that way for the last few days. Carlos mentioned that "something happened at home last week," but fell silent when the intake worker tried to engage him in a discussion of the occurrence. "Have you ever tried to hurt yourself or kill yourself?" the intake worker asked. Carlos did not say anything, but he looked at his left wrist, where there were several well-healed scars across the inside of his forearm. The intake worker asked when the injuries had happened (a year ago) and whether Carlos had required medical attention (he had, as well as a 2-day psychiatric inpatient stay). Carlos said he was not sure he would avoid hurting himself tonight if he had the opportunity.

Following standard detention center procedure for these circumstances, the intake worker assured Carlos that they were going to help him avoid the possibility of self-harm. Carlos was assigned to one of two one-person rooms nearest the staff area by the day room, where he could be observed at all times, and other standard suicide precautions were implemented. Carlos was also placed on the roster for meeting with the psychiatric consultant, who made weekly visits every Saturday morning, with instructions to the intake worker on the day shift to spend some time talking to Carlos on Friday morning to determine whether his mood had improved or whether the staff should seek an emergency psychiatric consultation.

ACKNOWLEDGMENTS

The MAYSI-2 was developed with grants from the William T. Grant Foundation, the John D. and Catherine T. MacArthur Foundation, and the Massachusetts Department of Mental Health through its Center for Mental Health Services Research at the University of Massachusetts Medical School.

REFERENCES

Achenbach, T. (1991). *Manual for the Child Behavior Checklist/4–18 and 1991 Profile.* Burlington: University of Vermont, Department of Psychiatry.

Archer, R. P., Stredny, R. V., & Mason, J. A. (2004). An examination and replication of the psychometric properties of the Massachusetts Youth Screening Instrument—Version 2 (MAYSI-2) among adolescents in detention settings. *Assessment, 11*, 1–13.

Chesney-Lind, M., & Sheldon, R. G. (1992). *Girls, delinquency, and juvenile justice.* Pacific Grove, CA: Brooks/Cole.

Cauffman, E. (2001). *Description of mental health symptoms as identified by the MAYSI-2 for the PCCD/JDCAP Mental Health Grant.* Pittsburgh, PA: Western Psychiatric Institute and Clinic, University of Pittsburgh.

Cauffman, E. (2004). A statewide screening of mental health symptoms among juvenile offenders in detention. *Journal of the American Academy of Child and Adolescent Psychiatry, 43*(4), 430–439.

Cocozza, J. J., & Skowyra, K. (2000). Youth with mental health disorders: Issues and emerging responses. *Juvenile Justice, 7*(1), 3–13.

Cruise, K. R., Dandreaux, D., & Marsee, M. (2004). Reliability and validity of the Massachusetts Youth Screening Instrument—Version 2 in incarcerated youth: A focus on critical items. In G. Vincent (Chair), *The Massachusetts Youth Screening Instrument—Version 2 (MAYSI-2): Utility and practical applications in juvenile justice.* Symposium conducted at the meeting of the American Psychology–Law Society, Scottsdale, AZ.

Espelage, D. L., Cauffman, E., Broidy, L., Piquero, A. R., Mazerolle, P., & Steiner, H. (2003). A cluster-analytic investigation of MMPI profiles of serious male and female juvenile offenders. *Journal of the American Academy of Child and Adolescent Psychiatry, 42*(7), 770–777.

Fisher, M. J. (2002). *Confirmatory factor analysis of the Massachusetts Youth Screening Instrument—Version 2 on a sample of conduct disordered males.* Unpublished manuscript, American International College, Springfield, MA.

Goldstein, N. E., Arnold, D. H., Weil, J., Mesiarik, C. M., Peuschold, D., Grisso, T., et al. (2003). Comorbid symptom patterns in female juvenile offenders. *International Journal of Law and Psychiatry, 26*(5), 565–582.

Grisso, T. (2004). *Double jeopardy: Adolescent offenders with mental disorders.* Chicago: University of Chicago Press.

Grisso, T., & Barnum, R. (2000). *Massachusetts Youth Screening Instrument—Second Version: User's manual and technical report.* Worcester: University of Massachusetts Medical School.

Grisso, T., & Barnum, R. (2003). *Massachusetts Youth Screening Instrument—Version 2: User's manual and technical report.* Sarasota, FL: Professional Resource Press.

Grisso, T., Barnum, R., Fletcher, K. E., Cauffman, E., & Peuschold, D. (2001). Massachusetts Youth Screening Instrument for mental health needs of juvenile justice youths. *Journal of the American Academy of Child and Adolescent Psychiatry,* *40*(5), 541–548.

Hathaway, S. R., & McKinley, J. (1967). *Minnesota Multiphasic Personality Inventory: Manual.* New York: Psychological Corporation.

Land, D. (1998). *Mental health screening of juveniles in the justice system: An evaluation of two screening instruments.* Unpublished report, Department of Criminal Justice Services, Richmond, VA.

Millon, T. (1993). *Millon Adolescent Clinical Inventory: Manual.* Minneapolis, MN: National Computer Systems.

Nordness, P. D., Grummert, M., Banks, D., Schindler, M. L., Moss, M. M., Gallagher, K., et al. (2002). Screening the mental health needs of youth in juvenile detention. *Juvenile and Family Court Journal, 53*(2), 43–50.

Rasmussen, A., Watt, K., & Diener, C. (2004a). *Concurrent validity of the MAYSI-2: Staff perceptions and MACI clinical subscales among youth in a county detention center.* Poster presented at the meeting of the American Psychology–Law Society, Scottsdale, AZ.

Rasmussen, A., Watt, K., & Diener, C. (2004b). MAYSI-2 subscales, institutional disciplinary measures, and mental health services. In A. Rasmussen (Chair), *Perspectives on delinquency and juvenile justice: Peers, parents, and mental health.* Symposium conducted at the meeting of the Society for Research on Adolescence, Baltimore.

Reppucci, N. D., & Redding, R. E. (2000). *Screening instruments for mental illness in juvenile offenders: The MAYSI and the BSI* (Juvenile Justice Fact Sheet). Charlottesville: Institute of Law, Psychiatry, and Public Policy, University of Virginia.

Steele, K. B. (2000). Dual symptomed juvenile offenders: A study of mental health and substance abuse symptoms within Washington state juvenile rehabilitation administration. *Dissertation Abstracts International, 61*(6).

Stewart, D., & Trupin, E. (2003). Clinical utility and policy implications of a statewide mental health screening process for juvenile offenders. *Psychiatric Services, 54*(3), 377–382.

Svoboda, S. (2001). *Identifying mental health needs of females in the juvenile justice system.* Unpublished manuscript, University of Missouri–Columbia.

Teplin, L. A., Abram, K. M., McClelland, G. M., Dulcan, M. K., & Mericle, A. A. (2002). Psychiatric disorders in youth in juvenile detention. *Archives of General Psychiatry, 59*(12), 1133–1143.

Warren, J. I., Aaron, J., Ryan, E., Chauhan, P., & DuVal, J. (2003). Correlates of adjudicative competence among psychiatrically impaired juveniles. *Journal of the American Academy of Psychiatry and the Law, 31*(3), 299–309.

Wasserman, G. A., McReynolds, L. S., Ko, S. J., Katz, L. M., Cauffman, E., Haxton, W., et al. (2004). Screening for emergent risk and service needs among incarcerated youth: Comparing MAYSI-2 and Voice DISC-IV. *Journal of the American Academy of Child and Adolescent Psychiatry, 43*, 629–639.

Wasserman, G. A., McReynolds, L. S., Lucas, C. P., Fisher, P., & Santos, L. (2002). The Voice DISC-IV with incarcerated male youths: Prevalence of disorder. *Journal of the American Academy of Child and Adolescent Psychiatry, 41*(3), 314–321.

CHAPTER 6

Problem-Oriented Screening Instrument for Teenagers

Richard Dembo
Amanda Anderson

PURPOSE

The Problem-Oriented Screening Instrument for Teenagers (POSIT; Rahdert, 1991) is a youth self-report screening instrument designed to identify potential psychosocial functioning in 10 areas requiring more thorough assessment. Results of an in-depth assessment would indicate the need for treatment or other intervention services. The POSIT was developed as a key component of the Adolescent Assessment/Referral System (AARS), undertaken by the National Institute on Drug Abuse (NIDA) in April 1987, under contract to the Pacific Institute for Research and Evaluation, Inc. (Rahdert, 1991). The POSIT was designed to be administered by a variety of assessors, including school personnel, court staff, medical care providers, and staff in alcohol or other drug abuse treatment programs.

Development of the POSIT was informed by the experience that troubled youths coming into contact with clinicians and a range of official agencies (e.g., school truancy offices, treatment programs, or juvenile justice authorities) often have problems in numerous areas of psychosocial functioning. Alcohol and other drug problems, for example, are highly prevalent among youths entering the juvenile justice system. Research has shown a strong positive association between drug use and crime (Dembo, Pacheco, Schmeidler, Fisher, & Cooper, 1997; National Institute of Justice, 2003). Arrested juveniles who use drugs are at considerable risk of continuing their involvement in crime and eventually entering the adult criminal justice system (Dembo, Williams, & Schmeidler, 1998; National Center on Addiction and Substance Abuse, 2002).

Research has shown that juvenile offenders experience problems in other areas as well, including physical abuse (Dembo et al., 1988; Dembo & Schmeidler, in press), sexual victimization (Dembo et al., 1989; Dembo & Schmeidler, in press; Mouzakitis, 1981), emotional/psychological functioning difficulties (Dembo & Schmeidler, 2003; Teplin, Abram, McClelland, Dulcan, & Mericle, 2002), and educational problems (Dembo, Williams, Schmeidler, & Howitt, 1991).

Development of the POSIT was also informed by the awareness that many points of agency contact for troubled youths lack resources for clinical assessment, and not all youths have problems of sufficient magnitude to require such assessment. Hence the instrument's intent is to identify youths with potential problems in psychosocial functioning, who can then receive essential in-depth assessments in areas with the highest potential for functioning difficulties.

BASIC DESCRIPTION

The POSIT is a self-administered questionnaire with 139 "yes–no" items, for use with male and female adolescents (12–19 years of age). The instrument has 10 scales, probing these areas of psychosocial functioning: (1) Substance Use/Abuse, (2) Physical Health, (3) Mental Health, (4) Family Relations, (5) Peer Relations, (6) Educational Status, (7) Vocational Status, (8) Social Skills, (9) Leisure/Recreation, and (10) Aggressive Behavior/Delinquency. The POSIT is worded at a fifth-grade reading level, is available in English and Spanish, and requires 20–30 minutes for youths to complete.

The instrument consists of a POSIT questionnaire, POSIT scoring templates, and a POSIT scoring sheet. No special qualifications are needed to administer the instrument, and its format is very clear and straightforward. Generally, youths are permitted to answer the instrument on their own, with the test administrator being available to answer any questions they may have. The administrator may read the questions to youths with reading problems. Since the POSIT is a self-report instrument, it is important to include collateral information to help validate the youths' answers. The current scoring system includes empirically based cutoff scores indicating low, middle, or high risk in each of the problem areas. A youth's total raw score in each problem area determines the level of risk for that area.

A computerized (CD-ROM) version of the POSIT is available in English or Spanish, which permits the youth to enter "yes" or "no" to each question. Alternatively, an audio option is available in either English or Spanish (this is an added feature of the CD-ROM version), and youths click "yes" or "no" answers to the items (*Power*Train, Inc., 1998).

Computerized scoring takes a few seconds. Scoring templates placed over the paper-and-pencil versions of the POSIT allow examiners to complete noncomputerized scoring in 2–5 minutes. Table 6.1 lists the 10 life areas probed by the scales of the POSIT, with sample questions from each. Also available is a follow-up version of the POSIT that screens for potential change in 7 of the 10 problem areas (i.e., Substance Use/Abuse, Physical Health, Mental Health, Family Relations, Peer Relations, Social Skills, and Leisure/Recreation).

TABLE 6.1. POSIT Functional Areas

Functional areas	Item examples
Substance Use/Abuse	"Do you get into trouble because you use drugs or alcohol at school?"
	"Have you started using more and more drugs or alcohol to get the effect you want?"
Physical Health	"Do you have trouble with stomach pain or nausea?"
	"Do you have less energy than you think you should?"
Mental Health	"Do you get easily frightened?"
	"Do you feel sad most of the time?"
Family Relations	"Do your parents or guardians usually agree about how to handle you?"
	"Do your parents or guardians and you do lots of things together?"
Peer Relations	"Do you have friends who damage or destroy things on purpose?"
	"Do your friends cut school a lot?"
Educational Status	"Do you get A's and B's in some classes and fail others?"
	"Are you good at math?"
Vocational Status (16 and over)	"Did you have a paying job last summer?"
	"Have you been frequently absent or late for work?"
Social Skills	"Is it hard for you to ask for help from others?"
	"Do people your own age like and respect you?"
Leisure/Recreation	"Is your free time spent just hanging out with friends?"
	"Do you participate in team sports which have regular practices?"
Aggressive Behavior/ Delinquency	"Have you stolen things?"
	"Do you get into fights a lot?"

HISTORY OF THE METHOD'S DEVELOPMENT

Development of the POSIT has proceeded through two major phases, referred to as the "development phase" and the "implementation and further development phase."

Development Phase: Late 1980s to Early 1990s

The AARS, of which the POSIT was a key component, was developed for NIDA under contract by Westover Consultants, Inc. (Washington, D.C.) and the Pacific Institute for Research and Evaluation (Bethesda, Maryland). Expert panels of clinical researchers and clinical practitioners guided the efforts of both groups. In particular, the expert panels strongly influenced selection of the 10 functional areas and formulation of the items probing them.

With respect to the original version of the POSIT, the expert clinical researchers helped establish a cutoff score for each functional area, and identified "red-flag" items. According to the score construction logic, an adolescent whose score exceeded the cutoff or who endorsed one or more red-flag items in a given functional area was felt to have a potential problem in need of further assessment. A preliminary assessment of the POSIT items' adequacy for tapping problem areas, and of the instrument's discriminant validity, was undertaken in a study involving 633 junior and senior high school students and 216 adolescents in substance abuse treatment programs. More youths in treatment were identified with a potential problem in each functional area than junior and senior high school students.

Implementation and Further Development Phase: Mid-1990s to Present

Several studies that examined use of the POSIT among different samples of youths documented the reliability and validity of the instrument. A number of facilities, programs, and agencies processing large numbers of youths began to adopt the POSIT. Some of these facilities included the Hillsborough County, Florida, Juvenile Assessment Center (JAC) in 1992; all juvenile assessment centers of the Kansas Youth Authority; and Maryland's statewide reporting system for all drug treatment programs.

At this point the POSIT was enhanced in several ways, including a new scoring algorithm and a user-friendly CD-ROM version of the instrument. Several new or revised POSIT instruments were developed, including (1) a POSIT follow-up; (2) the POSIT-for-Parents (POSIP); (3) revised Spanish versions of the POSIT, POSIT follow-up, and POSIP forms; and (4) a "mini-instrument" for assessing risk of HIV and sexually transmitted diseases, to be administered either alone or in combination with the POSIT. Furthermore, the "red-flag" items were eliminated and replaced with three-category risk ratings. No changes were made to the cutoff scores.

RESEARCH EVIDENCE

The POSIT has been used in a number of settings, including primary care settings, substance abuse treatment programs, and juvenile justice intake facilities. Selected studies reporting on the reliability and validity of the instrument are discussed below.

Internal Consistency and Reliability

Knight, Goodman, Pulerwitz, and DuRant (2001) studied the internal consistency and 1-week test–retest reliability of the POSIT among 193 medical patients receiving routine care who were 15–18 years of age. Results indicated that the Substance Use/Abuse, Mental Health, Educational Status, and Aggressive Behavior/Delinquency scales had adequate interitem consistency (alpha coefficients better than .70). Initial scores on all 10 functional areas had high intraclass correlations with scores received 1 week later (range from .72 to .88), although the correlations were lower for males than females on two of the scales (Family Relations and Leisure/Recreation). These repeat test administrations also indicated score reproducibility that was significantly better than chance (kappa = .42 to .73).

Another study examined test–retest reliability among 563 youths ages 12–19 who were processed at the Hillsborough County JAC on two or more occasions between May and December 1993 (Dembo, Schmeidler, et al., 1996). Results indicated that problem levels on the 10 POSIT scales, with few exceptions, were similar across gender, racial groups (African American vs. European American), and ethnicity groups (Hispanic vs. non-Hispanic) at both administrations. Dembo, Schmeidler, and colleagues (1996) reported concordance rates between Time 1 and Time 2 POSIT scores for the following intervals: (1) up to 2 weeks, (2) 3 to 4 weeks, (3) 5 to 8 weeks, (4) 9 to 12 weeks, and (5) 13 to 33 weeks. Concordance rates reflected the percentage of youths with no potential problem at either Time 1 or Time 2, or the percentage with a potential problem at both Time 1 and Time 2. Concordance rates between Time 1 and Time 2 remained high across all intervals of comparison, with concordance being highest for the shortest time intervals (especially up to 2 weeks). Kappa values indicated that agreement rates tended to be in the fair to good range (.40 to .75). At the same time, since the rates of problems were high, estimates of reliability were somewhat limited.

Validity

In one validation study, Hall, Richardson, Spears, and Rembert (1998) compared several social and behavioral characteristics of 21 adolescents who used drugs and 21 adolescents who abstained from drugs. The drug-using youths were recruited from residential and outpatient drug treatment centers. The abstaining youths were recruited from the social networks of the drug-using youths and from community agencies opposed to drug use. Nine of the 10 POSIT functional area scores for the drug-using youths were significantly greater (indicating higher risk) than for the abstaining youths, contributing to construct validity. Comparisons of the POSIT functional area scores with youths' scores on other instruments probing these domains indicated good concurrent validity.

Another validation study involved 2,027 delinquent youths ages 12–19 who were processed at the Hillsborough County JAC between May and December 1993 (Dembo, Turner, et al., 1996). Recidivism was recorded as the number of reentries to the JAC from the initial registration to the end of 1993. A cluster analysis of the 10 POSIT functional areas indicated the presence of four clusters ("types" of youths based on their pattern of POSIT scale scores): youths at low risk in all 10 areas (Cluster 1, $n = 770$); youths at moderate risk on all 10 POSIT areas (Cluster 2, $n = 794$); youths with severe problems, particularly in Substance Use/Abuse (Cluster 3, $n = 171$); and youths with severe problems, particularly in Mental Health and Educational Status (Cluster 4, $n = 292$).

The four clusters of youths were compared for their rates of return to the JAC. Overall, 30% of the youths were readmitted to the JAC following their first registration—18% once, 7% twice, and 5% three or more times. To account for time at risk, a recidivism rate was calculated; this rate was defined as the number of successive JAC registrations divided by the square root of the number of months between the initial registration and the end of the follow-up period. Thus youths who did not return to the JAC received negative recidivism scores. Recidivism scores ranged from –0.70 to 0.75, with an average of –0.10 ($SD = 0.63$). The clusters of youths with severe levels of problems (Clusters 3 and 4) had significantly higher rates of recidivism (see Table 6.2) than the lower-risk clusters; however, they did not differ significantly from each other. These results indicated preliminary promise for the POSIT classification scheme as a conceptual tool to practitioners making intervention decisions involving youths processed at the JAC.

TABLE 6.2. Recidivism for the Four Cluster Groups

	Cluster 1: Low risk	Cluster 2: Medium risk	Cluster 3: Severe problems— Substance Use/Abuse	Cluster 4: Severe problems— Mental Health and Educational Status
n	770	794	171	292
Mean recidivism rate	–0.18[a]	–0.10[a]	0.08[b]	–0.04[b]
SD	0.57	0.64	0.68	0.67

Note. Recidivism rates = number of JAC registrations / $\sqrt{\text{number of months follow-up}}$. Groups with different subscripts were significantly different from each other, $F(4, 2023) = 10.01$, $p < .001$. From Dembo, Turner, et al. (1996, Table 4, p. 317). Copyright 1996 by CRC Press, Boca Raton, Florida. Adapted with permission.

APPLICATION

The POSIT is a public domain instrument. Since its first appearance in the early 1990s, the POSIT has received increasing use in various states among different adolescent populations, including components of the juvenile justice system, drug treatment programs, schools, and medical and mental health service providers. It is generally used as a screening instrument in juvenile justice settings, followed by referral (if indicated) for an in-depth assessment with appropriate referrals to needed services. The POSIT is most helpful at points of intake into the juvenile justice system, such as juvenile assessment centers or pretrial detention centers. The POSIT can save considerable staff and financial resources at these intake points by directing more intensive evaluations to the subset of youths in most need of them.

The AARS manual (Rahdert, 1991), which includes the POSIT, is available free of charge from the National Clearinghouse for Alcohol and Drug Information (stock no. BKD-59, P.O. Box 2345, Rockville, MD 20847-2345; 800-729-6686). The CD-ROM version of the POSIT is available for purchase from *Power*Train, Inc. (8201 Corporate Drive, Suite 1080, Landover, MD 20785; 301-731-0900).

The POSIT should not be administered on a group basis. No special qualifications are needed to administer the instrument, but at the same time, it is important to maintain quality control over the administration of the POSIT. To facilitate this, we recommend that the POSIT be administered on an individual basis in a quiet location to permit focused attention. Collateral information that will help validate youths' answers is especially needed in the juvenile justice system—particularly in juvenile assessment centers, where youths can be expected to underreport problems with drug use. Routine drug testing is strongly recommended in these settings. Furthermore, users of the instrument should be aware that the instrument may work differently for different sociodemographic subgroups of youths, such as youths from different ethnic backgrounds. More research is needed to examine this important issue.

CASE EXAMPLE

The POSIT is being used in a clinical trial funded by the Center for Substance Abuse Treatment, involving youths placed in a juvenile justice diversion program in Florida Judicial Circuit 13, located in Hillsborough County. The following case example describes the use of the POSIT in this context. It is important to reiterate that the POSIT is used as a screening tool to target youths in need of more thorough assessments, and generally is not used to guide treatment planning. However, since the Hillsborough County project employed a licensed mental health clinician who assisted the staff in formulating intervention plans, it was possible to use the POSIT in this manner. Therefore, the following case illustrates an "extended" use of the POSIT, not its typical use as an intake screening tool to identify youths for further assessment.

Nina, a 16-year-old white female, was admitted to the Arbitration Intervention Program at the county courthouse in the spring of 2003, following charges of possession of marijuana and drug paraphernalia. Nina was skipping school with friends and went to smoke marijuana in one of the other students' backyards. The marijuana smoke drifted into a neighbor's yard, and the neighbor called the police. When the police officer arrived, Nina was the only one holding the marijuana and the paraphernalia.

An Arbitration Intervention Worker (AIW) contacted Nina's mother by telephone to schedule the first home visit for the Arbitration Intervention Program. She was very willing and eager for her and her daughter to start receiving this assistance. The initial home visit was scheduled for the following week. The first 3 weeks of home visits consisted of assessments and evaluations. One of the assessment tools the AIW utilized was the POSIT. From this assessment, it became apparent that Nina had many issues that were negatively affecting her life. Of the 10 POSIT problem areas, Nina obtained a high-risk score in three (Physical Health, Mental Health, and Vocational Status) and a moderate-risk score in six (Substance Use/Abuse, Family Relations, Peer Relations, Educational Status, Leisure/Recreation, and Aggressive Behavior/Delinquency).

On the basis of the POSIT results, the AIW offered Nina and her family certain referrals and other services related to attainable goals in each of the relevant problem areas. With respect to the Substance Use/Abuse score, Nina was ordered into the Satisfy Program during her initial hearing. This program provides substance use/abuse treatment, random drug screens, and case management services. While in this program, Nina independently contacted the agency on a daily basis to determine whether it was her day for a random drug screen. Nina also scored in the high-risk range in the Mental Health functional area of the POSIT. After reviewing Nina's case file, the AIW discovered that she had a history of, and was currently dealing with, mental health issues. She had been diagnosed at age 13 with depression and at age 15 with bipolar disorder. She had been seeing the same psychiatrist and counselor for approximately 6 months. At the beginning of her treatment, Nina had not been truthful with either the psychiatrist or the counselor about her substance use or emotional feelings. Once Nina became truthful with both of them, her medications were adjusted accordingly, and they were able to make a positive change in her mental health status.

When the AIW reviewed Nina's answers in the Physical Health category, she noticed that Nina indicated she slept too much and had less energy than she thought she should have. In the Peer Relations functional area, Nina revealed that she felt alone most of the time, even though she had numerous friends. After some discussion, Nina told the AIW that she had many "acquaintances" with whom she spent her time, but that when she was really pressed to think about it, she realized that the people she thought were her friends were not really "friends" at all. Nina told the AIW that she did have one very close friend who was perhaps her best ever. When asked about her free time in the Leisure/Recreation functional area, Nina answered that she spent her free time "just hanging out with friends." After discussing these results with Nina, the AIW determined that she was not active enough during the day, that she did not have a positive peer support group, and that she did not use her free time in an organized manner. The AIW and Nina set an activity goal in which she was to participate in a structured leisure activity at least once per week. Nina was apprehensive about this at first, but she soon started to enjoy herself. She stopped "just hanging out" with her friends who were using drugs, and she started to attend these activities with different, non-substance-using people. She got summer passes to the local pool, an amusement park, and the library.

In the Vocational Status functional area of the POSIT, Nina responded that she had never had a job and did not have a valid driver's license. After discussing this area with Nina, the AIW found that she was not filling out job applications correctly. The AIW made up a "job-seeking skills packet" that contained information on filling out applications, the interview process, and résumé writing. Over approximately a 6-week period, the AIW and Nina reviewed this information and completed the worksheets that accompanied the packet. At the completion of this packet, Nina was given information on how to obtain a Florida state identification card, as well as information on the local bus system.

In the Family Relations functional area on the POSIT, Nina indicated that her parents did not know what she was really thinking or feeling. She told the AIW that she and her mother would talk, but not about the things that were important to her. In the Aggressive Behavior/Delinquency functional area, Nina indicated that she was suspicious of other people and that she screamed a lot. When questioned about her answers, Nina told the AIW that she was only outwardly aggressive with her mother, because "She is always changing the rules, and she always brings up the negative things that I have done in the past." Nina also told the AIW that her previous substance use made her more aggressive and defensive than she had been in the past. The AIW set a goal for Nina and her mother to participate in a family activity— any activity that promoted communication—at least once per week. Nina and her mother did many activities that they had been accustomed to doing when she was younger. Nina's mother told the AIW that she still wanted to do these activities with her daughter, but it never seemed that there was enough time. Now that they were encouraged to do so, interacting was a lot easier. The communication between mother and daughter reportedly got much better. They now had thoughts and ideas to discuss about the positive and exciting activities they were going to do or had done together in the past. Finally, Nina scored in the moderate-risk category for Educational Status. Nina's risk status and recent drop in her grades were due in part to substance use, skipping school, and mental health issues. From the results of this assessment, it was clear how imperative it was for Nina to attend and participate in class. She also needed to study more, to complete all makeup and currently required assignments, and to discuss her career goals and how she would work toward achieving them with the AIW.

Nina complied with the goals that were set by the AIW, and she also complied with the substance use/abuse treatment program to which she was assigned. All of her random drug screen results came back negative. Nina successfully completed the Arbitration Intervention Program after 16 weeks of participation. While in this program, Nina obtained the knowledge and skills needed to become more aware of herself and to become a more productive person.

ACKNOWLEDGMENTS

Preparation of this chapter was supported by Grant No. TI12834 from by the Center for Substance Abuse Treatment. We are grateful for this support. The research results reported and the views expressed in the chapter do not necessarily imply any policy or research endorsement by our funding agency.

REFERENCES

Dembo, R., Pacheco, K., Schmeidler, J., Fisher, L., & Cooper, S. (1997). Drug use and delinquent behavior among high risk youths. *Journal of Child and Adolescent Substance Abuse, 6*, 1–25.

Dembo, R., & Schmeidler, J. (2003). A classification of high-risk youths. *Crime and Delinquency, 49*, 201–230.

Dembo, R., & Schmeidler, J. (in press). Correlates of male and female abuse experiences. *Violence and Victims*.

Dembo, R., Schmeidler, J., Borden, P., Turner, G., Sue, C. C., & Manning, D. (1996). Examination of the reliability of the Problem-Oriented Screening Instrument for Teenagers (POSIT) among arrested youths entering a juvenile assessment center. *Substance Use and Misuse, 31*, 785–824.

Dembo, R., Turner, G., Schmeidler, J., Sue, C. C., Borden, P., & Manning, D. (1996). Development and evaluation of a classification of high risk youths entering a juvenile assessment center. *International Journal of the Addictions, 31*, 303–322.

Dembo, R., Williams, L., Berry, E., Getreu, A., Washburn, M., Wish, E. D., et al. (1988). The relationship between physical and sexual abuse and illicit drug use: A replication among a new sample of youths entering a juvenile detention center. *International Journal of the Addictions, 23*, 1101–1123.

Dembo, R., Williams, L., La Voie, L., Berry, E., Getreu, A., Wish, E. D., et al. (1989). Physical abuse, sexual victimization and illicit drug use: Replication of a structural analysis among a new sample of high risk youths. *Violence and Victims, 4*, 121–138.

Dembo, R., Williams, L., & Schmeidler, J. (1998). A theory of drug use and delinquency among high risk youths. In A. R. Roberts (Ed.), *Juvenile justice: Policies, programs and services* (2nd ed., pp. 273–311). Chicago: Nelson-Hall.

Dembo, R., Williams, L., Schmeidler, J., & Howitt, D. (1991). *Tough cases: School outreach for at-risk youth*. Washington, DC: U.S. Department of Education, Office of the Assistant Secretary for Educational Research and Development.

Hall, J. A., Richardson, B., Spears, J., & Rembert, J. K. (1998). Validation of the POSIT: Comparing drug using and abstaining youth. *Journal of Child and Adolescent Substance Abuse, 8*, 29–61.

Knight, J. R., Goodman, E., Pulerwitz, T., & DuRant, R. H. (2001). Reliability of the Problem-Oriented Screening Instrument for Teenagers (POSIT) in adolescent medial practice. *Journal of Adolescent Health, 29*, 125–130.

Mouzakitis, C. M. (1981). Inquiry into the problem of child abuse and juvenile delinquency. In R. J. Hunner & Y. E. Walker (Eds.), *Exploring the relationship between child abuse and delinquency* (pp. 220–232). Montclair, NJ: Allanheld, Osmun.

National Center on Addiction and Substance Abuse. (2002). *Trends in substance use and treatment needs among inmates* (Final Report to the National Institute of Justice). New York: Author.

National Institute of Justice. (2003). *2000 arrestee drug abuse monitoring: Annual report*. Washington, DC: U.S. Department of Justice, Office of Justice Programs.

*Power*Train, Inc. (1998). *Computerized POSIT*. Landover, MD: Author.

Rahdert, E. R. (1991). *The Adolescent Assessment/Referral System*. Rockville, MD: National Institute on Drug Abuse.

Teplin, L., Abram, K., McClelland, G., Dulcan, M., & Mericle, A. (2002). Psychiatric disorders in youth in juvenile detention. *Archives of General Psychiatry, 59*, 1133–1143.

CHAPTER 7

Child and Adolescent Functional Assessment Scale

Kay Hodges

PURPOSE

The Child and Adolescent Functional Assessment Scale (CAFAS; Hodges, 2000a) was developed to assess impairment in day-to-day functioning in children or adolescents who have, or may be at risk for developing, psychiatric, psychological, emotional, behavioral, mental health, or substance use problems. It assesses youths' functioning across different settings (i.e., school, work, home, community, social interactions) and indicates whether functioning is affected by various problems that may require specialized services (i.e., mood disturbance, self-harmful behavior, substance use, or thinking problems). The CAFAS can be used in any referral source or service agency (e.g., mental health, education, social services, juvenile justice, public health, adoption). It is also an outcome evaluation tool because it can be administered repeatedly over time.

The CAFAS is useful in determining the intensity and type of services needed for a youth; in generating a service or treatment plan that matches the youth's needs to appropriate interventions; and in evaluating the youth periodically while he or she is receiving services, to determine whether interventions are being effective. The CAFAS can help determine the need for evaluation or treatment by providers in various areas, including education, mental health, and child welfare, and can be used to monitor the youth's progress in these areas. These uses are critical for youths in the juvenile justice system because of the known high rates of psychiatric disorders and poor academic achievement and vocational adjustment in this population (Teplin, Abram,

McClelland, Dulcan, & Mericle, 2002). At the program or system level, the CAFAS is used to determine programmatic needs and to advocate for youths under the care of juvenile justice. The scores for the CAFAS can be aggregated across youths to generate various reports that address such issues as type and extent of impairment of youths seeking services, outcome by client type, relationship between services received and outcome gains, and predictors of successful outcome.

As an outcome measure that assesses functioning, the CAFAS helps to address two needs that have emerged over the last decade. The first is the expectation that measures of change should assess everyday functioning in real-world contexts, to provide evidence that change is *clinically* significant and not just *statistically* significant (Kazdin & Kendall, 1998). Second, identification of impairments in functioning has become an important concept in mental health and juvenile justice. A "diagnosis" consists of a constellation of symptoms, whereas "impairment" reflects the consequences or effects of symptoms on day-to-day functioning. Research on community samples over the past decade has demonstrated that the presence of a diagnosis is not equivalent to impairment or need for treatment (Bird et al., 1990). The concept of impairment is included in the fourth edition of the *Diagnostic and Statistical Manual of Mental Disorders* (DSM-IV; American Psychiatric Association, 1994) and its text revision (DSM-IV-TR; American Psychiatric Association, 2000). It is also included in the definition of "serious emotional disturbance" (SED) used by the Substance Abuse and Mental Health Services Administration (SAMHSA), which oversees federal mental health monies given to the states. SED is defined as (1) the presence of a diagnosis and (2) impairment that substantially interferes with or limits the child's role or functioning in family, school, or community activities (Friedman, Katz-Leavy, Manderscheid, & Sondheimer, 1996). Research has shown that impairment is a robust predictor of service cost and utilization, school attendance, trouble with the law, and recidivism (Hodges, 2004a). These are the target goals for most funders and legislators.

BASIC DESCRIPTION

The CAFAS can be used with youths old enough to be in a full-day school program (i.e., kindergarten through 12th grade). A version for young adults (18–24 years old) is also available, because it was developed for follow-up studies of juvenile justice samples. The CAFAS is behaviorally based; it consists of concrete descriptions of behaviors written in common terms, such as "chronic truancy resulting in negative consequences (e.g., loss of course credit, failing courses or tests, parents notified)."

The behavioral descriptors in the CAFAS are categorized according to eight subscales that assess a youth and two optional subscales that assess a

TABLE 7.1. Description of the CAFAS Subscales

Subscales assessing the youth

School/Work	Ability to function satisfactorily in a group educational environment.
Home	Extent to which youth observes reasonable rules and performs age-appropriate tasks.
Community	Respect for the rights of others and their property and conformity to laws.
Behavior Toward Others	Appropriateness of youth's daily behavior toward others, including adults and peers.
Moods/Emotions	Modulation of the youth's emotional life.
Self-Harmful Behavior	Extent to which the youth can cope without resorting to self-harmful behavior or verbalizations.
Substance Use	Substance use and the extent to which it is maladaptive, inappropriate, or disruptive to functioning.
Thinking	Ability of youth to use rational thought processes.

Subscales assessing the caregiver

Material Needs	The extent to which the caregiver has difficulties in providing for the youth's material needs (e.g., housing), such that there is a negative impact on the youth's level of functioning.
Family/Social	The extent to which the caregiver has difficulties in providing a home setting that is free of known risk factors (e.g., abuse, parental alcoholism) or in providing for the youth's developmental needs (e.g., monitoring of youth's activities).

caregiver's ability to provide for the youth adequately (see Table 7.1). Within each of these subscales, behavioral descriptors are grouped according to four levels of impairment: "severe," "moderate," "mild," and "minimal or no impairment." In other words, there is a set of items describing behaviors for each severity level within each subscale. There are, on average, five items for each severity level on each subscale. A rater reviews items in the severe impairment categories first. If any one item describes the level of the youth's functioning, the level of impairment for the subscale is severe. If no items at the severe level characterize the youth, the rater continues to the moderate level and progresses downward through the remainder of the severity levels until the level of functioning can be described for each subscale. Thus level of impairment is determined for each subscale according to the behavioral descriptor that the rater selects as describing the most severe behavior displayed by the examinee during the rating period.

Each subscale is also accompanied by a list of positive characteristics. Contained in the School/Work subscale, for example, are the descriptors "attends regularly" and "gets along okay with teachers." These positive behavioral descriptions can be coded as strengths for youths with the characteristics, or as goals for youths without the behaviors. Thus raters can select one or more problem behaviors for each domain, as well as strengths and goals. Although the endorsement of goals and strengths is optional, most raters use them because they are helpful in developing outcome-driven, strengths-based treatment plans. Detailed descriptions of how to use the CAFAS for clinical assessment, to design treatment plans, and to link the CAFAS to evidence-based treatments are available elsewhere (Hodges, 2003b, 2004b, 2004c).

In order to rate youths and to delineate their strengths and goals, raters must obtain enough information about the youths' current functioning in various settings. A youth is rated on the CAFAS based on a rater's observations and the youth's, caregiver's, and other informant's reports about the youth's behavior during the past 3 months (or other time period chosen by the user). This information is typically collected as part of a routine intake. The actual rating of the CAFAS takes about 10 minutes, because a rater need only identify one item on each subscale; however, the rater typically indicates all items that pertain to an examinee at the selected impairment level, to better inform the treatment plan. The following forms were developed to assist in obtaining information about the youth:

- The CAFAS Parent Report (Hodges, 1994) is a 30- to 40-minute structured interview that obtains all of the information needed to rate the CAFAS. It can be administered via phone or in person (Hodges, 1995c) and is available in Spanish.
- The CAFAS Checklist for Adult Informants (Hodges, 1995a) also obtains all of the information needed to score the CAFAS, but consists of a series of statements that are scored as "yes" (true) or "no" (false). Items relevant to each CAFAS subscale appear on a separate page, so that any given informant (e.g., teacher, therapist, foster parent) can complete one or more subscales.
- The CAFAS Checklist for Youths (Hodges, 1995b) obtains information about problems that may not be known to the caregiver and consists of four subscales: Community (i.e., delinquency), Substance Use, Mood, and Self-Harmful Behavior. These questions are asked of the youth in an interview format.
- The CAFAS Screener (Hodges, 2003a) is a shortened version of the CAFAS Parent Report that takes about 15–20 minutes and was developed to determine the need for referral to community services or for more comprehensive assessment.
- The Advanced Child Management Skills Scale for CAFAS (Hodges, 2002) assesses a caregiver's skills at managing a youth's behavior (e.g., reinforcing good behavior, disciplining appropriately, and monitoring activities).

Raters can generate quantitative subscale scores according to the levels of impairment by using assigned scores: severe = 30, moderate = 20, mild = 10, and minimal or no impairment = 0. A total score can be computed for each examinee by totaling the scores on the eight youth subscales. Total scores range from 0 to 240, with higher scores indicating greater impairment. A calibration of clinical significance is inherent in the CAFAS, because normative behavior is defined by the "minimal or no impairment" severity level. Furthermore, behaviors assessed on the CAFAS relate to day-to-day functioning in the real world. Both the CAFAS total and subscale scores gauge how far the youth is from this standard.

A youth's scores across the subscales can be charted on a bar graph, as shown in Figure 7.1. In addition, the accompanying report typically includes a description of the youth's behavior that supports the CAFAS subscale scores and indicates whether any risk behaviors are present. Risk behaviors, such as suicidal, aggressive, sexual, fire-setting, runaway, dangerous substance use, and psychotic behaviors, are flagged on the CAFAS because they require special consideration when service providers are creating a treatment plan.

A software version of the CAFAS allows clinicians to rate youth functioning, strengths, and goals on a computer to generate a clinical interpretive report and a treatment plan for each CAFAS. In addition, the CAFAS Computer System generates two administrative reports that collapse data across clients for a time period specified by users. The software also exports data files that can be analyzed in common software packages, including SPSS. Other information collected in the computer program includes variables that have been identified as predictors of service cost and utilization. Thus the program serves as a modest management information system.

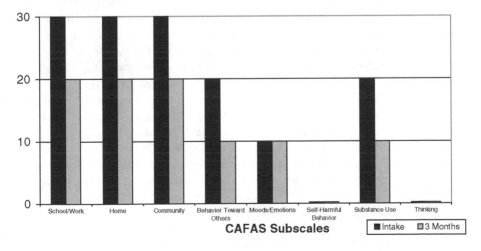

FIGURE 7.1. Case example of Lauren's CAFAS subscale scores at intake and 3 months.

HISTORY OF THE METHOD'S DEVELOPMENT

The precursor to the CAFAS was the Child Assessment Schedule (CAS), a semistructured clinical interview that I developed in 1978 to determine the presence of common psychiatric diagnoses in children. This interview was organized into areas of functioning, resulting in the following "content scales": School, Friends, Activities, Family, Fears, Worries and Anxieties, Self-Image, Depression, Physical Complaints, Expression of Anger (including delinquent and substance use behaviors), and Reality-Testing (i.e., thinking). The format for the interview was designed to facilitate good rapport with the youth, yet the questions and response options were standardized. The content reflected a traditional clinical interview for children, with items added to inquire about child functioning and presence–absence of specific diagnostic criteria for disorders typically arising in childhood and adolescence. Substantial reliability and validity data were generated for the CAS (Hodges, 1993; Hodges, McKnew, Cytryn, Stern, & Kline, 1982), including psychometric data on the diagnostically related items (Hodges, Saunders, Kashani, Hamlett, & Thompson, 1990) and on diagnostically unrelated items that inquired about general functioning (Hodges & Saunders, 1989). These studies culminated in ample evidence that the content scale scores provided valuable information about youths' functioning and outcome over time.

A new measure, the CAFAS, was developed in 1989 to assess the impact of diagnoses, problems, and symptoms on child functioning. The CAFAS incorporated items from the original content scales that had the highest internal consistency and test–retest reliability, and I consulted the research on child development, child psychopathology, and assessment of functioning in adults (Hodges, Bickman, & Kurtz, 1991; Hodges & Gust, 1995). In 1990, the CAFAS was included in the Fort Bragg Evaluation Study, which included a large battery of state-of-the-art assessment tools and a sample of 1,000 youths and their families (Breda, 1996). The CAFAS was found to be the best predictor of service cost and utilization (Hodges & Wong, 1996, 1997).

The Fort Bragg study and input from experts helped shape the 1994 revision of the CAFAS. I sent the CAFAS to 360 experts in three waves of 120. The first wave consisted of persons with expertise in a variety of diagnostic areas; the second included researchers who published in the areas of child development, juvenile justice, abuse, or education; and the third included researchers who studied ethnic minority issues or were themselves members of ethnic minority groups. Modifications based on their criticisms were resubmitted to every respondent for further feedback. The 1994 version of the CAFAS differed from the 1989 version by including eight (instead of five) subscales and an expanded and modified set of items.

The revision establishing the current version of the CAFAS was prompted by use of the 1994 version in the national evaluation of the demonstration service grants federally funded by the Center for Mental Health Services (CMHS) branch of SAMHSA. Since the purpose of these grants was to develop integrated care, the samples included referrals from various child-serving agencies, including juvenile justice, social services, education, and mental health. The studies generated from these ongoing national projects revealed the need to clarify scoring rules for children in residential settings. With data collected for the state of Michigan (Hodges, Xue, & Wotring, 2004b) and feedback from users in other states, the scoring rules and a few items were modified. These proposed changes were circulated to selected users for 3 years in order to solicit feedback before the current version was finalized in 2000.

RESEARCH EVIDENCE

Internal Consistency and Reliability

High interrater reliability has been reported for the CAFAS for both nonprofessional staff and clinical raters (Hodges & Wong, 1996) using criterion scores. With both types of raters, high correlations (.92 to .96) were observed for total scores, as well as individual subscales (.73 to .99). Intraclass correlations examining the consistency across raters, while ignoring the criterion answers, produced comparable results (Hodges & Wong, 1996). Good test–retest reliability was demonstrated in a study in which lay interviewers rated the 1994 CAFAS after administering the CAFAS Parent Report via the telephone (Hodges, 1995c). Two raters interviewed parents on separate occasions across intervals ranging from 3 to 14 days. Test–retest correlations for CAFAS total scores were .91 (.79 to 1.00 for individual subscales).

Validity

Support for the validity of the CAFAS has been provided by studies of subgroups of youths who presumably should differ in their extent of impairment. For example, inpatients scored significantly higher than youths receiving home-based services or day treatment, who scored significantly higher than youths in outpatient care (Hodges & Wong, 1996). Children living with their parents or in regular foster care were significantly less impaired than youths in various residential placements, and youths in therapeutic foster care scored in between these two groups (Hodges, Doucette-Gates, & Liao, 1999). Youths with more serious psychiatric disorders were more impaired than youths diagnosed with less serious disorders, such as adjustment or anxiety disorders (Hodges et al., 1999). The CAFAS also has strong concurrent validity, with higher impairment scores being associated with problems in social relationships (Hodges & Wong, 1996), involvement with juvenile justice (Doucette-Gates, Hodges, & Liao, 1998; Hodges et al., 1999; Hodges & Wong, 1996), school-related problems (Doucette-Gates et al., 1998; Hodges et al., 1999; Hodges & Wong, 1996), and child and family risk factors (Manteuffel, Stephens, & Santiago, 2002).

Other studies have demonstrated that youths referred from juvenile justice are as impaired (Walrath, dosReis, et al., 2001) or more impaired

(Walrath, Mandell, & Leaf, 2001; Walrath, Nickerson, Crowel, & Leaf, 1998; Walrath, Sharp, Zuber, & Leaf, 2001) than youths referred from mental health, social services, or education, even after controlling for the effects of sex, age, and ethnicity. Furthermore, among youths referred to mental health, those who had recently engaged in delinquent behavior were found to be more impaired than youths without delinquent behavior (Hodges, Xue, & Wotring, 2004a; Rosenblatt, Rosenblatt, & Biggs, 2000). Again, this difference was not due to demographic variables (i.e., age, gender, ethnicity) and remained true even after scores were adjusted by omitting the Community subscale of the CAFAS, which captures delinquency. However, despite the high levels of impairment, the youths with histories of delinquency were able to make statistically and clinically meaningful treatment gains (Hodges et al., 1999, 2003; Walrath, Mandell, & Leaf, 2001).

Other studies have examined the CAFAS's predictive validity, with favorable results. CAFAS scores at intake predict subsequent services utilization, cost for services, truancy, and contact with the law. In the Fort Bragg study, a higher CAFAS total score at intake predicted more restrictive care, higher costs, more bed days, and more days of services at 6 and 12 months postintake (Hodges & Wong, 1997). The CAFAS had more predictive power than other measures used in that study, including presence of specific psychiatric diagnoses (e.g., conduct disorder). The national evaluation of CMHS-funded sites found that the CAFAS predicted restrictiveness of living arrangements and days out of family care (Hodges, Doucette-Gates, & Kim, 2000). In addition, youths with higher impairment at intake were significantly more likely to have contact with the law or the courts and to have poor school attendance at 6 months postintake (Hodges & Kim, 2000). With regard to youths served by the juvenile justice system, Quist and Matshazi (2000) found that CAFAS functioning was significantly related to recidivism for 1 year after discharge from a juvenile rehabilitation group home. A youth's CAFAS score at discharge was a stronger predictor than age at discharge and prior offenses.

The CAFAS is sensitive to change over time, as demonstrated with a variety of youths. Statistically significant reductions in CAFAS total scores and moderate to large effect sizes were observed from intake to 6 and 12 months postintake in a study of youths referred for mental health services (Hodges & Wong, 1996; Hodges, Wong, & Latessa, 1998). In the evaluation study of the CMHS-funded sites, the CAFAS total score decreased significantly after 6 months (Hodges et al., 1999) and 2 years after intake (Manteuffel et al., 2002). Outcomes for individual CMHS-funded sites have revealed significant reductions in youth impairment (Resendez, Quist, & Matshazi, 2000; Rosenblatt & Furlong, 1998). Results from a large outcome study conducted for the state of Michigan found a significant reduction in impairment on the total and subscale scores, primarily demonstrating moderate to large effects (Hodges et al., 2004).

"Generalizability" refers to whether a measure performs similarly across various subgroups of examinees. The CAFAS has been studied with youths referred from a variety of agencies; with youths ranging in age from 3 to 18 years; with samples including 35% to 50% girls; and with different racial groups (i.e., African American, Asian, European American, Hispanic, and multiracial; Hodges & Wong, 1997; Hodges et al., 2004; Mak & Rosenblatt, 2002; Walrath et al., 2001). Age effects are typical, with older youths having higher impairment scores, as would be expected. No differences in overall impairment between boys and girls have been observed (Hodges & Wong, 1996). The only consistent race effect has been higher impairment among European Americans (Hodges & Wong, 1997; Mak & Rosenblatt, 2002).

APPLICATION

More than 25 states use the CAFAS as one component for determining whether a child is eligible for SED services or for assessing treatment outcomes among youths in child welfare or juvenile justice systems (Georgetown University National Technical Assistance Center for Children's Mental Health, 2002). The CAFAS is copyrighted and is published by Functional Assessment Systems (see *http://www.CAFAS.com* for contact information). Thus others may not reproduce, disseminate, modify, or make derivative versions of the instrument.

Although the CAFAS was originally developed within the mental health field, professionals from other child-serving agencies easily learn to rate the CAFAS by using the training materials. Professionals who have been successfully trained include juvenile justice staff members who conduct intake assessments or counseling, probation officers, group home staffers, child protection workers, school counselors, mental health workers, and teachers. Extensive training and support materials are available. The *CAFAS Self-Training Manual* (Hodges, 2000b) is used to train raters to be reliable. It contains instructions for scoring, demonstration vignettes with answers, and vignettes for establishing rater reliability. New employees can work through the manual on their own. Simple criteria for judging reliability are given in the *Manual for Training Coordinators, Clinical Administrators, and Data Managers* (Hodges, 2003b).

In a juvenile justice setting, the CAFAS can be used to generate a plan for services and to evaluate progress. It is particularly well suited for evaluating youths who are court-ordered to receive services in the community (e.g., intensive community programs, probation) or in residential settings. It can also be used at discharge to plan aftercare or step-down services. For example, in an urban county in Michigan, every youth who is convicted of a criminal or status offense receives an evaluation that includes the CAFAS to generate individualized plans of action. The facts and judgments contained in these evaluations, along with other information, are used to make decisions about security, level of care, and treatment recommendations. Treatment plans typically prioritize the areas for intervention, suggest how to utilize the youth's strengths, and indicate whether further evaluations or specialized services may be needed. Because the CAFAS comments on functioning across a variety of domains, it provides both an objective measurement of functioning and a practical guide for prioritizing interventions. The CAFAS has been used in detention settings; however, in most cases time constraints do not permit adequate data collection. As an alternative, the CAFAS Screener can be used to determine whether youths need a comprehensive evaluation and whether they could benefit from local community services.

As is true with any assessment tool, the CAFAS should not be used as the sole determinant for any disposition. In addition, use of the CAFAS total score in any strict application of "cutoff scores" is unwise, since the subscale profile, strengths, presence of risk behaviors, and assessment of the caregiving environment are all important components in interpreting the CAFAS. Also, only trained raters should use the CAFAS.

CASE EXAMPLE

Lauren was a 15-year-old girl charged with assaulting her mother. She became involved with the court's status offender unit at an early age, and she had a long history of status offenses, including home truancy. Lauren was referred to a juvenile justice assessment center for treatment planning in the community. A master's-level staff member of the juvenile justice office conducted a routine interview with the youth and her mother in their home.

Lauren's mother was a nurse at a hospital in a neighboring community. Her mother worked hard to provide for Lauren and was the primary financial support for the family. Lauren had a poor relationship with her father, from whom the mother was divorced. Lauren had missed school with regularity since seventh grade and was missing credits because of poor attendance, inattentiveness to homework, and suspensions. She tested at a ninth-grade reading level and a seventh-grade math level. Lauren's mother reported that Lauren was smart; she just did not apply herself. At home, Lauren defied her mother's rules regarding boys, sexual activity, curfew, and behavioral expectations. Lauren's mother had not been able to account for Lauren's whereabouts after school and in the early evening for some time. She had left home for 3 to 14 days without permission on numerous occasions. Lauren had a small group of intimate friends with whom she shared secrets. Other than these relationships, she had very poor relationships with adults and other young women. She was frequently volatile with others when she felt angry. Lauren had a low sense of self-worth, but her mother and Lauren both denied that she was depressed, overly anxious, or self-harmful. From Lauren's comments, it appeared that she might have been sexually or emotionally abused in past relationships with older boyfriends. She used marijuana and alcohol on Friday and Saturday nights. There was no evidence of bizarre behavior or thought disturbance in her history.

The evaluator used the information collected during the routine intake interview to rate the CAFAS. The most severe items endorsed at intake for each subscale (presented in abbreviated format) were as follows: School, chronic truancy (severe); Home, run away from home (severe); Community, involvement with juvenile justice system because of physical assault (severe); Behavior Toward Others, frequent display of anger towards others and poor judgment (moderate); Moods/Emotions, very self-critical, low self-esteem (mild); Self-Harmful Behavior, not indicative of self-harm (no impairment); Substance Use, high or intoxicated once or twice a week, and vulnerable to injury or date rape (moderate); and Thinking, thought not disordered (no impairment). Lauren's total score was 140, indicating a need for intensive treatment. The solid bars in Figure 7.1 represent Lauren's profile at intake.

A treatment plan was then designed, based on the behavioral items endorsed on the CAFAS and the goals and strengths endorsed for each sub-scale. The CAFAS software automatically generated the format for the treat-ment plan, including a grid for each of the subscales. Figure 7.2 depicts this grid for the School/Work subscale. Raters simply write in the specifics under the heading "Plan" (see Figure 7.2). Although not shown here, the remainder of the treatment plan in this case included home-based counseling with Lauren and her mother for 8 weeks to establish clearer rules and better monitoring of Lauren's activities, as well as to encourage discussion between mother and daughter regarding sexual issues; installation of a motion detector to deter runaway behavior; weekly drug testing and attendance at a substance use pro-gram; participation in an after-school drama program to enhance self-esteem; and weekly contact with her case manager to monitor treatment progress and effectiveness.

	Item	Item description	Impairment
Problem	006	Chronic truancy resulting in negative consequences	Severe (30)
Strengths	S20	Likes to read	
Goals	G3 G16	Attends regularly Completes schoolwork	
Plan		1. Enroll Lauren in Stoney Creek alternative public school (which provides door-to-door pickup by school bus) to ensure attendance, close supervision, remedial educational services (i.e., in math), after-school activities, and weekly contact with parents and probation officer regarding behavior and academic performance. 2. Teacher to reinforce Lauren for her excellent reading skills. 3. During home-based counseling services, counselor checks with mother to see whether she is supervising schoolwork and giving Lauren rewards and consequences, as per agreement with school personnel.	

FIGURE 7.2. Excerpt from Lauren's Treatment Plan: CAFAS School/Work sub-scale.

The gray bars in Figure 7.1 represent 3-month follow-up ratings for Lauren after intensive services, which was done by staff from the juvenile justice assessment center, although it could also have been done by her therapist or case manager. Lauren's score decreased by 50 points from intake to 3 months, showing significant improvement. As services continue, Lauren's progress can be continuously charted on the CAFAS profile so that the judge, other court workers, Lauren, her parents, and the rest of her treatment team can use it to inform decisions regarding her care.

REFERENCES

American Psychiatric Association. (1994). *Diagnostic and statistical manual of mental disorders* (4th ed.). Washington, DC: Author.

American Psychiatric Association. (2000). *Diagnostic and statistical manual of mental disorders* (4th ed., text rev.). Washington, DC: Author.

Bird, H. R., Yager, T. J., Staghezza, B., Gould, M. S., Canino, G., & Rubio-Stipec, M. (1990). Impairment in the epidemiological measurement of childhood psychopathology in the community. *Journal of the American Academy of Child and Adolescent Psychiatry, 29,* 796–803.

Breda, C. S. (1996). Methodological issues in evaluating mental health outcomes of a children's mental health managed care demonstration. *Journal of Mental Health Administration, 23,* 40–50.

Doucette-Gates, A., Hodges, K., & Liao, Q. (1998, March). *Using the Child and Adolescent Functional Assessment Scale: Examining child outcomes and service use patterns.* Paper presented at the 11th annual research conference: A System of Care for Children's Mental Health: Expanding the Research Base, University of South Florida, Tampa, FL.

Friedman, R. M., Katz-Leavy, J. W., Manderscheid, R. W., & Sondheimer, D. L. (1996). Prevalence of serious emotional disturbance in children and adolescents. In R. W. Manderscheid & M. A. Sonnerschein (Eds.), *Mental health, United States* (pp. 71–89). Tiburon, CA: CentraLink.

Georgetown University National Technical Assistance Center for Children's Mental Health. (2002). *Evaluation initiative.* Retrieved from *http://www.georgetown.edu/research/gucdc/eval.html*

Hodges, K. (1993). Structured interviews for assessing children. *Journal of Child Psychology and Psychiatry, 34,* 49–65.

Hodges, K. (1994). *CAFAS Parent Report.* Ann Arbor, MI: Functional Assessment Systems.

Hodges, K. (1995a). *CAFAS Checklist for Adult Informants.* Ann Arbor, MI: Functional Assessment Systems.

Hodges, K. (1995b). *CAFAS Checklist for Youths.* Ann Arbor, MI: Functional Assessment Systems.

Hodges, K. (1995c, March). *Psychometric study of a telephone interview for the CAFAS using an expanded version of the scale.* Paper presented at the 8th annual research conference: A System of Care for Children's Mental Health: Expanding the Research Base, University of South Florida, Tampa, FL.

Hodges, K. (2000a). *Child and Adolescent Functional Assessment Scale* (3rd ed.). Ypsilanti: Eastern Michigan University.

Hodges, K. (2000b). *Child and Adolescent Functional Assessment Scale self-training manual* (3rd ed.). Ypsilanti, MI: Eastern Michigan University.

Hodges, K. (2002). *Advanced Child Management Skills Scale for CAFAS.* Ann Arbor, MI: Functional Assessment Systems.

Hodges, K. (2003a). *CAFAS Screener: Adult Information Version.* Ann Arbor, MI: Functional Assessment Systems.

Hodges, K. (2003b). *Manual for training coordinators, clinical administrators, and data managers* (2nd ed.). Ann Arbor, MI: Functional Assessment Systems.

Hodges, K. (2004a). The Child and Adolescent Functional Assessment Scale (CAFAS). In M. E. Maruish (Ed.), *The use of psychological testing for treatment planning and outcomes assessment* (3rd ed., pp. 405–441). Mahwah, NJ: Erlbaum.

Hodges, K. (2004b). *Guide for matching CAFAS profiles to evidence based treatments.* Ann Arbor, MI: Functional Assessment Systems.

Hodges, K. (2004c) Using assessment in everyday practice for the benefit of families and practitioners. *Professional Psychology: Research and Practice, 35,* 449–456.

Hodges, K., Bickman, L., & Kurtz, S. (1991, February). *Multidimensional measure of level of functioning for children and adolescents.* Paper presented at the 4th annual research conference: A System of Care for Children's Mental Health: Expanding the Research Base, University of South Florida, Tampa, FL.

Hodges, K., Doucette-Gates, A., & Kim, C. S. (2000). Predicting service utilization with the Child and Adolescent Functional Assessment Scale in a sample of youths with serious emotional disturbance served by Center for Mental Health Services-funded demonstrations. *Journal of Behavioral Health Services and Research, 27,* 47–59.

Hodges, K., Doucette-Gates, A., & Liao, Q. (1999). The relationship between the Child and Adolescent Functional Assessment Scale (CAFAS) and indicators of functioning. *Journal of Child and Family Studies, 8,* 109–122.

Hodges, K., & Gust, J. (1995). Measures of impairment for children and adolescents. *Journal of Mental Health Administration, 22,* 403–413.

Hodges, K., & Kim, C. S. (2000). Psychometric study of the Child and Adolescent Functional Assessment Scale: Prediction of contact with the law and poor school attendance. *Journal of Abnormal Child Psychology, 28,* 287–297.

Hodges, K., McKnew, D., Cytryn, L., Stern, L., & Kline, J. (1982). The Child Assessment Schedule (CAS) diagnostic interview: A report on reliability and validity. *Journal of the American Academy of Child Psychiatry, 21,* 468–473.

Hodges, K., & Saunders, W. B. (1989). Internal consistency of a diagnostic interview for children: The Child Assessment Schedule. *Journal of Abnormal Child Psychology, 17,* 691–701.

Hodges, K., Saunders, W. B., Kashani, J., Hamlett, K., & Thompson, R. J. (1990). Internal consistency of DSM-III diagnoses using the symptom scales of the Child Assessment Schedule. *Journal of the American Academy of Child and Adolescent Psychiatry, 29,* 635–641.

Hodges, K., & Wong, M. M. (1996). Psychometric characteristics of a multidimensional measure to assess impairment: The Child and Adolescent Functional Assessment Scale (CAFAS). *Journal of Child and Family Studies, 5,* 445–467.

Hodges, K., & Wong, M. M. (1997). Use of the Child and Adolescent Functional Assessment Scale to predict service utilization and cost. *Journal of Mental Health Administration, 24,* 278–290.

Hodges, K., Wong, M. M., & Latessa, M. (1998). Use of the Child and Adolescent Functional Assessment Scale (CAFAS) as an outcome measure in clinical settings. *Journal of Behavioral Health Services and Research, 25,* 325–336.

Hodges, K., Xue, Y., & Wotring, J. (2004a). *Predicting outcome for delinquent youth served by public mental health.* Manuscript under review.

Hodges, K., Xue, Y., & Wotring, J. (2004b). Use of the CAFAS to evaluate outcome for youths with SED served by public mental health. *Journal of Child and Family Studies, 13,* 325–339.

Kazdin, A. E., & Kendall, P. C. (1998). Current progress and future plans for developing effective treatments: Comments and perspectives. *Journal of Clinical Child Psychology, 27,* 217–226.

Mak, W., & Rosenblatt, A. (2002). Demographic influences on psychiatric diagnoses among youth served in California systems of care. *Journal of Child and Family Studies, 11,* 165–178.

Manteuffel, B., Stephens, R., & Santiago, R. (2002). Overview of the national evaluation of the Comprehensive Community Mental Health Services for Children and Their Families Program and summary of current findings. *Children's Services: Social Policy, Research, and Practice, 5,* 3–20.

Quist, R., & Matshazi, D. (2000). The Child and Adolescent Functional Assessment Scale (CAFAS): A dynamic predictor of juvenile recidivism. *Adolescence, 35*(137), 181–192.

Resendez, M. G., Quist, R. M., & Matshazi, D. G. M. (2000). A longitudinal analysis of empowerment of families and client outcomes. *Journal of Child and Family Studies, 9,* 449–460.

Rosenblatt, J. A., & Furlong, M. (1998). Outcomes in a system of care for youths with emotional and behavioral disorders: An examination of differential change across clinical profiles. *Journal of Child and Family Studies, 7,* 217–232.

Rosenblatt, J. A., Rosenblatt, A., & Biggs, E. E. (2000). Criminal behavior and emotional disorder: Comparing youth served by the mental health and juvenile justice systems. *Journal of Behavioral Health Services and Research, 27,* 227–237.

Teplin, L. A., Abram, K. M., McClelland, G. M., Dulcan, M. K., & Mericle, A. A. (2002). Psychiatric disorders in youth in juvenile detention. *Archives of General Psychiatry, 59,* 1133–1143.

Walrath, C. M., dosReis, S., Miech, R., Liao, Q., Holden, W., DeCarolis, G., et al. (2001). Referral source differences in functional impairment levels for children served in the Comprehensive Community Mental Health Services for Children and Their Families Program. *Journal of Child and Family Studies, 10,* 385–397.

Walrath, C. M., Mandell, D., & Leaf, P. J. (2001). Responses of children with different intake profiles to mental health treatment. *Psychiatric Services, 52,* 196–201.

Walrath, C. M., Nickerson, K. J., Crowel, R. L., & Leaf, P. J. (1998). Serving children with serious emotional disturbance in a system of care: Do mental health and non-mental health agency referrals look the same? *Journal of Emotional and Behavioral Disorders, 6,* 205–213.

Walrath, C. M., Sharp, M. J., Zuber, M., & Leaf, P. J. (2001). Serving children with SED in urban systems of care: Referral agency differences in child characteristics in Baltimore and the Bronx. *Journal of Emotional and Behavioral Disorders, 9,* 94–105.

PART III

Unidimensional Screening Tools

Anyone working with youthful offenders will confirm that certain mental health conditions are of especially great concern both for youths' welfare and for juvenile justice objectives. Among these are drug and alcohol abuse/dependence, posttraumatic stress disorder (PTSD), and attention-deficit/hyperactivity disorder (ADHD). These conditions are disproportionately represented in juvenile justice populations. They frequently contribute to the initiation and maintenance of juvenile delinquency, pose tremendous challenges to juvenile justice facilities charged with managing dangerous behaviors, and interfere with the long-term rehabilitation of juvenile offending.

The scales included in Part III focus on the assessment of these three conditions. They are suitable for screening purposes, but in contrast to the multidimensional tools in Part II, each of them is unidimensional, focusing on clinical characteristics associated with a single mental health condition. These instruments can be employed across a range of juvenile justice entry points and can be part of broader assessments of youths, as discussed in Chapter 3.

Part III begins with Miller and Lazowski's review of the Substance Abuse Subtle Screening Inventory for Adolescents—Second Version (SASSI-A2) in Chapter 8. This scale offers value in distinguishing between youths who exhibit a high or low probability of having a substance use disorder. Some forms of substance misuse appear to influence delinquency by increasing the likelihood that youths will place themselves in high-risk situations, often with other high-risk youths. Substance misuse impairs an adolescent's already immature judgment and impulse control. Furthermore, it can function as a numbing agent for family problems and the symptoms of other mental health conditions. This type of clinical information is useful to detention center staff members concerned with medical withdrawal complications of a recently admitted youth, as well as to a forensic examiner assessing delinquency recidivism risk in an evaluation of a youth who has been adjudicated delinquent and requires a treatment and rehabilitation plan.

In Chapter 9, Wolpaw and colleagues review the Trauma Symptom Checklist for Children (TSCC). The TSCC measures the emotional, behavioral, and cognitive effects of trauma exposure that can be relevant to several juvenile justice concerns. PTSD resulting from experiences such as childhood physical and sexual abuse, exposure to family violence, and involvement in gang violence appears to be more prevalent in delinquent groups. Trauma-related difficulties are especially salient for America's growing number of female juvenile offenders. Research suggests that female delinquents are traumatized at a much higher rate than community girls and are more likely to be diagnosed with PTSD than male delinquents. Thus, for example, information from scales like the TSCC can help staff members to determine whether a female offender with PTSD resulting from paternal sexual abuse should undergo suicide monitoring by a male correctional staffer, whose mere presence might inadvertently trigger serious emotional and behavioral difficulties.

In Chapter 10, the final chapter in Part III, Loney and Counts review three different instruments that briefly but comprehensively evaluate ADHD symptoms in youths: the Conners Rating Scales—Revised, the ADHD Rating Scale–IV, and the Attention Deficit Disorders Evaluation Scale—Second Edition. These instruments can help front-line staff members to manage myriad negative behaviors often seen in youths with ADHD in secure settings. In addition, research has firmly established that the combination of ADHD hyperactivity–impulsivity and early-onset delinquent behavior is related to serious offending into adolescence and adulthood. Successful identification and treatment of ADHD difficulties can reap long-standing benefits in the form of decreased recidivism, especially violent recidivism.

CHAPTER 8

Substance Abuse
Subtle Screening Inventory
for Adolescents—Second Version

Franklin G. Miller
Linda E. Lazowski

PURPOSE

The Substance Abuse Subtle Screening Inventory for Adolescents—Second Version (SASSI-A2; Miller & Lazowski, 2001) is a brief, easily administered screening measure that helps identify youths ages 12–18 who are likely to require further assessment and possible treatment for substance use disorders—specifically, substance abuse and substance dependence. Substance misuse is pervasive among juvenile offenders. In the nine major metropolitan sites included in the National Institute of Justice's *Arrestee Drug Abuse Monitoring (ADAM) 2000 Annualized Site Reports*, the percentage of juveniles who tested positive for the presence of any drug ranged from 35.2% to 68.3% (National Institute of Justice, 2001). Of those detained, 53% had been under the influence of drugs at the time of their arrest (see also Belenko & Dembo, 2003). Therefore, it is important to identify those with substance-related problems and refer them to appropriate services in order to reduce recidivism.

Identifying individuals in need of treatment for substance misuse is complicated by the need to distinguish between problematic and nonproblematic substance use. Alcohol consumption is a pervasive aspect of many social milieus. Even use of illicit drugs is a substantial part of our culture. The difficulty of distinguishing between problematic and nonproblematic usage is compounded in screening adolescents, because experimentation with substance use during adolescence is a common phenomenon. Furthermore, substance use is not stable through the course of an individual's life; peaks of usage that may evolve during the course of adolescence may decline during the normal course of maturation (see Jones, 1990; Kandel & Logan, 1984; Leccese & Waldron, 1994; Phillips, 1995). However, for some adolescents, heavy use evolves into a progressive disorder that can have a devastating impact on the individuals themselves, their family members, and society.

Because problematic substance use can be defined in a variety of ways, it is important to proceed with a clear understanding of the "target" of the screening. Diagnoses according to the American Psychiatric Association's (1994) *Diagnostic and Statistical Manual of Mental Disorders*, fourth edition (DSM-IV) were chosen as the target or criterion variables in developing the SASSI-A2, because they are the diagnostic classifications that are most commonly used for purposes of treatment planning. Thus the purpose of the SASSI-A2 is to screen for the likelihood of the presence of the two DSM-IV substance use disorders, substance abuse and substance dependence.

Substance abuse is defined by the presence of at least one of four criteria that address ongoing problematic use of alcohol or other drugs:

1. Recurrent use despite impaired work, school, or family functioning.
2. Recurrent use despite physical hazards.
3. Recurrent substance-related legal problems.
4. Continued use despite recurrent social problems.

Substance dependence is defined by the presence of at least three of seven criteria suggesting loss of control in usage:

1. Tolerance.
2. Withdrawal.
3. Greater use than intended.
4. Unsuccessful efforts to control use.
5. Excessive time spent in substance-related activities.
6. Impairment of social, occupational, or recreational functioning by substance use.
7. Continued use despite recurrent psychological or physical problems.

Other considerations in the development of the SASSI-A2 were brevity, cost effectiveness, ease of scoring, and ability to identify some teens unable or unwilling to acknowledge substance misuse (e.g., due to denial or lack of insight and awareness).

BASIC DESCRIPTION

The SASSI-A2 is available as a single-page, paper-and-pencil questionnaire that can be hand-scored. The paper-and-pencil version comes with a profile sheet that is used to graph the individual scale scores and derive the test classification. Software versions provide automated administration and/or scoring of the instruments via desktop computer. For large-volume usage, there is an optical scanning version. All software versions produce an assessment overview, including the results of the SASSI-A2 decision rule that classifies adolescents as having a high or low probability of having a substance use disorder, as well as the scores of the individual scales that are used to determine the results. Several versions of the software also generate a brief interpretive report that provides supplemental clinical information pertaining to acknowledged substance misuse, attitudes toward usage, defensiveness, emotional pain, acting out, and treatment considerations. Support materials include a *User's Guide* containing easy-to-understand instructions for administering, scoring, and interpretation, and a *Manual* providing comprehensive information on development, reliability, and validity. In addition, the SASSI Institute maintains a toll-free clinical support line for help in administering, scoring, and interpreting the adult and adolescent versions of the SASSI.

The SASSI-A2 requires approximately 15 minutes to administer and can be scored in 5 minutes. It has a reading grade level of 4.4. An audiocassette is available to aid in administering the SASSI-A2 to those with vision or reading difficulties. An adult version is available for individuals 18 years and older. The SASSI Institute has also developed and conducted validation research on a Spanish version of the SASSI; however, it has not been validated for use with adolescents.

One side of the SASSI-A2 questionnaire contains 72 "true–false" questions. There are four types of true–false questions:

- Symptom-related items, which provide a direct measure of acknowledged substance misuse.
- Risk items, measuring the degree to which the adolescent's family and social environment might create a relatively high risk for substance misuse.
- Attitudinal items, providing an indication of the adolescent's attitudes and beliefs about alcohol and other drug use.
- Subtle items, which seem unrelated to substance use. These enable the SASSI-A2 to identify some youths with alcohol and other drug problems, even if they do not acknowledge substance misuse or symptoms associated with it.

The second side of the questionnaire has 28 questions asking adolescents to report how frequently they have experienced specified problems related to substance misuse (e.g., using more than intended, using to cope with problems, negative consequences of usage). Generally, it is useful to obtain information pertaining to the adolescent's entire history of substance misuse. However, in some circumstances a 6-month period prior to or just after an important event may be more helpful. For example, a program may have admission criteria that focus on recent use, or an assessment may focus on substance misuse following treatment or incarceration. Therefore, one can specify various time frames for responding to the frequency items: (1) the client's lifetime, (2) the past 6 months, or (3) the 6 months preceding or following a significant event.

The SASSI-A2 yields a test classification with two possible outcomes: "high probability" or "low probability" of having a substance use disorder. Obtaining the results of the dichotomous test classification requires determining numerical scores for each of nine scales. When the instrument is being hand-scored, the scale scores are transferred to a profile sheet that is provided with the questionnaire. On the right side of the profile sheet are nine rules that ask whether particular scale scores exceed empirically determined cutoffs. If any of the nine rules is answered "Yes," the adolescent is classified as having a high probability of having a substance use disorder. For those with such a result, the Secondary Classification Scale (SCS) can then be used to provide additional information regarding whether DSM-IV substance abuse or substance dependence is more likely. If all of the nine rules are answered "No," the adolescent is classified as having a low probability of having a substance use disorder.

The nine scales that are used to classify the adolescent's probability of having a substance use disorder are as follows:

1. FVA (Face-Valid Alcohol)—acknowledged problematic use of alcohol.
2. FVOD (Face-Valid Other Drugs)—acknowledged problematic use of other drugs.
3. FRISK (Family and Friends Risk)—involvement in a family/social system that is likely to enable substance misuse.
4. ATT (Attitudes toward Substance Use)—attitudes and beliefs regarding substance use.
5. SYM (Symptoms of Substance Misuse)—consequences of substance misuse and loss-of-control in usage.
6. OAT (Obvious Attributes)—characteristics commonly associated with substance misuse.
7. SAT (Subtle Attributes)—personal style similar to that of people with substance dependence.
8. DEF (Defensiveness)—lack of forthright disclosure not necessarily related to substance use.
9. SAM (Supplemental Addiction Measure)—supplements other scales in some decision rules.

Two additional scales are used to refine the test classifications:

1. VAL (Validity Check)—identifies some individuals for whom further evaluation may be of value, even though they are classified as having a low probability of a substance use disorder.
2. SCS (Secondary Classification Scale)—helps distinguish between substance abuse and dependence.

The COR (Correctional) scale is also included in the SASSI-A2, but is not used in test classification. It measures the extent to which the individual responds to the SASSI-A2 similarly to adolescents involved with the juvenile justice system.

HISTORY OF THE METHOD'S DEVELOPMENT

The original adolescent version of the SASSI (the SASSI-A) was published in 1990 (Miller, 1990). Items were chosen and the decision rules were formulated to maximize the extent to which the results would match a criterion variable, or "gold standard." Research on the SASSI-A2 began in 1998, using a similar focus on correspondence to a criterion variable (or variables). There were two key considerations underlying the development of the SASSI-A2: (1) choice of the criterion variables and (2) content domain.

Choice of Criterion Variables

When both the original adult version of the SASSI and the SASSI-A were developed, the common clinical practice was to refer people to residential or inpatient treatment for what was then termed "chemical dependence," largely on the basis of evidence of an extensive history of negative consequences. Therefore, the criterion used to develop and validate the original SASSI-A was admission to residential or inpatient treatment, and the adolescents were classified as having a high or low probability of being "chemically dependent." Miller (1990) reported that the SASSI-A correctly identified 83% of the chemically dependent teens, but missed the other 17% of the teens with chemical dependence. In other words, the instrument was found to have a sensitivity of 83% and a false-negative rate of 17%. Seventy-two percent of the nondependent teens were correctly classified in the *low-probability* category, meaning that the instrument misclassified 28% of the nondependent teens. In other words, the instrument was found to have a specificity of 72% and a false-positive rate of 28%.

Subsequent to its publication, various other criterion variables were used in research on the SASSI-A. Risberg, Stevens, and Graybill (1995) found that 79% of a sample of 107 adolescents who had been admitted to a chemical abuse treatment program were test-positive on the SASSI-A (i.e., sensitivity = 79%). This study did not include any cases in which the teens were not in treatment, and therefore it was unable to provide an estimate of the specificity of the SASSI-A in correctly identifying nondependent teens. Bauman, Merta, and Steiner's (1999) criterion variable was a DSM-IV diagnosis of substance dependence, and they found that the Adolescent SASSI-A correctly identified 94% of the adolescents who had substance dependence. The data in the Bauman and colleagues study did not allow an assessment of the accuracy of the SASSI-A in identifying adolescents who had DSM-IV substance abuse or adolescents who did not have any substance use disorder. Piazza (1996) examined the correspondence between diagnoses of substance use disorders and SASSI-A results in a sample of 203 adolescents in an acute care psychiatric treatment facility. The SASSI-A yielded 86% sensitivity and 93% specificity. Rogers, Cashel, Johansen, Sewell, and Gonzalez (1997) did not use either admission for treatment or diagnoses as the criterion variable in their research on the accuracy of the SASSI-A. Rather, they conducted archival reviews on select portions of the clinical records of 311 adolescents in a dual-diagnosis inpatient unit and found evidence of *regular* substance abuse in 292 of the 311 reports. The authors classified those 292 participants as "chemically dependent," and the SASSI-A was test-positive in 265 of those cases (i.e., 91% sensitivity). Of the 19 adolescents who were in the dual-diagnosis inpatient unit and were nevertheless classified as "nonusers" by the authors, 15 were test-positive on the SASSI-A (i.e., 21% specificity).

The choice of the criterion variable(s) used to develop and validate a screening instrument determines the target(s) of the screening, and, thereby, the clinical utility of the instrument. As illustrated by the many criterion variables used in research on the original SASSI-A, the range of problems associated with adolescent substance misuse precludes a single or simple answer to the question "What constitutes an appropriate target for screening?" Within the context of the many unresolved issues underlying identification and treatment of substance-related problems among adolescents, criteria for admission to treatment for substance-related problems have become increasingly specific, with greater emphasis on DSM-IV diagnoses. Therefore, in formulating and validating the SASSI-A2, clinically derived diagnoses of both DSM-IV substance dependence and substance abuse were used as the criterion variables.

Content Domain

A review of the literature on the etiology, assessment, and treatment of substance misuse among adolescents identified new items that would enhance the accuracy of the SASSI-A2, leading to 45 experimental items. These were added to the original SASSI-A items in the research version of the SASSI-A2. Statistical analyses led to selection of items that were most effective in identifying adolescents with substance use disorders. These new items, included in the SASSI-A2, address three issues: (1) the extent to which a youth is part of a family/social system that is likely to foster substance misuse (e.g., "Many of my friends drink or get high regularly"); (2) the youth's attitudes and beliefs regarding substance use (e.g., "Drugs help people to be creative"); and (3) the consequences of substance misuse and loss of control in usage (e.g., "My drinking or other drug use causes problems between my family and me").

Research to test the SASSI-A2 used data from 1,244 adolescents who were being assessed for substance-related problems. The data from each adolescent included a completed copy of the research version and a diagnosis based on DSM-IV criteria. Half of the cases were randomly selected to be used to develop the decision rules, and the remaining half were reserved to evaluate the accuracy of the test classifications.

RESEARCH EVIDENCE

The following is a summary of the data that were used to develop and test the accuracy of the SASSI-A2 (Miller & Lazowski, 2001).

Reliability

Seventy junior high and high school students were administered the research version of the SASSI-A2 twice, so as to determine the stability of the results. Findings indicated highly significant agreement between test classifications on the first and second administrations in 94% of the cases. Test–retest reliability coefficients (a statistical measure of the stability of clients' responses over time) for the nine scales used for test classification and for two of the supplemental scales were all above .80 (with that for the COR scale being .71).

Validity

Half of the cases were used to formulate a scoring system that yielded 94% correspondence between the test classifications and clinical diagnoses of DSM-IV substance use disorders, with sensitivity of 94% and specificity of 92%. When the scoring system was applied to cases that were reserved to evaluate the accuracy of the test classifications, sensitivity was 96%, specificity was 87%, and overall accuracy was 95%. When all of the available cases were used, the SASSI-A2 was found to be sensitive in identifying 93% of youths with substance abuse and 97.5% with substance dependence.

These results were obtained in a study of 920 male and 307 female adolescents between the ages of 12 and 18, with educational levels ranging from 4th through 12th grades. Four types of programs provided data: (1) addictions treatment, (2) inpatient general psychiatric, (3) outpatient behavioral health, and (4) juvenile corrections. The sample consisted of 56% European Americans, 12% Hispanic Americans, 10% African Americans, 9% Native Americans, 2% Asian Americans, and 11% other or unknown ethnicity. Accuracy of SASSI-A2 test classification was not affected by gender, age, educational level, type of program, or ethnicity.

Seven hundred and ninety-one respondents came from juvenile justice programs, and the prevalence of substance use disorders in that sample was 86%. The SASSI-A2 was accurate for 737 (93.2%) of those cases (95% sensitivity, 85% specificity). Also, 84% of all respondents reported a history of legal problems, and the accuracy of SASSI-A2 test classifications was not affected by legal history.

As noted earlier, the SCS is a SASSI-A2 scale indicating the relative likelihood that a high-probability adolescent will be diagnosed as having substance abuse versus substance dependence. In the combined development and cross-validation sample, 76% of the test-positive cases with an SCS score at or above the empirically determined cutoff of 16 had been diagnosed with substance dependence, and only 24% were diagnosed with substance abuse. By contrast, among the test-positive cases that had an SCS score less than 16, 57% had been diagnosed as having substance abuse, 39% were diagnosed with substance dependence, and 4% were false positives. None of the false-positive cases had an SCS score of 16 or greater. Thus the SCS was found to be of potential value in refining the test classification and determination of the relative suitability of treatment options.

Also as noted earlier, the COR scale was developed empirically to identify individuals with response patterns similar to those of adolescents with histories of involvement in the juvenile justice system. COR scores for adolescents who reported having been in trouble with the law were found to be significantly higher than the COR scores of those who had not had legal difficulties. Eighty-eight percent of the adolescents who scored at or above a T-score of 60 on COR were from juvenile justice settings, and the figure rose to 95% for those who scored at or above a T-score of 70. Thus, depending on the context and goals of the assessment, elevated scores on the COR scale can be used to identify some adolescents for further assessment of relatively high risk of becoming involved with the juvenile justice system. However, the COR scale is not intended to serve as a source of information about the cause or nature of youths' delinquent behaviors.

APPLICATION

Since its publication in 2001, the SASSI-A2 has been used in approximately 2,500 programs throughout the United States and Canada, including juvenile justice programs, probation offices, drug courts, and both private and public youth service agencies. The SASSI-A2 is available from the SASSI Institute. It is a copyrighted instrument and should not be modified or duplicated.

Individuals who have had training and/or experience in assessment are qualified to obtain the SASSI-A2 from the SASSI Institute. For individuals who do not have specialized training and/or experience in assessment, and for anyone wishing to have training in the use of the SASSI-A2, the SASSI Institute sponsors two training programs throughout the United States and Canada—one on administration and scoring, and one on clinical interpretation and feedback. The questionnaire itself can be administered and scored by any staff member under the supervision of a qualified user.

The SASSI-A2 is intended and designed to serve as one component of a broader assessment process. It provides objective information regarding the likelihood of a substance use disorder; it is therefore useful as part of a screening process to identify problems to be considered for further assessment and possible treatment. Examination of responses on the face-valid scales provides information regarding (1) loss of control in usage, (2) preoccupation with alcohol and other drugs, (3) usage to overcome negative feelings, (4) negative consequences related to substance use, (5) involvement in family and social groups that support a pattern of misuse, and (6) attitudes and beliefs that promote substance misuse. Feedback on SASSI-A2 results can be useful in engaging adolescents in the assessment and treatment process.

The SASSI-A2 is not an infallible index of the presence of a substance use disorder. It should be used as a source of information that is taken into account and integrated with all of the other data gathered during the course of assessment. It is not intended to identify all substance-related problems, and the results obtained in the development and validation of the SASSI-A2 may not generalize to all populations. Although the SASSI-A2 is largely composed of subtle items that are resistant to underreporting of substance-related problems, the instrument also includes face-valid items that address substance misuse in an apparent manner. Thus it is possible for adolescents either to overreport or to underreport substance-related problems on the SASSI-A2.

CASE EXAMPLE

Rob was a 16-year-old European American male who was arrested, charged with violation of probation and incorrigibility, and transported to the youth shelter at 2:30 A.M.. During the admission procedure, he expressed anger that he was being detained, but he was cooperative and gave no signs of intoxication or other impaired functioning. Rob had had two prior arrests—one in which he was caught passing around a marijuana cigarette after school, and one in which he was part of a group of adolescents apprehended at a state park for illegal consumption. The second incident also included a charge of incorrigibility, because he had left his home against his parents' instructions (contrary to the terms of his probation). On the night of the current incident, Rob's parents called the police to report Rob for incorrigibility and violation of the conditions of his probation. Rob had become belligerent, kicked a hole in the wall, and stormed out of the house when his parents denied him permission to "go and hang out" with his friends.

The morning following Rob's arrest, a staff member began the assessment process. Rob expressed a willingness to participate and acknowledged that he was wrong to have acted violently. However, he deflected responsibility from himself by focusing on the unreasonableness of his parents' refusal to allow him to be with his friends. He denied using alcohol or other drugs that evening, and he agreed to submit to a urine test.

The shelter's assessment protocol includes the SASSI-A2 for all youths whose presenting problems or histories include substance misuse. The time frame for the FVA and FVOD scales is "your entire life," and the staff member examines the responses to the items on the face-valid scales prior to interviewing the youths about their alcohol and other drug consumption.

Rob was classified by the SASSI-A2 with a high probability of having substance abuse or substance dependence (see his profile sheet, Figure 8.1). Five of the nine rules were marked "Yes." Rob's SCS score was 17, indicating that he was more likely to have substance dependence than substance abuse. The profile sheet also revealed that Rob had scores above the 85th percentile for five scales—FRISK, ATT, SAT, DEF, and COR. The elevated score on FRISK suggested the likelihood that Rob was part of a family and/or social system that might support rather than discourage substance use/misuse. The ATT score was indicative of attitudes likely to promote substance use. The elevated SAT and DEF scores indicated that Rob was likely to be defensive and also to have difficulty perceiving that his substance use was causing him problems. Finally, the COR scale suggested that Rob's responses were similar to those of other adolescents with a history of involvement in the juvenile justice system. It was also important to note that Rob's scores on the three scales measuring consequences of substance misuse (FVA, FVOD, and SYM) were not elevated. Viewed in the context of the overall SASSI-A2 profile, this suggested that Rob was likely to underreport his substance misuse during the assessment.

Rob reported that he had first used alcohol and marijuana in the 10th grade. He denied regular usage, indicating that it was just something he and his friends did once in a while. When pressed, Rob reported that they drank and/or used drugs on weekends about three times a month—not every week. He said that he had used on weekdays, but only once or twice. On one occasion he had smoked marijuana before coming to school, but he insisted that he was not using at the time he was arrested. He claimed that after his arrest and the initiation of urine screens by his probation officer, he had not used marijuana; however, he acknowledged he had been drinking on the night of his second arrest. He indicated that he planned to resume marijuana usage when he was no longer subject to urine screens.

Rob's parents reported that that they believed he had been using marijuana, but they had no clear evidence other than the positive urine screen conducted after his first arrest. Subsequent urine screens did not reveal evidence of marijuana usage. They expressed extreme concern over Rob's escalating defiance and the fact that his grades had declined from a B+ to a C average. They said the current incident was the only time when Rob had acted out his anger in a violent manner. Although his parents expressed tolerance regarding experimentation with substance use, they believed that Rob's problems were likely to be caused or made worse by his usage. They insisted that he remain abstinent. There was no history of alcohol or other drug problems in their family.

The assessment yielded a number of areas of concern with regard to the possibility of a progressive problem related to substance misuse. As noted ear-

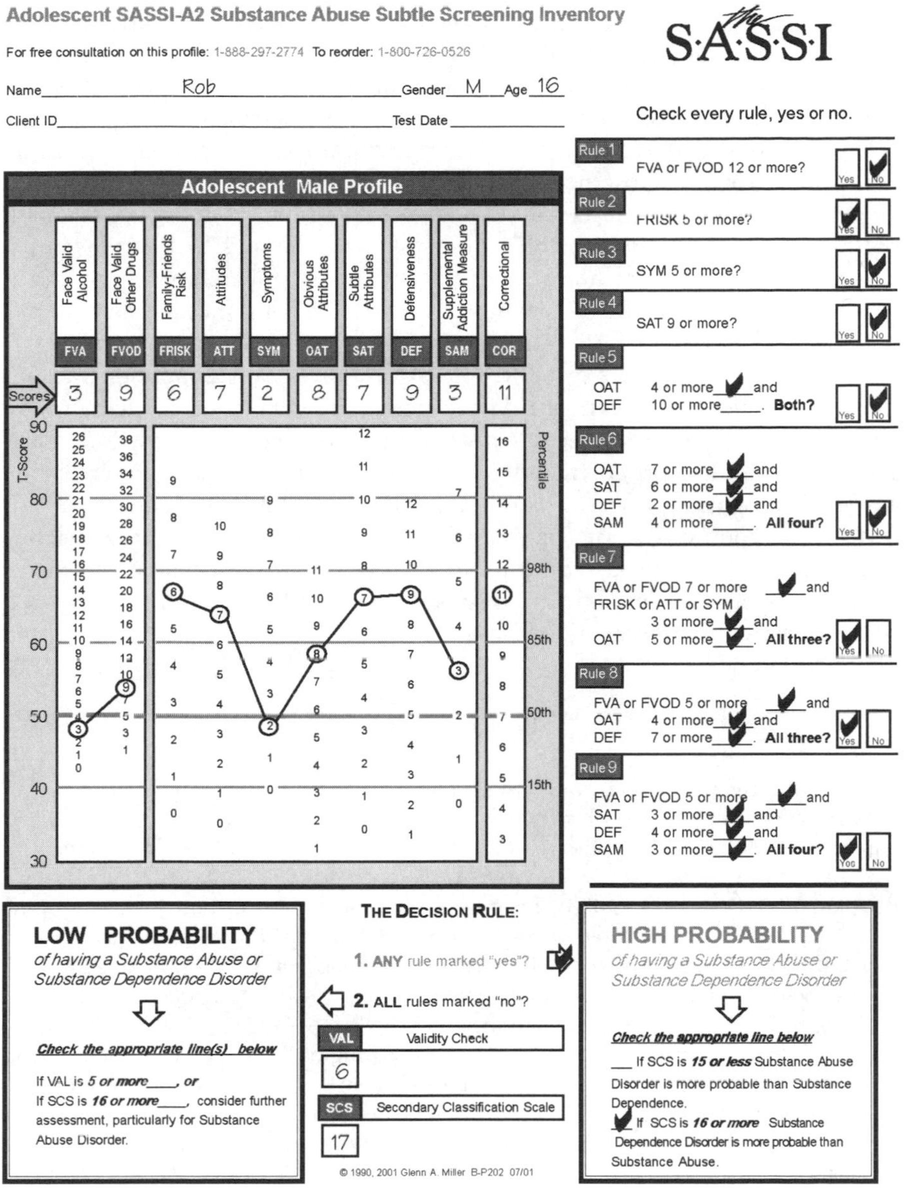

Adolescent SASSI-A2 Substance Abuse Subtle Screening Inventory

For free consultation on this profile: 1-888-297-2774 To reorder: 1-800-726-0526

S·A·S·S·I

Name ___Rob___ Gender __M__ Age _16_

Client ID_____ Test Date _____

Check every rule, yes or no.

Rule 1 — FVA or FVOD 12 or more? [Yes] [✓ No]

Rule 2 — FRISK 5 or more? [✓ Yes] [No]

Rule 3 — SYM 5 or more? [Yes] [✓ No]

Rule 4 — SAT 9 or more? [Yes] [✓ No]

Rule 5
OAT 4 or more ✓ and
DEF 10 or more ____. **Both?** [Yes] [✓ No]

Rule 6
OAT 7 or more ✓ and
SAT 6 or more ✓ and
DEF 2 or more ✓ and
SAM 4 or more ____. **All four?** [Yes] [✓ No]

Rule 7
FVA or FVOD 7 or more ✓ and
FRISK or ATT or SYM 3 or more ✓ and
OAT 5 or more ✓. **All three?** [✓ Yes] [No]

Rule 8
FVA or FVOD 5 or more ✓ and
OAT 4 or more ✓ and
DEF 7 or more ✓. **All three?** [✓ Yes] [No]

Rule 9
FVA or FVOD 5 or more ✓ and
SAT 3 or more ✓ and
DEF 4 or more ✓ and
SAM 3 or more ✓. **All four?** [✓ Yes] [No]

Adolescent Male Profile

	FVA	FVOD	FRISK	ATT	SYM	OAT	SAT	DEF	SAM	COR
Scores	3	9	6	7	2	8	7	9	3	11

LOW PROBABILITY
of having a Substance Abuse or Substance Dependence Disorder
⬇
Check the appropriate line(s) below
If VAL is *5 or more*____, or
If SCS is *16 or more*____, consider further assessment, particularly for Substance Abuse Disorder.

THE DECISION RULE:
1. **ANY** rule marked "yes"?
2. **ALL** rules marked "no"?

VAL	Validity Check
6	

SCS	Secondary Classification Scale
17	

© 1990, 2001 Glenn A. Miller B-P202 07/01

HIGH PROBABILITY
of having a Substance Abuse or Substance Dependence Disorder
⬇
Check the appropriate line below
____ If SCS is *15 or less* Substance Abuse Disorder is more probable than Substance Dependence.
✓ If SCS is *16 or more* Substance Dependence Disorder is more probable than Substance Abuse.

FIGURE 8.1. Rob's SASSI-A2 profile sheet.

lier, the SASSI-A2 classified Rob as having a high probability of having a substance use disorder. Rob's scale scores suggested that he might be defensive and lack awareness and insight regarding the impact of substance misuse on his life, leading to possible underreporting in the assessment process. SASSI-A2 results also suggested that Rob's treatment was likely to be complicated by his attitudes toward substance use and his involvement in a social and/or family system supporting substance use. The SASSI results were consonant with the fact that subsequent to Rob's onset of usage he had had three arrests, experienced problems at home, and performed inadequately in school, suggesting that he met DSM-IV diagnostic criteria for substance abuse.

On the basis of the SASSI-A2 results and the preliminary diagnostic interviews, the staff member referred Rob to a substance abuse counselor for continued assessment and treatment. The treatment plan included participation in an after-school group for teens with substance-related problems, individual sessions to monitor progress, and continued supervision and urine screens by a juvenile probation officer. The initial goals for treatment included (1) abstinence, (2) modification of cognitions and attitudes regarding psychoactive substances, (3) improved school performance, (4) increased involvement in school activities, (5) development of positive peer influence, and (6) increased compliance with parental supervision.

REFERENCES

American Psychiatric Association. (1994). *Diagnostic and statistical manual of mental disorders* (4th ed.). Washington, DC: Author.

Bauman, S., Merta, R., & Steiner, R. (1999). Further validation of the adolescent form of the SASSI. *Journal of Child and Adolescent Substance Abuse, 9*(1), 51–71.

Belenko, S., & Dembo, R. (2003). Treating adolescent substance abuse problems in the juvenile drug court. *International Journal of Law and Psychiatry, 26*, 87–110.

Jones, R. L. (1990). Evaluation of drug use in the adolescent. In L. M. Haddad & J. F. Winchester (Eds.), *Clinical management of poisoning and drug overdose* (2nd ed., pp. 679–687). Philadelphia: Saunders.

Kandel, D. B., & Logan, J. A. (1984). Patterns of drug use from adolescence to young adulthood: I. Periods of risk for initiation, continued use, and discontinuation. *American Journal of Public Health, 74*(7), 660–666.

Leccese, M., & Waldron, H. B. (1994). Assessing adolescent substance use: a critique of current measurement instruments. *Journal of Substance Abuse Treatment, 11*(6), 554–563.

Miller, F. G., & Lazowski, L. E. (2001). *The Adolescent Substance Abuse Subtle Screening Inventory-A2 (SASSI-A2) manual.* Springville, IN: SASSI Institute.

Miller, G. A. (1990). *The Substance Abuse Subtle Screening Inventory (SASSI) adolescent manual.* Bloomington, IN: SASSI Institute.

National Institute of Justice. (2001). *Arrestee drug abuse monitoring (ADAM) 2000 annualized site reports.* Rockville, MD: Author.

Phillips, R. O. (1995, January–February). Issues in substance abuse and adolescence. *The Counselor*, pp. 18–22.

Piazza, N. J. (1996). Dual diagnosis and adolescent psychiatric inpatients. *Substance Use and Misuse, 31*(2), 215–223.

Risberg, R. A., Stevens, M. J., & Graybill, D. F. (1995). Validating the adolescent form of the Substance Abuse Subtle Screening Inventory. *Journal of Child and Adolescent Substance Abuse, 4*(4), 25–41.

Rogers, R., Cashel, M. L., Johansen, J., Sewell, K. W., & Gonzalez, C. (1997). Evaluation of adolescent offenders with substance abuse: Validation of the SASSI with conduct-disordered youth. *Criminal Justice and Behavior, 24*, 114–128.

CHAPTER 9

Trauma Symptom Checklist for Children

Jennifer Meltzer Wolpaw
Julian D. Ford
Elana Newman
Joanne L. Davis
John Briere

PURPOSE

The Trauma Symptom Checklist for Children (TSCC; Briere, 1996) is widely used by mental health clinicians because it provides an efficient, standardized measure of both posttraumatic and associated symptomatology. In juvenile justice settings, screening and assessment often have tight time constraints and must cover a wide range of psychosocial and dispositional issues. Therefore, the assessment of traumatic stress symptoms must be concise, versatile, and accurate, as well as sufficiently "value-added," in order to be included in evaluations conducted in juvenile justice settings. The TSCC was developed to assess trauma-related symptoms among children (ages 8–16) who have been exposed to traumatic life events. Unlike previous instruments available to assess specific trauma-related symptoms in particular subgroups (e.g., Wolfe, Gentile, Michienzi, Sas, & Wolfe, 1991), the TSCC is designed to assess a wide range of youths and symptoms, and was standardized on large clinical and nonclinical groups (Briere, 1996). The TSCC has been increasingly used in forensic settings, because recent research suggests that traumatic stress symptoms play a role in juvenile offending and responsiveness to rehabilitation (e.g., Newman, 2002).

The correct identification and classification of posttraumatic stress disorder (PTSD) symptoms will enhance the development of a treatment and rehabilitation plan designed to fit the unique needs of each particular youth. Unfortunately, although trauma and PTSD are highly prevalent in the juvenile justice population, assessment of trauma exposure and its psychological consequences is often overlooked (McMackin, Morrissey, Newman, Erwin, & Daly, 1998; Newman, 2002). Historically, trauma was evaluated in children and adolescents primarily through clinical observation and through parental and/or teacher report of a child's symptoms. Instruments that specifically assessed trauma in children had not been developed; therefore, adult measures of trauma and PTSD were often administered to children. In the 1980s, PTSD became more widely recognized and was formally codified with adults. Tragedies such as school shootings, along with an increase in public and professional awareness of the prevalence of and harm caused by child abuse, prompted an increase in attention to PTSD in children. Since that time, many PTSD instruments have been adapted or specifically designed for children and adolescents (Nader, 1997).

"Traumatic stressors" are defined by the American Psychiatric Association (2000) as follows: "the person experienced, witnessed, or was confronted with an event or events that involved actual or threatened death or serious injury, or a threat to the physical integrity of self or others," and "the person's response involved intense fear, helplessness, or horror" (p. 467). Youths in the juvenile justice system are often exposed to physical abuse, sexual abuse, or family or community violence (e.g., gang- or crime-related violence) that is psychologically traumatic for them. They may also witness or be confronted with serious accidents, disasters, or illness. Most youths in juvenile justice settings have experienced at least one, and often several, traumatic events (Carrion & Steiner, 2000; Ruchkin, Schwab-Stone, Koposov, Vermeiren, & Steiner, 2002; Steiner, Garcia, & Matthews, 1997).

PTSD occurs when a person who has experienced traumatic stress has subsequent problems with daily functioning that are results of not being able to recover from the emotional shock of the trauma. PTSD involves three types of symptoms: (1) persistent unwanted memories of traumatic event(s); (2) avoidance of trauma memories (including avoidance through substance use or impulsive/risky behavior), and feeling emotionally numb and detached even in close relationships; and (3) problems with sleep, anger, and mental concentration as a result of feeling persistently tense, on edge, and unsafe. Almost anyone who experiences a traumatic stressor will have some of these symptoms for a short time afterward. Dissociation (feeling and acting "spaced out," or as if "on automatic pilot," or even "in a dream") is not formally part of the diagnostic criteria, though it often occurs with PTSD, especially when the trauma involves prolonged exposure to sexual or physical abuse.

PTSD prevalence estimates in the juvenile justice population range widely, depending on several factors (Abram et al., 2004). Instruments that base PTSD diagnosis on symptoms related only to the adolescent's worst traumatic experience tend to yield lower prevalence estimates than instruments that reference the symptoms to any (or all) traumatic experience(s). Diagnoses also differ when based upon child report versus parent report. PTSD prevalence estimates based upon the current month or past year are lower than those based upon the child's lifetime experience of symptoms. Given these factors, PTSD prevalence estimates in the juvenile justice population range between 3% and 50% (Arroyo, 2001; Cauffman, Feldman, Waterman, & Steiner, 1998; Garland et al., 2001; Teplin, Abram, McClelland, Dulcan, & Mericle, 2002; Wasserman, McReynolds, Lucas, Fisher, & Santos, 2002). These rates are up to eight times as high as in community samples of similar-age peers (Giaconia et al., 1995; Saigh, Yasik, Sack & Koplewicz, 1999; Saltzman, Pynoos, Layne, Steinberg, & Aisenberg, 2001). PTSD prevalence rates for girls in juvenile justice settings are higher than those for boys. One study reported that as many as two-thirds of all such girls may have PTSD, compared to about one-third of boys (Cauffman et al., 1998); however, Abram and colleagues (2004) recently reported a prevalence of PTSD for girls in urban detention centers to be only slightly higher than that for boys.

BASIC DESCRIPTION

The TSCC is a 54-item self-report questionnaire that assesses emotional, behavioral, and cognitive effects of trauma exposure. The TSCC has clinical scales for Anxiety, Depression, Posttraumatic Stress, Dissociation (Overt and Fantasy subscales), Anger, and Sexual Concerns (Preoccupation and Distress subscales). The TSCC is also available in a 44-item alternate version (TSCC-A) that excludes the Sexual Concerns subscale items. Two validity scales (Underresponse and Hyperresponse) assess the child's tendency to deny or overrespond to symptom items. Eight critical items indicate potential problems warranting further assessment with regard to suicidality, self-injury, desire to harm others, concern about sexual abuse, fear of men or women, fear of death, and involvement in fights.

The TSCC presents a list of feelings, thoughts, and behaviors, asking respondents to rate each on a 4-point scale from "never" (0) to "almost all the time" (3). Administration usually takes 15–20 minutes. Scoring and profiling require another 5–10 minutes (Briere, 1996). The TSCC is appropriate for either individual or group administration. Group administration requires precautions to preserve confidentiality and minimize peer biasing of responses. Although this occurs infrequently, youths may become distressed by the questions, so it is advisable to have a mental health professional available to assist if needed (Briere, 1996). Items may be read aloud to children who have difficulty reading, although this procedural modification differs from that used in normative studies and should be noted in reports. Readability for TSCC items is approximately at the fourth-grade level, as determined by the Flesch–Kincaid method. The TSCC does not assess specific trauma events, so it is best to administer it in conjunction with a trauma history assessment.

Based on a standardization sample, raw scores are transformed to *T*-scores (mean = 50, standard deviation = 10), with separate norms for younger

(8- to 12-year-old) and older (13- to 16-year-old) males and females. A *T*-score of 65 or above is defined as clinically significant, except on Sexual Concerns, which uses a *T*-score of 70 for clinical significance. (For a description of *T*-scores, see Chapter 4 of this volume.)

HISTORY OF THE METHOD'S DEVELOPMENT

Development of the TSCC was approached with attention to several objectives for the screening and assessment of trauma history and PTSD: (1) clients' safety; (2) multiple assessment perspectives; (3) assessment format; (4) sensitivity to ethnocultural, socioeconomic, gender-related, and developmental factors; and (5) relevance to the juvenile justice context.

Safety is paramount not just for a child, but also for his or her family members and peers. Safety has both an objective dimension (e.g., determining whether the child or caregiver is currently experiencing, or at imminent risk for, further trauma experiences) and a subjective dimension (e.g., the child's and caregiver's sense of personal safety) (Newman, 2002). In juvenile justice settings, safety also involves maintaining clear boundaries about confidentiality and limits on the sharing of clinical information (e.g., mandated reports or requests for information by courts, correctional staff members, child welfare workers, or probation officers).

Multiperspective assessment reduces the likelihood that unintended bias or distortion will be created by information obtained from any individual informant. The youth's perspective is important, because other informants (e.g., caregiver, teacher, peers) may either overreport symptoms or mainly report overt symptoms (e.g., acting-out behaviors) while overlooking more covert, internalizing symptoms (e.g., anxiety or depression) (Cashel, 2003). However, other informants are vital, because children who are traumatized may underreport symptoms that caregivers recognize as problematic (Newman, 2002).

This multiperspective consideration is reflected in the wide range of current approaches to the assessment of trauma and posttraumatic sequelae in children and adolescents. Three such approaches are worth description; each of these has been used to some extent with youths in juvenile justice settings.

First, several instruments are designed to measure traumatic experiences directly (e.g., Daviss et al., 2000; Ford et al., 2000). Interviews include the Clinician Administered PTSD Scale for Children and Adolescents for DSM-IV (Newman et al., in press), the Childhood PTSD Interview (Fletcher, 1996a), the Child PTSD Inventory (Saigh, 1989), the UCLA PTSD Index for DSM-IV (Pynoos, Rodriguez, Steinberg, Stauber, & Frederick, 1998), and a cartoon-based method to assess PTSD symptoms and associated features in children ages 6–11 (Praver & Pelcovitz, 1996). Self-report instruments include the Child and Adolescent Trauma Survey (March, Amaya-Jackson, Murray, & Schulte, 1998), the Childhood PTSD Reaction Index (Nader, 1996), Child's Reaction to Traumatic Events Scale (Jones, 1994), Impact of Event Scale

(Dyregrov, Kuterovac, & Barath, 1996), the Los Angeles Symptom Checklist (King, 1996), the TSCC (Briere, 1996), and When Bad Things Happen Scale (Fletcher, 1996b).

Second, several omnibus child diagnostic instruments include PTSD sub-scales. Such instruments evaluate the presence of PTSD symptoms, but in the context of other items addressing a broad range of psychiatric conditions. These include the Anxiety Disorders Interview Schedule for DSM-IV: Child Version (Albano & Silverman, 1996), the Child and Adolescent Psychiatric Assessment (Angold et al., 1995), the Diagnostic Interview Schedule for Children (Costello, Edelbrock, Dulcan, Kalas, & Klaric, 1984; Shaffer, Fisher, Piacentini, Schwab-Stone, & Wicks, 1992), the Diagnostic Interview for Children and Adolescents—Revised (Reich, Shayka, & Taibleson, 1991), and the Schedule for Affective Disorders and Schizophrenia for School-Age Children—Present and Lifetime Version (Kaufman et al., 1997).

Third, several instruments assess symptoms that are not trauma-specific, but may reflect symptoms of traumatic stress or clinical issues that often co-occur with PTSD. For example, specific measures are available to assess disso-ciation (Carrion & Steiner, 2000; Putnam, Helmers, & Trickett, 1993), anxi-ety (March, Parker, Sullivan, Stallings, & Conners, 1997), and depression (Kovacs, 1985).

Assessment format also requires consideration, because of children's and parents' or other caregivers' reactions to different assessment approaches and contexts. For example, a child's answers to structured interviews in which both the child or caregiver and the assessor can probe for clarification may be more complete than with a self-report questionnaire—but interviews may be biased if a respondent feels that certain answers are "expected" by an inter-viewer. In addition, children interviewed in a group may answer in ways that they think conform to their peers' or caregivers' expectations. Efforts should be made to interview children individually for this reason.

Developmental, socioeconomic, gender-related, and ethnocultural factors should be considered when evaluators are establishing rapport with and gath-ering assessment data from children and their caregivers. The optimal delivery of questions varies for children of different ages, genders, developmental lev-els, and ethnic backgrounds. What constitutes a "symptom" (as opposed to expected, age-appropriate behavior) may vary for youths of different ages and different socioeconomic and ethnocultural contexts. For example, carrying a weapon to school may be viewed as a necessary precaution to conform to peer or gang pressures or to protect against retaliation in some settings. However, others in that same school or community may deem such an action unaccept-able and view it as an antisocial symptom. Children of each gender and of dif-ferent ages and sociocultural backgrounds may also respond differently to interview and questionnaire formats, as well as to assessors with different styles and backgrounds (Cohen, Deblinger, Mannarino, & De Arellano, 2001).

Finally, the juvenile justice context is important to consider, because youths in this context are often encountered soon after they are exposed to traumatic events (their own victimization, or their victimization of others) associated with the offenses for which they have been apprehended. In addition, the juvenile justice context can influence a youth's or caregiver's willingness and ability to disclose information about traumatic experiences or posttraumatic symptoms. Underreporting and overreporting are both potential concerns.

Given these considerations, development of the TSCC began with 75 items derived from clinical experience to assess anxiety, depression, anger, posttraumatic stress, dissociation, and sexual concerns. After consultation with several child psychologists, 54 items were retained and tested in several clinical samples. A nonclinical standardization sample was then obtained, including children from a wide range of racial groups, geographical areas, and socioeconomic groups. The sample of 3,008 children included 2,399 school children in Illinois and Colorado (Singer, Anglin, Song, & Lunghofer, 1995), 387 Colorado school children (Evans, Briere, Boggiano, & Barrett, 1994), and 222 children at the Mayo Clinic in Minnesota who were relatives of patients or were undergoing minor or routine medical care themselves (Friedrich, 1995).

Preliminary statistical analyses of the TSCC reported in the instrument's manual revealed that children ages 8 through 12 scored higher than children ages 13 through 16 on the TSCC scales measuring Anxiety, Depression, and Posttraumatic Stress, while the older youths scored higher on the Underresponse scale (Briere, 1996). In addition, scores for males decreased with age on several of the TSCC scales, and younger and older girls scored somewhat differently on two scales. The TSCC manual recommends, therefore, that assessors refer to the separate norms provided for preadolescents and adolescents in the standardization sample, as well as the appropriate gender, when interpreting each individual child's scores (Briere, 1996). The decision to standardize the TSCC on the basis of both age and gender is a strength of the instrument; it accurately reflects the current understanding about the role of development and gender on susceptibility to and expression of trauma-related symptoms (e.g., Cauffman et al., 1998).

Approximately 55% of the normative sample was identified as belonging to an ethnic minority (i.e., African American, Hispanic, Asian, or other). Small differences were found by race, but these were not sufficient to require separate profiles. More research is needed with members of minority groups, including Native Americans and self-identified multiethnic individuals (Briere, 1996).

Concerning the two validity scales, the Underresponse scale was formed by selecting the 10 items least likely to receive a 0 response in the normative sample. The Hyperresponse scale was created by selecting the 8 items most rarely endorsed with a 3.

Based on statistical analyses of the responses from several surveys using the TSCC, two subscales were created within scales. The Overt and Fantasy subscales of the Dissociation scale help assessors distinguish youths who have the classic symptoms of dissociation described above (e.g., "spacing out" or having blackouts) from those who are aware of their behavior but tend to withdraw into a fantasy world. The Preoccupation and Distress subscales of the Sexual Concerns scale distinguish youths who are overly drawn to sexual activity (preoccupied) from those who avoid and are highly distressed by any involvement in sexual activities.

RESEARCH EVIDENCE

Psychometric studies indicate that the TSCC is internally consistent, meaning that all of the items tend to contribute to a single meaningful score. From a research standpoint, this is shown by the alpha statistic's exceeding .80 for all scales but Sexual Concerns (which tends to have an alpha of .65–.75) (Briere, 1996). TSCC scales and subscales for Posttraumatic Stress, Dissociation, Anxiety, Depression, and Sexual Concerns tend to be consistent with scores from similar measures (Crouch, Smith, Ezzell, & Saunders, 1999; Friedrich, Jaworski, Huxsahl, & Bengtson, 1997; Sadowski & Friedrich, 2000). TSCC scores are also higher for youths who have PTSD (Mertin & Mohr, 2002) or who have been victimized (Hastings & Kelley, 1997; Johnson et al., 2002; Singer et al., 1995; Wolfe, Scott, Wekerle, & Pittman, 2001) than for youths without these problems. Finally, TSCC scores tend to improve as a result of therapy (Cohen & Mannarino, 2000; Greenwald, 2002; Lanktree & Briere, 1995), as well as of improved forensic (Elliott & Briere, 1994) and child protection (Henry, 1997) status (i.e., reduced delinquent behavior).

Song, Singer, and Anglin (1998) examined the role of exposure to violence and emotional trauma as precursors to adolescent violent behavior with a large sample of public high school students in Ohio and Colorado (48% male, 52% female; 35% African American, 33% European American, and 23% Hispanic). TSCC total scores, combined with a history of violence exposure, accounted for 50% of boys' and girls' reports of violent behavior. Anger was the most commonly reported TSCC symptom. These findings indicated that adolescents who perpetrated violence were likely to have been victimized in the past and to report PTSD symptoms, particularly anger.

With the same sample of adolescents, Flannery, Singer, and Webster (2001) identified a dangerously violent subgroup and a matched sample of controls (age range = 14–19; 72% male, 28% female; 45% African American, 27% Hispanic, and 20% European American). Dangerously violent girls were more likely than female controls to display clinically elevated TSCC scores (especially anger, depression and suicidal ideation). Thus the TSCC may be useful in preventive screening to identify and provide services for adolescents at risk for violent behavior, particularly females.

Another study administered the TSCC and several measures of dissociation to males convicted of sex offenses and to psychiatric patients of both genders (Friedrich et al., 2001). The sample of males with sex offenses was 59% European American, 32% African American, 4% Native American, 3% Asian

American, and 3% Hispanic. The mean age of the sample was 15.9 years (*SD* = 1.5). The psychiatric sample was 96% European American, 2% African American, and 2% Asian American. The mean age of this sample was 15.1 years (*SD* = 1.6). Total TSCC scores were not associated with other measures of dissociation in the sex offenses group, but there were significant correlations between TSCC subscale scores for emotional abuse, domestic violence, and sexual abuse and the other measures. Dissociation was especially related to sexual and emotional abuse and to domestic violence.

Several doctoral dissertation studies have examined the TSCC. Berg-Sonne (2002) compared TSCC scores for violent and nonviolent female adolescents in the juvenile justice system, finding no significant differences between the two groups. However, the sample size was small, and the TSCC was completed as part of a broader forensic test battery (which may have limited the adolescents' sense of confidentiality and willingness to provide candid responses to the TSCC). Leite (2001) found that community violence and TSCC Posttraumatic subscale scores were correlated with scores from a validated anger measure among 75 adjudicated adolescents in residential placements. Valentine (2001) examined the relationship between depression, self-esteem, trauma, and psychopathy among 25 male and 36 female adolescents in a residential treatment facility for inner-city youths who were diagnosed with conduct disorder. Significant correlations were found between several of the measured variables (e.g., depressive and posttraumatic symptoms and self-esteem).

APPLICATION

The TSCC is probably the most frequently used of all standardized trauma symptom measures in the United States and Canada, in both clinical and forensic settings. The TSCC manual (Briere, 1996) is copyrighted and must be purchased from the publisher, Psychological Assessment Resources, Inc. Materials include a manual, test booklets, and age- and sex-appropriate profile forms. The publisher also provides technical assistance and computer scoring, as well as free software updates. Purchase of the manual requires a degree from a 4-year college or university in psychology or a related field, plus acceptable completion of coursework in test interpretation or a related course, or a license/certification from an agency that requires training and experience in the ethical and competent use of psychological tests. Formal training or clinical experience is not required for administration of the TSCC, although a thorough understanding of the information presented in the manual is highly recommended. The TSCC manual recommends that the interpretation of the protocols be performed by individuals with graduate training in a mental-health-related field and appropriate training or coursework in interpreting psychological tests.

The TSCC manual includes empirical data from studies of changes in TSCC scale scores after therapy and over time, to facilitate interpretation of scores when the TSCC is readministered (e.g., to monitor the effects of treatment or rehabilitation services). The separate versions of the TSCC allow for flexibility in using the measure when there is concern about asking questions related to sexual issues. The TSCC enables clinicians or researchers to efficiently assess several symptom areas that have a common connection to trauma, rather than using several measures. The TSCC is also not limited to any type of trauma, so it is appropriate for a general juvenile justice population that is likely to have experienced a wide variety, and multiple types, of traumatic and stressful experiences. The TSCC's empirically based profiles by gender and age (8–12, 13–16) provide a degree of precision in identifying the severity of trauma symptoms that is relevant to each youth's gender and age group.

The TSCC has the same limitations as other self-report psychometric measures. In addition, TSCC scores should never be used to infer that trauma has (or has not) occurred for a respondent. The TSCC provides an indication of the type and severity of trauma symptoms and is recommended for clinical use primarily within a battery of assessment measures in the multimodal approach described earlier.

CASE EXAMPLE

Roberto was a 15-year-old Hispanic boy who lived with his mother and her fiancé. Roberto's father had passed away, following a prolonged illness, when Roberto was just 9 years old. Until that time, Roberto had lived with his parents and his paternal grandmother. After his father died, Roberto began to be involved with a neighborhood gang. He stayed on the fringes of the gang, because his grandmother, who had remained with the family to assist in rearing the children (including a younger sister and two older brothers), "made me stay in school and told me I could make something of my life." Three years ago, tensions between Roberto's mother and grandmother led Roberto's mother to ask his grandmother to move out, and Roberto now saw his grandmother only once a month. Roberto had been a B student until about 2 years ago, when his teachers reported that he became unfocused in class, didn't do the work, and was often truant. Roberto was seldom disruptive to the class; instead, he tended to "zone out" or to fall asleep.

Two months ago, Roberto was picked up by the police, along with several gang members who were suspected of dealing drugs to elementary school children. The police report that Roberto pulled a knife on them and had to be restrained forcibly. Although his mother was very angry when she learned of Roberto's arrest, she said that she didn't know anything about any gang activity, and that Roberto was "just looking for attention and lazy." The judge was considering sending Roberto to a high-security juvenile correctional facility, but Roberto's probation officer felt there was more to the situation and recommended a psychological evaluation prior to any placement.

Traumatic stress could be playing a role in Roberto's psychosocial difficulties in several ways. He had been exposed to and participated in numerous incidents of violence as a gang member, including firing a handgun wildly during a gang fight and having to go to the local hospital's emergency department after being assaulted with a knife by a rival gang member while walking home alone one night. Roberto had also experienced two potentially traumatic losses: (1) his father's illness and death, and (2) separation from the person (his grandmother) who had been one of his primary caregivers.

Roberto's behavior was consistent with "traumatic grief" (Prigerson et al., 1999), which is a combination of traumatic stress and unresolved grief that is distinct from, but often co-occurs with, depression. Roberto denied any distress related to his violence history or family issues, but he scored in or near the clinical range on the TSCC Posttraumatic Stress, Depression, Anxiety, and Dissociation scales. He scored low on the TSCC Anger subscale, but scored high on the Underresponse scale (the TSCC validity scale that measures denial or minimization). Thus Roberto's fatigue, truancy, and inattention could reflect difficulty in managing posttraumatic stress, emotional numbing due to suppressing anger, and unresolved grief. None of these posttraumatic problems were even considered until the TSCC was administered.

The TSCC findings could inform the placement and service plan for Roberto. Sending him to a high-security correctional setting would be likely to increase rather than reduce PTSD symptoms, given the exposure to real danger and to a peer group encouraging violence and callous disregard for people and the law. On the other hand, placement in a secure residential treatment program could begin to provide necessary mental health treatment addressing his PTSD symptoms and family losses, which were probably contributing factors to his future violence and delinquency risk. Counseling and group activities could teach Roberto practical skills for dealing with the unwanted memories of violence he experienced. In counseling, it would be possible to determine more clearly whether Roberto's apparent indifference and lack of motivation were due to anxiety, unwanted memories, or dissociation—as opposed to the more obvious possibility that he was simply "antisocial." Family counseling also could help his mother to empathize with Roberto's sense of loss and his need for emotional support from caregivers, and to be more consistent and supportive. Family counseling also might help his mother manage her own stress responses when she felt angry with Roberto or his grandmother. Psychiatric evaluation could also determine whether medication could help with Roberto's depression and PTSD symptoms.

REFERENCES

Abram, K. M., Teplin, L. A., Charles, D. R., Longworth, S. L., McClelland, G. M., & Dulcan, M. K. (2004). Posttraumatic stress disorder and trauma in youth in juvenile detention. *Archives of General Psychiatry, 61,* 403–410.

Albano, A. M., & Silverman, W. (1996). *Anxiety Disorders Interview Schedule for DSM-IV: Child Version*. San Antonio, TX: Psychological Corporation.

American Psychiatric Association. (2000). *Diagnostic and statistical manual of mental disorders* (4th ed., text rev.). Washington, DC: Author.

Angold, A., Prendergast, M., Cox, A., Harrington, R., Simonoff, E., & Rutter, M. (1995). The Child and Adolescent Psychiatric Assessment (CAPA). *Psychological Medicine, 25*, 739–753.

Arroyo, W. (2001). PTSD in children and adolescents in the juvenile justice system. *Review of Psychiatry, 20*(1), 59–86.

Berg-Sonne, P. (2002). *A comparison of violent and nonviolent female juvenile offenders using the Trauma Symptom Checklist for Children*. Unpublished doctoral dissertation, Chicago School of Professional Psychology.

Briere, J. (1996). *Trauma Symptom Checklist for Children (TSCC): Professional manual*. Odessa, FL: Psychological Assessment Resources.

Carrion, V., & Steiner, H. (2000). Trauma and dissociation in delinquent adolescents. *Journal of the American Academy of Child and Adolescent Psychiatry, 39*, 353–359.

Cashel, M. (2003). Validity of self-reports of delinquency and socio-emotional functioning among youth on probation. *Journal of Offender Rehabilitation, 37*, 11–23.

Cauffman, E., Feldman, S., Waterman, J., & Steiner, H. (1998). Posttraumatic stress disorder among female juvenile offenders. *Journal of the American Academy of Child and Adolescent Psychiatry, 37*(11), 1209–1216.

Cohen, J. A., Deblinger, E., Mannarino, A. P., & De Arellano, M. A. (2001). The importance of culture in treating abused and neglected children: An empirical review. *Child Maltreatment, 6*, 148–157.

Cohen, J. A., & Mannarino, A. P. (2000). Predictors of treatment outcome in sexually abused children. *Child Abuse and Neglect, 24*, 983–994.

Costello, A., Edelbrock, L,, Dulcan, M., Kalas, R., & Klaric, S. (1984). *Report on the NIMH Diagnostic Interview Schedule for Children (DISC)*. Bethesda, MD: National Institute of Mental Health.

Crouch, J. L., Smith, D. W., Ezzell, C. E., & Saunders, B. E. (1999). Measuring reactions to sexual trauma among children: Comparing the Children's Impact of Events Scale and the Trauma Symptom Checklist for Children. *Child Maltreatment, 4*, 255–263.

Daviss, W. B., Racusin, R., Fleischer, A., Mooney, D., Ford, J. D., & McHugo, G. (2000). Acute stress disorder symptomatology during hospitalization for pediatric injury. *Journal of the American Academy of Child and Adolescent Psychiatry, 39*, 569–575.

Dyregrov, A., Kuterovac, G., & Barath, A. (1996). Factor analysis of the Impact of Event Scale with children in war. *Scandinavian Journal of Psychology, 37*, 339–350.

Elliott, D. M., & Briere, J. (1994). Forensic sexual abuse evaluations of older children: Disclosures and symptomatology. *Behavioral Sciences and the Law, 12*, 261–277.

Evans, J. J., Briere, J., Boggiano, A. K., & Barrett, M. (1994). *Reliability and validity of the Trauma Symptom Checklist for Children in a normal sample*. Paper presented at the San Diego Conference on Responding to Child Maltreatment, San Diego, CA.

Flannery, D. J., Singer, M. I., & Webster, K. (2001). Violence exposure, psychological trauma, and suicide risk in a community sample of dangerously violent adolescents. *Journal of the American Academy of Child and Adolescent Psychiatry, 40*(4), 435–442.

Fletcher, K. E. (1996a). Psychometric review of Childhood PTSD Interview. In B. H. Stamm (Ed.), *Measurement of stress, trauma, and adaptation* (pp. 87–92). Lutherville, MD: Sidran Press.

Fletcher, K. E. (1996b). Psychometric review of When Bad Things Happen Scale. In B. H. Stamm (Ed.), *Measurement of stress, trauma, and adaptation* (pp. 435–437). Lutherville, MD: Sidran Press.

Ford, J. D., Racusin, R., Daviss, W. B., Reiser, J., Fleischer, A., & Thomas, J. (2000). Child maltreatment, other trauma exposure, and posttraumatic symptomatology among children with oppositional defiant and attention deficit hyperactivity disorders. *Child Maltreatment, 5*, 205–217.

Friedrich, W. N. (1995). Unpublished raw dataset, Mayo Clinic, Rochester, MN.

Friedrich, W. N., Gerber, P. N., Koplin, B., Davis, M., Giese, J., Mykelbust, C., & Franckowiak, D. (2001). Multimodal assessment of dissociation in adolescents: Inpatients and juvenile sex offenders. *Sexual Abuse: A Journal of Research and Treatment, 13*(3), 167–177.

Friedrich, W. N., Jaworski, T. M., Huxsahl, J. E., & Bengtson, B. S. (1997). Dissociative and sexual behaviors in children and adolescents with sexual abuse and psychiatric histories. *Journal of Interpersonal Violence, 12*, 155–171.

Garland, A. F., Hough, R. L., McCabe, K. M., Yeh, M., Wood, P. A., & Aarons, G. A. (2001). Prevalence of psychiatric disorders in youths across five sectors of care. *Journal of the American Academy of Child and Adolescent Psychiatry, 40*, 409–418.

Giaconia, R., Reinherz, H., Silverman, A., Pakiz, B., Frost, A., & Cohen, E. (1995). Traumas and posttraumatic stress disorder in a community population of older adolescents. *Journal of the American Academy of Child and Adolescent Psychiatry, 34*, 1369–1380.

Greenwald, R. (2002). Motivation-adaptive skills-trauma resolution (MASTR) therapy for adolescents with conduct problems: An open trial. *Journal of Aggression, Maltreatment and Trauma, 6*(1), 237–261.

Hastings, T. L., & Kelley, M. L. (1997). Development and validation of the Screen for Adolescent Violence Exposure (SAVE). *Journal of Abnormal Child Psychology, 25*, 511–520.

Henry, J. (1997). System intervention trauma to child sexual abuse victims following disclosure. *Journal of Interpersonal Violence, 12*, 499–512.

Johnson, R. M., Kotch, J. B., Catellier, D. J., Winsor, J. R., Dufort, V., Hunter, W. M., et al. (2002). Adverse behavioral and emotional outcomes from child abuse and witnessed violence. *Child Maltreatment, 7*, 179–186.

Jones, R. T. (1994). *Child's Reaction to Traumatic Events Scale (CRTES): A self report traumatic stress measure.* (Available from R. T. Jones, Department of Psychology, 137 Williams Hall, Virginia Polytechnic Institute and State University, Blacksburg, VA 24061)

Kaufman, J., Birmaher, B., Brent, D., Rao, U., Flynn, C., Moreci, P., et al. (1997). Schedule for Affective Disorders and Schizophrenia for School-Age Children— Present and Lifetime Version (K-SADS-PL): Initial reliability and validity data. *Journal of the American Academy of Child and Adolescent Psychiatry, 36*(7), 980–988.

King, L. A. (1996). Psychometric review of the Los Angeles Symptom Checklist (LASC). In B. H. Stamm (Ed.), *Measurement of stress, trauma, and adaptation* (pp. 202–204). Lutherville, MD: Sidran Press.

Kovacs, M. (1985). The Children's Depression Inventory (CDI). *Psychopharmacology Bulletin, 21,* 995–998.

Lanktree, C. B., & Briere, J. (1995). Outcome of therapy for sexually abused children: A repeated measures study. *Child Abuse and Neglect, 19,* 1145–1155.

Leite, S. S. (2001). *Community-based trauma and anger expression in adjudicated adolescents.* Unpublished doctoral dissertation, University of Hartford.

March, J. S., Amaya-Jackson, L., Murray, M. C., & Schulte, A. (1998). Cognitive behavioral psychotherapy for children and adolescents with posttraumatic stress disorder after a single incident stressor. *Journal of the American Academy of Child and Adolescent Psychiatry, 37,* 585–593.

March, J. S., Parker, J., Sullivan, K., Stallings, P., & Conners, C. K. (1997). The Multidimensional Anxiety Scale for Children (MASC): Factor structure, reliability, and validity. *Journal of the American Academy of Child and Adolescent Psychiatry, 36*(4), 554–565.

McMackin, R. A., Morrissey, C., Newman, E., Erwin, B., & Daly, M. (1998). Perpetrator and victim: Understanding and managing the traumatized young offender. *Corrections Management Quarterly, 2,* 35–44.

Mertin, P., & Mohr, P. B. (2002). Incidence and correlates of posttrauma symptoms in children from backgrounds of domestic violence. *Violence and Victims, 17,* 555–567.

Nader, K. O. (1996). Psychometric review of Childhood PTSD Reaction Index (PTSD-RI). In B. H. Stamm (Ed.), *Measurement of stress, trauma, and adaptation* (pp. 83–86). Lutherville, MD: Sidran Press.

Nader, K. O. (1997). Assessing traumatic experiences in children. In J. P. Wilson & T. M. Keane (Eds.), *Assessing psychological trauma and PTSD* (pp. 291–348). New York: Guilford Press.

Newman, E. (2002). Assessment of PTSD and trauma exposure in adolescents. *Journal of Aggression, Maltreatment and Trauma, 6,* 59–77.

Newman, E., Weathers, F., Nader, K., Kaloupek, D., Pynoos, R. S., Blake, D. D., & Kriegler, J. (in press). *Clinician Administered PTSD Scale for Children and Adolescents for DSM-IV: Manual.* Los Angeles: Western Psychological Services.

Praver, F., & Pelcovitz, D. (1996). Psychometric review of Angie/Andy Child Rating Scales: A Cartoon Based Measure for Post Traumatic Stress Responses to Chronic Interpersonal Abuse. In B. H. Stamm (Ed.), *Measurement of stress, trauma, and adaptation* (pp. 65–70). Lutherville, MD: Sidran Press.

Prigerson, H. G., Shear, M. K., Jacobs, S. C., Reynolds, C. F., III, Maciejewski, P. K., Davidson, J. R. T., et al. (1999). Consensus criteria for traumatic grief: A preliminary empirical test. *British Journal of Psychiatry, 174*(1), 67–73.

Putnam, F. W., Helmers, K., & Trickett, P. K. (1993). Development, reliability, and validity of a child dissociation scale. *Child Abuse and Neglect, 17,* 731–741.

Pynoos, R., Rodriguez, N., Steinberg, A., Stauber, M., & Frederick, C. (1998). *UCLA PTSD Index for DSM-IV: Child version.* Los Angeles: UCLA Trauma Psychiatry Service.

Reich, W., Shayka, J. J., & Taibleson, C. (1991). *Diagnostic Interview for Children and Adolescents (DICA)—Revised.* St. Louis, MO: Washington University.

Ruchkin, V., Schwab-Stone, M., Koposov, R., Vermeiren, R., & Steiner, H. (2002).

Violence exposure, posttraumatic stress, and personality in juvenile delinquents. *Journal of the American Academy of Child and Adolescent Psychiatry, 41*(3), 322–329.

Sadowski, C. M., & Friedrich, W. N. (2000). Psychometric properties of the Trauma Symptom Checklist for Children (TSCC) with psychiatrically hospitalized adolescents. *Child Maltreatment, 5*, 364–372.

Saigh, P. A. (1989). The development and validation of the Children's Posttraumatic Stress Disorder Inventory. *International Journal of Special Education, 4*, 75–84.

Saigh, P. A., Yasik, A. E., Sack, W. H., & Koplewicz, H. S. (1999). Child–adolescent posttraumatic stress disorder: Prevalence, risk factors, and comorbidity. In P. A. Saigh & J. D. Bremner (Eds.), *Posttraumatic stress disorder: A comprehensive text* (pp. 18–43). Boston: Allyn & Bacon.

Saltzman, W. R., Pynoos, R. S., Layne, C. M., Steinberg, A. M., & Aisenberg, E. (2001). Trauma- and grief-focused intervention for adolescents exposed to community violence: Results of a school-based screening and group treatment protocol. *Group Dynamics: Theory, Research, and Practice, 5*(4), 291–303.

Shaffer, D., Fisher, P., Piacentini, J., Schwab-Stone, M., & Wicks, J. (1992). *The Diagnostic Interview Schedule for Children (DISC)*. (Available from the authors, Columbia NIMH DISC Training Center, Division of Child and Adolescent Psychiatry—Unit 78, New York State Psychiatric Institute, 722 West 168th Street, New York, NY 10032)

Singer, M. I., Anglin, T. M., Song, L. Y., & Lunghofer, L. (1995). Adolescents' exposure to violence and associated symptoms of psychological trauma. *Journal of the American Medical Association, 273*, 477–482.

Song, L., Singer, M., & Anglin, T. M. (1998). Violence exposure and emotional trauma as contributors to adolescents' violent behaviors. *Archives of Pediatrics and Adolescent Medicine, 152*, 531–536.

Steiner, H., Garcia, I. G., & Matthews, Z. (1997). Posttraumatic stress disorder in incarcerated juvenile delinquents. *Journal of the American Academy of Child and Adolescent Psychiatry, 36*(3), 357–365.

Teplin, L. A., Abram, K. M., McClelland, G. M., Dulcan, M. K., & Mericle, A. A. (2002). Psychiatric disorders in youth in juvenile detention. *Archives of General Psychiatry, 59*, 1133–1143.

Valentine, I. S. (2001). The relationship between depression, self esteem, trauma, and psychopathy in understanding conduct disordered adolescents. *Dissertation Abstracts International, 61*(10), 5585B.

Wasserman, G. A., McReynolds, L. S., Lucas, C. P., Fisher, P., & Santos, L. (2002). The Voice DISC-IV with incarcerated male youths: Prevalence of disorder. *Journal of the American Academy of Child and Adolescent Psychiatry, 41*, 314–321.

Wolfe, D. A., Scott, K., Wekerle, C., & Pittman, A. L. (2001). Child maltreatment: Risk of adjustment problems and dating violence in adolescence. *Journal of the American Academy of Child and Adolescent Psychiatry, 40*, 282–289.

Wolfe, V. V., Gentile, C., Michienzi, T., Sas, L., & Wolfe, D. A. (1991). The Children's Impact of Traumatic Events Scales: A measure of post-sexual-abuse PTSD symptoms. *Behavioral Assessment, 13*(4), 359–383.

CHAPTER 10

Scales for Assessing Attention-Deficit/ Hyperactivity Disorder

Bryan R. Loney
Carla A. Counts

PURPOSE

Children exhibiting inattentive, hyperactive, and impulsive behaviors consistent with a diagnosis of attention-deficit/hyperactivity disorder (ADHD) are overrepresented in juvenile justice facilities (Foley, Carlton, & Howell, 1996; Garland et al., 2001). This is not surprising, given the established relationship between ADHD and chronic antisocial behavior in the juvenile delinquency research literature. The presence of pronounced hyperactivity and impulsivity symptoms has been associated with an earlier onset of conduct problems, greater severity and stability of antisocial behavior, and increased risk for criminality (Frick & Loney, 1999; Loeber, Farrington, Stouthamer-Loeber, Moffitt, & Caspi, 1998). As a consequence, ADHD symptoms—particularly impulsivity symptoms—have been included in various risk prediction models for violence and sexual offending in children (e.g., Borum, Bartel, & Forth, 2002; Hoge & Andrews, 2002; Prentky & Righthand, 2003) and adults (e.g., Quinsey, Harris, Rice, & Cormier, 1996; Webster, Douglas, Eaves, & Hart, 1997).

Recent research suggests that ADHD may only predict later delinquency when it is associated with pronounced oppositional behavior (Lahey, McBurnett, & Loeber, 2000). After all, it appears that the majority of children with ADHD do not exhibit later criminal behavior (Goldstein, 1997). Regardless, clinic-referred and nonreferred children exhibiting co-occurring conduct problems and ADHD symptoms have demonstrated varied neuropsychological, emotional, behavioral, and familial impairments (Abikoff & Klein, 1992; Frick, 1998). This has led to the speculation that the combination of ADHD and child conduct problems could be representative of a particularly virulent form of juvenile delinquency (Lynam, 1996) or a life-course-persistent trajectory of antisocial behavior (Moffitt, 1993).

The current ADHD diagnosis is described in the fourth edition of the *Diagnostic and Statistical Manual of Mental Disorders* (DSM-IV; American Psychiatric Association, 1994) and its text revision (DSM-IV-TR; American Psychiatric Association, 2000). It contains two symptom lists: (1) a nine-item inattention symptom list, including symptoms such as failing to give close attention to details, difficulty organizing tasks, and being easily distracted; and (2) a nine-item hyperactivity–impulsivity symptom list, including symptoms such as excessive fidgetiness, difficulty playing quietly, and frequent intrusion into others' conversations or activities. Children must exhibit at least six out of the nine symptom criteria from either symptom list, over at least a 6-month period, to receive a diagnosis of ADHD. In addition, there must be evidence that (1) some of the symptoms were present prior to age 7; (2) the current symptoms are present across two or more settings; and (3) the symptoms are associated with significant impairment related to social, academic, or occupational functioning. The majority of children receiving an ADHD diagnosis exhibit six or more symptoms from both lists and receive a diagnosis of ADHD, combined type. However, it is possible to receive a diagnosis of ADHD, predominant inattentive type, or ADHD, predominant hyperactive–impulsive type.

The relation between ADHD and juvenile delinquency has primarily been investigated in large-scale community and clinic-referred samples of children and adolescents (e.g., Christian, Frick, Hill, Tyler, & Frazer, 1997; Loeber et al., 1998). This research has focused almost exclusively on the use of ADHD symptoms to predict delinquent behavior. There is a lack of studies specifically examining the relation between ADHD symptoms and rehabilitation progress, completion, and recidivism (Vermeiren, de Clippele, & Deboutte, 2000). Preliminary investigations have linked elevated hyperactivity–impulsivity symptoms to failure to complete treatment (Kraemer, Salisbury, & Spielman, 1998) and greater recidivism rates (Miner, 2002; Vermeiron et al., 2000) among adolescents, as well as to institutional violence among adults (Wang & Diamond, 1999). However, these studies suffer from a number of limitations, including selective samples of juvenile offenders (e.g., those charged with sexual offenses) and the use of measures of hyperactivity–impulsivity that are not well established.

There are multiple points at which the screening of ADHD could inform the juvenile justice process. Currently, the assessment of ADHD has exhibited its greatest impact on the adjudication process, where it has been used to argue for reduced sentencing of juvenile offenders (Foley et al., 1996; Goldstein, 1997). Proper screening and assessment upon referral to juvenile justice agencies could allow documentation of potential mental health needs that could work against the rehabilitation and prevention of delinquent behavior. It has been argued that youths with ADHD do not require special treatment facilities, given the high levels of structure and consistency present in most juvenile correctional institutions (Goldstein, 1997). However, delinquent youths with prominent symptoms of ADHD could potentially benefit from empirically supported treatment modalities such as psychotropic medication (e.g., methylphenidate or other stimulants), behavioral parent training (Barkley, Edwards, & Robin, 1999), and multisystemic therapy (Henggeler, Melton, Brondino, Scherer, & Hanley, 1997).

The current chapter focuses specifically on narrow-band measures that comprehensively tap ADHD hyperactivity–impulsivity symptoms. The ADHD hyperactivity–impulsivity symptoms are typically viewed as a single dimension of behavioral functioning that is uniquely related to risk for delinquent behavior. Narrow-band measures are relatively brief and target a limited number of behavioral domains, in contrast with broad-band measures, which cover a wide variety of emotional and behavioral difficulties.

Several narrow-band ADHD rating scales may prove useful in evaluating youths in the juvenile justice system. Interested readers are referred to Kamphaus and Frick (2002) and to Collett, Ohan, and Myers (2003) for a more comprehensive and detailed comparison of the strengths and weaknesses of these various rating scales. The current review focuses on three instruments that arguably have the greatest promise for juvenile justice screening and assessment: the Conners Rating Scales—Revised (CRS-R; Conners, 1997), which are actually a package of scales (long and short versions for each of three different informants); the ADHD Rating Scale–IV (ADHD RS-IV; DuPaul, Power, Anastopoulos, & Reid, 1998); and the Attention Deficit Disorders Evaluation Scale—Second Edition (ADDES-2; McCarney, 1995a, 1995b). Information is provided separately for each instrument within each section of this review.

BASIC DESCRIPTION

All three of these instruments provide detailed coverage of ADHD symptoms, are based on large and ethnically diverse normative samples, and have demonstrated reliability and validity across child and adolescent age ranges. In selecting them, we also considered they are(1) frequently used in research and clinical settings, (2) relatively inexpensive and easy to obtain, and (3) require minimal training to administer and interpret. Table 10.1 contains a basic description and comparison of the selected instruments.

TABLE 10.1. A Description and Comparison of Selected ADHD Rating Scales

CRS-R	ADHD RS-IV	ADDES-2
Primary reference, publisher, and contact information		
Conners (1997) Multi-Health Systems (*http://www.mhs.com*)	DuPaul et al. (1998) Guilford Press (*http:// www.guilford.com*)	McCarney (1995) Hawthorne Educational Services (*http://www.hes-inc.com*)
Informants and ages assessed		
Parent and teacher report: Ages 3–17 Self-report: Ages 12–17	Parent and teacher report: Ages 5–18	Parent and teacher report: Ages 4–19
Response format and number of items		
4-point scale Parent = 80/27 items Teacher = 59/28 items Self = 87/27 items	4-point scale Parent = 18 items Teacher = 18 items	5-point scale Parent = 46 items Teacher = 60 items
Scale description		
Four to seven core subscales tapping ADHD symptoms and common associated difficulties such as conduct problems and anxiety	Total score and two subscales tapping inattention and hyperactivity–impulsivity symptoms	Total score and two subscales tapping inattention and hyperactivity–impulsivity symptoms
Administration time		
Long version = 15–20 minutes Short version = 5–10 minutes	5–10 minutes	15–20 minutes
Unique strengths		
Inclusion of norm-referenced self-report format; assessment of broader symptom content than other measures	One-to-one correspondence with DSM-IV ADHD diagnostic criteria; free and unlimited copies of the instrument	Very strong initial psychometric data; location-specific modifiers, increasing ecological validity of parent and teacher reports

Conners Rating Scales—Revised

The CRS-R are a well-established package of measures that met all of the selection criteria and are the only scales reviewed that include a youth self-report format. This is a strength, given that it can be difficult at various stages of the juvenile justice process to obtain information from other informants (Wasserman et al., 2003). The CRS-R tap ADHD symptoms along with common associated psychiatric difficulties (e.g., conduct problems and anxiety). There are separate short and long versions of the parent rating scale (27 items vs. 80 items) and the teacher rating scale (28 items vs. 59 items) for children and adolescents ages 3–17. There are also short and long versions of the self-report scale (27 items vs. 87 items) for adolescents ages 12–17.

The long versions of the CRS-R assess a broader spectrum of psychopathology and may arguably be better described as broad-band measures. Initial research indicated that the parent measure contains seven core subscales, while the teacher and self-report measures contain six core subscales. (See Table 10.2 for a listing of subscales and sample item content.) The majority of subscales contain item content that is closely aligned with the subscale labels. However, it should be noted that the Cognitive Problems subscale taps ADHD inattention symptoms and related learning difficulties. The developers of the instrument also created some additional scales from items contained on the core subscales that provide for more detailed coverage of ADHD symptoms. These include (1) two subscales directly corresponding to the DSM-IV inattention and hyperactivity–impulsivity criteria for ADHD; (2) an ADHD Index subscale, composed of items that have done a good job of differentiating diagnosed youths from matched controls in initial investigations; and (3) two additional subscales tapping restless–impulsive behavior and emotional lability that were developed as indexes of general psychopathology.

Each long version takes approximately 15–20 minutes to administer and allows for the calculation of standard scores referred to as "T-scores." These standard scores are derived from large normative samples and are associated with percentile rankings that indicate where a child's scores stand relative to those of same-age peers. When responses have been converted to standard scores, clinicians can quickly determine whether or not a child's score for a given subscale is elevated relative to age peers, as well as in relation to other standard scores on the same or different measures. An average T-score is 50, and a child is typically considered to have an elevated rating on a measure if his or her T-score is 65–70. These T-scores correspond to the 92nd and 98th percentiles, respectively.

The short versions of the CRS-R pull select item and scale content from the long versions of the instrument; this includes three of the core subscales contained on the parent, teacher, and self-report forms. These scales are asterisked in Table 10.2. The short versions also contain the ADHD Index subscale contained in the long versions of the instrument. These measures take approximately 5–10 minutes to administer.

TABLE 10.2. CRS-R Subscales and Sample Items

Core subscales	Sample items
	Parent and teacher report
Oppositional*	Actively defies or refuses to comply with adults' requests.
Cognitive Problems*	Difficulty engaging in tasks that require sustained mental effort.
Hyperactivity*	Is always "on the go" or acts as if driven by a motor.
Anxious–Shy	Timid, easily frightened.
Perfectionism	Everything must be just so.
Social Problems	Does not know how to make friends.
Psychosomatic (parent version only)	Gets aches and pains or stomachaches before school.
	Self-report
Family Problems	My parents do not really care about me.
Emotional Problems	I worry a lot about little things.
Conduct Problems*	I break rules and am easily led into trouble.
Cognitive Problems*	I have trouble keeping my thoughts organized.
Anger Control Problems	People bug me and get me angry.
Hyperactivity*	Sometimes I feel like I am driven by a motor.

Note. All of the subscales described in the table are contained in the long versions of the instrument. Asterisked subscales are contained in both the long and short versions. Copyright (c) 1997 Multi-Health Systems Inc. All rights reserved. In the USA, P.O. Box 950, North Tonawanda, NY 14120-0950, 1-800-456-3003. In Canada, 3770 Victoria Park Ave., Toronto, ON M2H 3M6, 1-800-268-6011. Internationally, +1-416-492-2627. Fax, +1-416-492-3343. Reproduced with permission.

Across all versions of the instrument, separate norms are available for each gender within 3-year age groupings (e.g., for adolescents, norms are broken down into separate 12–14 and 15–17 age groupings). The self-report version also includes separate norms for African American adolescents (Conners, 1997). The CRS-R are currently available in paper-and-pencil format, although a Windows-based version should be available for use in the near future. The CRS-R use a 4-point response format ranging from 0 for "not at all true" to 3 for "very much true." T-scores of 65 or greater are generally considered clinically significant. There are multiple options available for scoring the CRS-R: (1) the QuikScore format (consisting of multilayer "copies" that automatically translate raw scores into T-scores), (2) the ColorPlot format (documenting treatment response over time), (3) computer scoring software, (4) scores via facsimile service, and (5) scores via mail-in service. The CRS-R parent and teacher forms require a ninth-grade reading level, while the self-report versions require a sixth-grade reading level. French Canadian and Spanish translations are available.

ADHD Rating Scale–IV

The ADHD RS-IV is an 18-item paper-and-pencil measure that corresponds closely to the ADHD symptoms listed in the DSM-IV (DuPaul et al., 1998). The ADHD RS-IV is used for children ages 5–18 and contains separate Inattention and Hyperactivity–Impulsivity subscales. These subscales can be summed to form a total score. Home (parent report) and school (teacher report) versions are available. Items are assessed on a 4-point scale ranging from 0 for "never or rarely" to 3 for "very or often." Both versions take approximately 5–10 minutes to administer. Items are summed and converted to T-scores and percentile rankings by using tables contained in the manual. Different cutoffs are recommended, depending upon the subtype of ADHD being assessed (e.g., predominantly inattentive or combined) and whether the primary goal is to screen or diagnose for ADHD. Separate norms are available for each gender, with two adolescent age groupings (ages 11–13 and 14–18). No information is provided in the technical manual regarding the required reading level. The home version includes a Spanish translation.

Attention Deficit Disorders Evaluation Scale—Second Edition

The ADDES-2 is a paper-and-pencil inventory that assesses ADHD symptoms of children and adolescents ages 4–19 (McCarney, 1995a, 1995b). Similar to the ADHD RS-IV, it includes separate home and school versions (46 items and 60 items, respectively) and separate Inattention and Hyperactivity–Impulsivity subscales that can be combined into a total score. The ADDES-2 also provides location-specific descriptors (classroom or home) that assist in differentiating parent and teacher report formats and linking symptoms to real-life settings (Collett et al., 2003). A 5-point response format is used to rate each symptom on frequency, ranging from a score of 0 for "does not engage in behavior" to 4 for "one to several times per hour." The scales take approximately 15–20 minutes to administer. Responses can be translated into standard scores and percentile rankings. There are separate norms for gender and various age groups, with adolescent norms collapsed across ages 13–18 (McCarney, 1995a, 1995b).

A unique feature of the ADDES-2 is that *lower* scores signify *greater* levels of ADHD symptoms. This can be somewhat confusing, given the precedent for measures of psychopathology to be scored in the opposite direction. In addition, the ADDES-2 does not use T-scores. It uses a different type of standard score referred to as a "scaled score." Scaled scores range from 1 to 20. An average score is 10, and the ADDES-2 considers scores less than 4 to be indicative of serious concern. The ADDES-2 is scored by using tables included in the technical manuals or using a computer-based scoring program. No information is provided regarding the required reading level. There is a Spanish version of both the home and school versions.

HISTORY OF THE METHODS' DEVELOPMENT

Conners Rating Scales—Revised

The CRS-R have a long history, with initial research beginning in the 1960s (Conners, 1997). Collett and colleagues (2003) indicate that the earliest scales were primarily created to measure frequent child problem behaviors in clinical settings (e.g., difficulty eating, sleep instability, and social problems). Extension of the initial scales led to the creation of the Conners Parent Rating Scale–93 and the Conners Teacher Rating Scale–39, with the proposed use of examining medication efficacy in treatment studies. The scales became commonly used in the assessment and treatment of ADHD. However, there was difficulty obtaining reliable subscales, and the norms were based on a very small sample. Consequently, advancements in research led to the Conners Parent Rating Scale–48 and the Conners Teacher Rating Scale–28, but these scales still lacked adequate normative data (Collett et al., 2003). The CRS-R were developed in response to these problems and to be compatible with the ADHD diagnostic criteria contained in the DSM-IV.

The CRS-R were created to tap multiple emotional and behavioral difficulties in a variety of clinical, school, and research settings. Uses of the CRS-R include, but are not limited to, the screening of ADHD symptoms and assessment of treatment efficacy (Conners, 1997). The CRS-R were designed to be used in combination with other sources of information (e.g., interview and behavioral observations) to make clinical judgments (Conners, 1997). The development of the CRS-R largely occurred from 1992 to 1996. Items were initially created to tap features of the DSM-IV criteria. Subsequently, child assessment specialists examined the items, and pilot studies were performed to evaluate individual items and scale properties. Next, the items were revised, edited, and administered to a new sample in order to reassess item strength and psychometric properties. Finally, normative data were collected from a large (i.e., approximately 8,000 raters) and ethnically diverse sample (including African American, Hispanic, Asian, and Native American children) obtained from . nearly every state in the United States and 10 provinces in Canada (Conners, 1997). Manuals were developed and forms edited in order to increase the scales' functionality.

ADHD Rating Scale–IV

The ADHD RS-IV was created in response to the release of the DSM-IV (American Psychiatric Association, 1994) and is a revision of an original ADHD Rating Scale created by DuPaul and colleagues in 1991 (see DuPaul et al., 1998). It was designed to correspond closely to the ADHD diagnostic criteria, as the authors noted that many ADHD rating scales provided insufficient coverage of ADHD symptoms. According to DuPaul and colleagues (1998), the ADHD RS-IV is appropriate for use in screening and diagnosis of

ADHD in clinic and school settings. Normative data were derived from a mixed-gender and ethnically diverse normative sample. This included parent and teacher ratings of approximately 2,000 children and adolescents from various regions of the United States (DuPaul et al., 1998).

Attention Deficit Disorders Evaluation Scale—Second Edition

Similar to the ADHD RS-IV, the ADDES-2 was created in response to the release of the DSM-IV and is an update of an earlier scale created by McCarney in 1989. Items were developed to closely approximate DSM-IV ADHD symptoms, and were based on the recommendations of clinical experts, educators, and parents of children with ADHD (Collett et al., 2003; McCarney, 1995a, 1995b). The scale was developed to enhance the screening and assessment of ADHD symptoms and can be used for diagnostic purposes as part of a comprehensive assessment (McCarney, 1995a, 1995b). The ADDES-2 normative sample is large and ethnically diverse. It is a nationally representative sample containing both genders, parent ratings of approximately 2,500 children, and teacher ratings of approximately 5,800 children (McCarney, 1995a, 1995b).

RESEARCH EVIDENCE

All of the measures included in the current review provide for age-normative data based on large mixed-gender samples that are geographically and ethnically diverse. This is generally important and crucial for juvenile justice facilities, given that (1) minority youths are often disproportionately represented in forensic settings (Grisso & Underwood, 2003), and (2) female referrals have been steadily increasing across the past few decades (Loney & Lima, 2003). A primary consideration for the selection of measures was the amount of research evidence supporting their use in adolescent samples. Most ADHD rating scales have been developed largely for elementary-school-age samples and are based on diagnostic criteria that are arguably biased toward the behavior of preadolescent children (Collett et al., 2003).

Developmentally, researchers have documented that ADHD symptoms generally decrease across adolescence and young adulthood. This is particularly true of the hyperactivity–impulsivity symptoms and does not indicate that ADHD is simply a childhood phenomenon or that children uniformly "mature out of" the disorder. A portion of this decline appears to be due to developmental differences in the expression of hyperactivity–impulsivity symptoms in older children and adults (Barkley, 1997; Root & Resnick, 2003). For example, one of the ADHD hyperactivity–impulsivity symptoms pertains to running about or climbing excessively. This symptom, like others in the list, is geared toward younger children. Although the DSM-IV states that hyperactivity may be experienced as a subjective feeling of restlessness in adolescents and adults, "subjective restlessness" can be difficult to quantify. Fortunately, most of the ADHD symptoms are not qualified in that fashion.

Researchers are presently exploring the development of new ADHD symptom content and diagnostic criteria that may be more appropriate for adolescents and young adults. Meanwhile, it is important to note that some teenagers may fail to meet the number of symptoms needed for a diagnosis (e.g., six out of nine hyperactivity–impulsivity symptoms) despite meeting all other diagnostic criteria, including significant impairment in social, academic, and occupational functioning. Unlike the DSM-IV, rating scales control for developmental differences when the severity of symptom presentations is being determined. For example, the ADHD RS-IV contains separate norms for youths ages 11–13 and 14–18. A parent raw score of 16 on the Hyperactivity–Impulsivity scale for a boy corresponds to the 93rd percentile for the younger age grouping and the 98th percentile for the older grouping; the difference is probably due to greater levels of developmental immaturity in the younger children. The use of norm-referenced rating scales with adolescents assists in pinpointing potentially impairing levels of ADHD symptoms that may be missed by the DSM-IV criteria, which do not readily take into account typical changes in psychosocial maturity and circumstances. This supports the selection of rating scales that provide for the smallest, most refined age windows across childhood and adolescence.

Conners Rating Scales—Revised

The current review summarizes psychometric findings for the long and short versions of the CRS-R, given the similarity of findings across versions of the instrument. The adolescent age range is highlighted, except when only data collapsed across the child and adolescent age ranges are available.

In terms of reliability (or consistency) of CRS-R scores, all subscales of the CRS-R have met minimum requirements for internal consistency, with the majority of scales demonstrating internal-consistency estimates greater than .80 both within and across various age and gender groupings (Conners, 1997). In addition, the CRS-R have evidenced strong stability of test scores across a 6- to 8-week time interval (i.e., test–retest reliability), with the majority of subscale scores exhibiting test–retest correlations of .65 or greater (Conners, 1997). Finally, correlations between informants (e.g., parents and teachers) have been consistent with values obtained from the greater child and adolescent assessment literatures (Achenbach, McConaughy, & Howell, 1987; Kamphaus & Frick, 2002). For example, the majority of subscales tapping ADHD symptoms have generally exhibited informant correlations of .30 or greater.

In terms of validity, the CRS-R have exhibited significant correlations with performance measures of inattention and impulsivity (e.g., continuous-performance tests) and other ADHD rating scales (Collett et al., 2003; Conners, 1997). Moreover, Conners and colleagues (Conners, 1997; Conners,

Sitarenios, Parker, & Epstein, 1998a, 1998b) have documented that the CRS-R do a good job of differentiating children diagnosed with ADHD from matched control groups. Initial research indicates that children with clinician-based diagnoses are typically characterized by ADHD scale elevations (i.e., T-scores = 65 or greater), and children without an ADHD diagnosis are typically characterized by low scores. The parent rating scale has done the best job of matching scale elevations to diagnostic status.

Collett and colleagues (2003) note that the CRS-R have been used in a wide variety of clinical and research applications. For example, the CRS-R have been used in treatment studies examining their sensitivity in assessing medication effects, as well as in assessing the psychosocial impairments associated with female ADHD diagnoses (Rucklidge & Tannock, 2001). There is a notable absence of published research studies using the CRS-R or previous versions of the instrument within the juvenile justice system. This is a limitation of all three of the reviewed measures, on which we will comment further after discussing the research support for the other measures.

The investigation of gender and ethnic differences in CRS-R reports has uncovered some important findings in need of further research. Consistent with prior research (Collett et al., 2003), males in the normative sample generally scored higher on scales assessing conduct problems and related acting-out behaviors. Females scored higher on scales assessing anxiety and related features of emotional distress. With respect to ethnic comparisons, there were minimal ethnic differences for the parent and teacher measures. However, comparisons of ethnic groups on the self-report measure indicated that Native American youth endorsed a greater number of hyperactivity symptoms than Caucasian and Asian groups. In addition, African American children endorsed a greater number of family problems, conduct problems, anger control problems, and ADHD symptoms than Caucasian children. There were a limited number of Native American youths in the normative sample, making it difficult to interpret related findings. The findings for African American youths suggest that caution should be taken in applying general norms to that ethnic group. This has led to the inclusion of separate African American norms for the self-report format.

ADHD Rating Scale–IV

The principal psychometric data for the ADHD RS-IV were derived from a sample of 71 children ages 5–17 recruited from two school districts in the northeastern United States (DuPaul et al., 1998). This introduces some bias into the psychometric data, as many of the reliability and validity data reviewed in the technical manual are based on a predominantly European American sample. This limited number of youths also prevents an inspection of reliability, specifically within the adolescent age range. Despite this limitation, the initial reliability evidence is impressive. The home and school versions of the instrument exhibited strong internal consistency, with all coefficients greater than .85. Stability of scores across a 4-week interval was similarly impressive, with test–retest correlations approximating .80 to .90. Finally, correlations between parent and teacher ratings ranged from .40 to .45 across subscales (DuPaul et al., 1998).

As described in the technical manual, initial validity investigations have documented strong correlations with related rating scales, such as earlier versions of the Conners rating scales and significant correlations with direct observations of classroom behavior. Although limited psychometric data other than the information presented in the manual are available, researchers are currently using the ADHD RS-IV to investigate age, gender, and ethnic trends in ADHD reporting (e.g., Reid et al., 1998, 2000). In addition, Power and colleagues (1998) have used the measure to investigate how well the parent and teacher ratings predict clinician-based diagnoses. Collett et al. (2003) have indicated that the parent and teacher ratings on the ADHD RS-IV have exhibited suboptimal agreement with clinician-based diagnoses. Preliminary research suggests that isolated use of the ADHD RS-IV is best suited for ruling out an ADHD diagnosis (Power et al., 1998). This means that more confidence can be placed in low scores revealing no diagnosis than in high scores revealing the presence of a diagnosis.

With respect to gender and ethnic trends, boys in the normative sample generally exhibited greater numbers of inattention and hyperactive/impulsive symptoms than girls. Ethnic comparisons were limited to African American, Caucasian, and Hispanic youths, given a paucity of other ethnic groups in the normative sample. Parents and teachers generally endorsed a greater number of ADHD symptoms for African American youths than for the comparison groups. This particular finding has led the authors of the instrument to caution against using the norm-referenced data with African American children, in order to avoid overidentification of ADHD cases (i.e., false positives). The ADHD RS-IV does not contain separate norms based on ethnicity.

Attention Deficit Disorders Evaluation Scale—Second Edition

The ADDES-2 is commonly used in clinical and school settings, but Collett and colleagues (2003) indicate that it is not commonly cited in the research literature, and there are few psychometric studies other than the information provided in the technical manuals. Although this is clearly a limitation of the instrument, the initial psychometric data for the ADDES-2 are quite impressive and are generally viewed as among its strengths (Collett et al., 2003). For example, reliability data derived from the normative sample included internal-consistency estimates ranging from .96 to .99 for the parent and teacher scales, with 30-day test–retest correlations approaching a similar magnitude (i.e., $r = .88–.97$). Correlations between different informants on the same measure (e.g., two different parents on the parent measure) were extremely high ($r = .80–.90$ across the adolescent age range), in comparison to what is usually found ($r = .60$) for the child assessment methods (Achenbach et al., 1987).

Validity data are limited with the ADDES-2. However, the ADDES-2 has demonstrated strong correlations with related measures, such as earlier versions of the Conners scales. Initial investigation has indicated that the ADDES-2 scales are effective at discriminating clinic-referred children diagnosed with ADHD from community control participants (McCarney, 1995a, 1995b). Although boys are generally characterized by higher scores on the ADDES-2 subscales, no ethnic comparisons are presented in the technical manual. The ADDES-2 is the weakest measure in terms of sensitivity to how psychosocial maturity factors may influence interpretations from normative data (i.e., it collapses normative data across ages 13–18).

APPLICATION

All of the measures reviewed are easy to obtain through the publisher and contact information listed in Table 10.1. They are relatively inexpensive, require minimal training to administer, and tap symptom content that is particularly relevant to the juvenile justice process (e.g., impulsive behaviors, social problems, and anger control problems). In addition, the selected measures are brief. This is important, given that juvenile justice staff may have as little as 10–15 minutes to administer screenings or assessments during various stages of the juvenile justice process (Grisso & Underwood, 2003). The current review argues that measures of ADHD are easy to administer within the juvenile justice system and could contribute significantly to the prevention and rehabilitation of delinquent behavior. However, the potential benefits of these measures must be weighed against a number of limitations.

First, there is less research than is desirable regarding the psychometric properties and clinical utility of the reviewed measures within the juvenile justice system. Although it is likely that norm-referenced ADHD rating scales could contribute to the prediction of institutional adjustment and recidivism, the use of the reviewed ADHD measures for this purpose is not supported by the current research literature. The research that has been conducted on ADHD within the juvenile justice system has typically not used norm-referenced measures such as those reviewed in this chapter. This makes it difficult to estimate how common the use of narrow-band, norm-referenced measures is in juvenile justice facilities. However, the current status of the research literature suggests that very few facilities are using such measures to assist with diagnostic and rehabilitation decisions.

Second, there is currently very little research on the utility of the self-report of ADHD symptoms. There are some promising initial research findings supporting the reliability of self-reported ADHD symptoms (e.g., Conners, 1997; Smith, Pelham, Gnagy, Molina, & Evans, 2000). However, validity studies have not been conducted in forensic settings, where a number of factors may compromise the veracity of responding. For example, juvenile offenders may underreport ADHD symptoms because of poor judgment, limited insight, and the potential negative implications of sentencing (e.g., incarceration) (Grisso & Underwood, 2003).

Finally, there has been limited research with juvenile justice samples that explores ethnic differences in the reporting and predictive utility of ADHD symptoms. The research currently available suggests that certain minority groups may score relatively higher on ADHD measures. Although the clinical significance of these elevations is uncertain, they raise the possibility of unacceptable rates of false-positive test scores. This should lead to a particularly cautious approach to using ADHD measures for the screening and diagnosis of minority youths.

Despite these limitations, juvenile justice staff members are encouraged to integrate ADHD measures into the broader mental health screening process. Rates of ADHD are clearly elevated in the juvenile justice system, and research suggests that ADHD symptoms may play a causal role in the development of stable offending. Early detection and treatment of ADHD could assist in the reduction of risk and severity of antisocial behavior during and after contact with the juvenile justice system. It is recommended that ADHD measures be routinely administered during the initial intake and pretrial detention phase, when juvenile justice staffers are most likely to obtain information from multiple informants. It can be difficult to obtain information from caregivers at other points in the system. For example, research suggests that more than 60% of youth in the juvenile justice system are not visited by their parents or other caregivers, regardless of the length of their sentences (Wasserman et al., 2003).

Elevations on ADHD subscales could trigger review by a staff clinician, who would then determine whether to refer the youth for a comprehensive mental health evaluation. Pending the results of initial screening and assessment efforts, subsequent testing can occur at different points to monitor rehabilitation progress. Teacher versions of the instruments reviewed here would be the most appropriate version of the instruments to administer to staff members, as they were designed to be completed by an adult authority figure outside the home environment. The CRS-R show particular promise for the juvenile justice system, given the availability of both long and short versions, as well as the provision of a self-report format (which is lacking in the other measures). If possible, the long versions of the CRS-R could be administered at intake, in order to screen for a wider variety of emotional (e.g., anxiety) and behavioral (e.g., anger control and social problems) concerns that may go undetected if the focus is specifically on ADHD symptoms. The long version could subsequently be augmented with periodic reassessment using the short versions of the instrument.

Successful detection of an ADHD diagnosis could lead to the introduction of empirically supported treatment modalities (e.g., medication and cognitive-behavioral interventions) before, during, and after contact with the juvenile justice system. Treatment could be tethered to appropriate conduct disorder intervention strategies, such as multisystemic therapy (Henggeler et al., 1997), to exert the greatest potential impact on delinquency recidivism.

CASE EXAMPLE

Jordan was a 14-year-old Caucasian male who was detained on a burglary charge. He was accused of stealing over $1,000 worth of goods from a local apartment complex with some of his friends. Upon arriving at a local detention center, Jordan and his mother were interviewed by a staff member and asked to complete a number of background forms. They were then asked several questions pertaining to Jordan's medical and mental health history. This included the administration of long versions of the CRS-R parent and self-report rating scales. Jordan's mother spontaneously told the intake interviewer that Jordan had always been an energetic and somewhat difficult child, but he was not a criminal. She stated that he had experienced particular difficulty since moving to the city approximately 6 months ago. Jordan moved after his parents' contentious divorce; he maintained no contact with his biological father. Jordan's mother indicated that her son's grades had dropped dramatically since the move; he had been in multiple fights at school; and he was having difficulty making friends. She described his few friends as bad influences.

Jordan's responses to the CRS-R resulted in scale elevations (i.e., T-scores > 65) on the Family Problems, Conduct Problems, Anger Control Problems, and Hyperactivity subscales. This was consistent with his mother's interview information and report on the CRS-R parent scale, which revealed similar elevations on the Cognitive Problems, Oppositional, Hyperactivity, and Social Problems subscales. The intake worker observed that Jordan was quite distractible, fidgeting in his seat and frequently asking for questions to be repeated.

Following an initial court appearance, Jordan was placed on home detention. He soon appeared again in court and was adjudicated delinquent on the burglary charge. Based on the intake screening data, Jordan was court-ordered to participate in a comprehensive psychological evaluation to assist with sentencing and rehabilitation decisions. The psychologist conducting the evaluation reviewed the intake screening instruments to help guide the assessment. For example, based on information derived from the CRS-R parent and self-report forms, the psychologist administered a CRS-R teacher rating scale to one of Jordan's ninth-grade teachers. The teacher scale revealed elevations on the Cognitive Problems, Oppositional, and Social Problems subscales. The psychologist also administered a rating scale measure of depression to Jordan, which revealed a number of potential concerns related to his emotional functioning. No learning impairments were detected upon inspection of achievement and intelligence testing.

The results of the psychological evaluation supported separate diagnoses of ADHD and an adjustment disorder with mixed disturbance of emotions and conduct. Jordan's current school difficulties were attributed to difficulty in sustaining attention to and completing tasks secondary to these emotional and behavioral issues. The psychologist indicated that chronic stressors associated with the divorce appeared to have worked in concert with Jordan's developmental immaturity in impulse control to overload his coping capacities. Therefore, the poor judgment he showed by engaging in the delinquent conduct was likely to have been influenced by the confluence of these psychiatric and developmental factors.

Following the psychological evaluation, Jordan again appeared in court and was sentenced to 2 years of probation. Jordan was not sentenced to rehabilitation in a correctional facility for several reasons: This was his first referral; he displayed remorse and accepted responsibility for his actions; and it became clear during the deliberation process that he did not initiate the crime. Jordan was required to complete 100 hours of community service, and to make restitution for damages. He and his mother were also ordered to attend therapy sessions to assist with managing Jordan's conduct problems, peer difficulties, and adjustment to the divorce. Jordan was referred for a psychiatric consultation and placed on stimulant medication to help address the hyperactivity and impulse control problems related to his ADHD diagnosis. Reassessment of ADHD symptoms was conducted 3 months later with the short versions of the CRS-R measures, which revealed a significant drop in hyperactivity and conduct problem symptoms (i.e., T-scores for all parent, teacher, and self-report ratings were below 65).

REFERENCES

Abikoff, H., & Klein, R. G. (1992). Attention deficit hyperactivity and conduct disorder: Comorbidity and implications for treatment. *Journal of Consulting and Clinical Psychology, 60,* 881–892.

Achenbach, T. M., McConaughy, S. H., & Howell, C. T. (1987). Child/adolescent behavioral and emotional problems: Implications of cross-informant correlations for situational specificity. *Psychological Bulletin, 101,* 213–232.

American Psychiatric Association. (1994). *Diagnostic and statistical manual of mental disorder* (4th ed.). Washington, DC: Author.

American Psychiatric Association. (2000). *Diagnostic and statistical manual of mental disorder* (4th ed., text rev.). Washington, DC: Author.

Barkley, R. A. (1997). *ADHD and the nature of self-control.* New York: Guilford Press.

Barkley, R. A., Edwards, G. H., & Robin, A. L. (1999). *Defiant teens: A clinician's manual for assessment and family intervention.* New York: Guilford Press.

Borum, R., Bartel, P., & Forth, A. (2002). *Manual for the Structured Assessment for Violence Risk in Youth (SAVRY).* Tampa: Florida Mental Health Institute, University of South Florida.

Christian, R. E., Frick, P. J., Hill, N. L., Tyler, L., & Frazer, D. R. (1997). Psychopathy and conduct problems in children: II. Implications for subtyping children with conduct problems. *Journal of the American Academy of Child and Adolescent Psychiatry, 36*, 233–241.

Collett, B. R., Ohan, J. L., & Myers, K. M. (2003). Ten-year review of rating scales: V. Scales assessing attention-deficit/hyperactivity disorder. *Journal of the Academy of Child and Adolescent Psychiatry, 42*, 1015–1037.

Conners, C. K. (1997). *Conners Rating Scales—Revised: Technical manual.* North Tonawanda, NY: Multi-Health Systems.

Conners, C. K., Sitarenios, G., Parker, J. D. A., & Epstein, J. N. (1998a). The revised Conners Parent Rating Scale (CPRS-R): Factor structure, reliability, and criterion validity. *Journal of Abnormal Child Psychology, 26*, 257–268.

Conners, C. K., Sitarenios, G., Parker, J. D. A., & Epstein, J. N. (1998b). Revision and standardization of the Conners Teacher Rating Scale (CTRS-R): Factor structure, reliability, and criterion validity. *Journal of Abnormal Child Psychology, 26*, 279–291.

DuPaul, G. J., Power, T. J., Anastopoulos, A. D., & Reid, R. (1998). *ADHD Rating Scale–IV: Checklists, norms, and clinical interpretation.* New York: Guilford Press.

Foley, H. A., Carlton, C. O., & Howell, R. J. (1996). The relationship of attention deficit hyperactivity disorder and conduct disorder to juvenile delinquency: Legal implications. *Bulletin of the American Academy of Psychiatry and Law, 24*, 333–343.

Frick, P. J. (1998). *Conduct disorders and severe antisocial behavior.* New York: Plenum Press.

Frick, P. J., & Loney, B. (1999). Outcomes of oppositional defiant disorder and conduct disorder. In H. C. Quay & A. E. Hogan (Eds.), *Handbook of disruptive behavior disorders* (pp. 507–524). New York: Plenum Press.

Garland, A. F., Hough, R. L., McCabe, K. M., Yeh, M., Wood, P. A., & Aarons, G. A. (2001). Prevalence of psychiatric disorders in youths across five sectors of care. *Journal of the American Academy of Child and Adolescent Psychiatry, 40*, 409–418.

Goldstein, S. (1997). Attention-deficit/hyperactivity disorder: Implications for the criminal justice system. *FBI Law Enforcement Bulletin, 66*, 11–16.

Grisso, T., & Underwood, L. (2003, January). *Screening and assessing mental health and substance use disorders among youth in the juvenile justice system* (Research and Program Brief). Delmar, NY: National Center for Mental Health and Juvenile Justice.

Henggeler, S. W., Melton, G. B., Brondino, M. J., Scherer, D. G., & Hanley, J. H. (1997). Multisystemic therapy with violent and chronic juvenile offenders and their families: The role of treatment fidelity in successful dissemination. *Journal of Consulting and Clinical Psychology, 65*, 821–833.

Hoge, R., & Andrews, D. (2002). *The Youth Level of Service/Case Management Inventory.* Toronto: Multi-Health Systems.

Kamphaus, R. W., & Frick, P. J. (2002). *Clinical assessment of child and adolescent personality and behavior* (2nd ed.). Boston: Allyn & Bacon.

Kraemer, B. D., Salisbury, S. B., & Spielman, C. R. (1998). Pretreatment variables associated with treatment failure in a residential juvenile sex-offender program. *Criminal Justice and Behavior, 25*, 190–203.

Lahey, B. B., McBurnett, K., & Loeber, R. (2000). Are attention-deficit/hyperactivity disorder and oppositional defiant disorder developmental precursors to conduct disorder? In A. J. Sameroff, M. Lewis, & S. M. Miller (Eds.), *Handbook of developmental psychopathology* (2nd ed., pp. 431–446). New York: Kluwer Academic/Plenum.

Loeber, R., Farrington, D. P., Stouthamer-Loeber, M., Moffitt, T. E., & Caspi, A. (1998). The development of male offending: Key findings from the first decade of the Pittsburgh Youth Study. *Studies on Crime and Crime Prevention, 7*, 141–171.

Loney, B. R., & Lima, E. N. (2003). The classification and assessment of conduct disorders. In C. A. Essau (Ed.), *Conduct and oppositional defiant disorders: Epidemiology, risk factors, and treatment* (pp. 3–31). Mahwah, NJ: Erlbaum.

Lynam, D. R. (1996). The early identification of chronic offenders: Who is the fledgling psychopath? *Psychological Bulletin, 120*, 209–234.

McCarney, S. B. (1995a). *The Attention Deficit Disorders Evaluation Scale—Home Version: Technical manual* (2nd ed.). Columbia, MO: Hawthorne Educational Service.

McCarney, S. B. (1995b). *The Attention Deficit Disorders Evaluation Scale—School Version: Technical manual* (2nd ed.). Columbia, MO: Hawthorne Educational Service.

Miner, M. H. (2002). Factors associated with recidivism in juveniles: an analysis of serious juvenile sex offenders. *Journal of Research in Crime and Delinquency, 39*, 421–436.

Moffitt, T. E. (1993). Adolescent-limited and life-course persistent antisocial behavior: A developmental taxonomy. *Psychological Review, 100*, 674–701.

Power, T. J., Andrews, T. J., Eiraldi, R. B., Doherty, B. J., Ikeda, M. J., DuPaul, G. J., & Landau, S. (1998). Evaluating attention deficit hyperactivity disorder using multiple informants: The incremental utility of combining teacher with parent reports. *Psychological Assessment, 10*, 250–260.

Prentky, R., & Righthand, S. (2003). *Manual for the Juvenile Sex Offender Protocol–II (J-SOAP-II)*. Boston: F&P Associates.

Quinsey, G., Harris G., Rice, M., & Cormier, C. (1996). *Violent offenders: Appraising and managing risk*. Washington, DC: American Psychological Association.

Reid, R. DuPaul, G. J., Power, T. J., Anastopoulos, A. D., Rogers-Adkinson, D., Noll, M., & Riccio, C. (1998). Assessing culturally different students for attention deficit hyperactivity disorder using behavior rating scales. *Journal of Abnormal Child Psychology, 26*, 187–198.

Reid, R., Riccio, C. A., Kessler, R. H., DuPaul, G. J., Power, T. J., Anastopoulos, A. D., et al. (2000). Gender and ethnic differences in ADHD as assessed by behavior ratings. *Journal of Emotional and Behavioral Disorders, 8*, 38–48.

Root, R. W., & Resnick, R. J. (2003). An update on the diagnosis and treatment of attention-deficit/hyperactivity disorder in children. *Professional Psychology: Research and Practice, 34*, 34–41.

Rucklidge, J. J., & Tannock, R. (2001). Psychiatric, psychosocial, and cognitive functioning of female adolescents with ADHD. *Journal of the American Academy of Child and Adolescent Psychiatry, 40*, 530–540.

Smith, B. H., Pelham, W. E., Gnagy, E., Molina, B., & Evans, S. (2000). The reliability, validity, and unique contributions of self-report by adolescents receiving treatment for attention-deficit/hyperactivity disorder. *Journal of Consulting and Clinical Psychology, 68*, 489–499.

Vermeiren, R., de Clippele, A., & Deboutte, D. (2000). Eight month follow-up of delinquent adolescents: Predictors of short-term outcome. *European Archives of Psychiatry, 250,* 133–138.

Wang, E. W., & Diamond, P. M. (1999). Empirically identifying factors related to violence risk in corrections. *Behavioral Sciences and the Law, 17,* 377–389.

Wasserman, G. A., Jensen, P. S., Ko, S. J., Cocozza, J., Trupin, E., Angold, A., et al. (2003). Mental health assessments in juvenile justice: Report on the Consensus Conference. *Journal of the American Academy of Child and Adolescent Psychiatry, 42,* 752–762.

Webster, C., Douglas, K., Eaves, D., & Hart, S. (1997). *HCR-20 Assessing Risk for Violence: Version II.* Burnaby, BC, Canada: Mental Health, Law and Policy Institute, Simon Fraser University.

PART IV

Comprehensive Assessment Instruments

Part IV reviews psychological instruments that are typically used for comprehensive assessments of youths who are thought to have special mental health needs. Each assesses a number of psychological characteristics within the domains of mental health problems, personality traits, and adaptive strengths. They typically require more time and resources than multidimensional or unidimensional screening instruments do. Nevertheless, some of them can be used as screening tools in settings that can afford the cost when applied to every youth at intake.

The comprehensive assessment tools reviewed here are of two types. Some are single instruments administered only to a youth. Others are actually "families" of instruments consisting of several different versions, which are administered to the youth and to collateral informants familiar with the youth's functioning (e.g., parents or teachers). Evaluation instruments that use several informants are especially useful for diagnoses requiring information about problem behaviors in two or more settings (e.g., home and school). Mental health practice is usually improved by obtaining clinical data from informants across several settings, although this is not possible in all juvenile justice contexts.

The first three chapters of Part IV describe "families" of assessment instruments (or tools belonging to such "families"). Chapter 11 presents Achenbach's review of the Achenbach System of Empirically Based Assessment (ASEBA). The ASEBA instruments assess a broad spectrum of behavioral, emotional, and social problems in children, adolescents, and young adults. The three primary ASEBA questionnaires are the Youth Self-Report (YSR), the Child Behavior Checklist (CBCL), and the Teacher's Report Form (TRF), which are filled out by the youth, parent, and teacher, respectively. The YSR by itself is sufficiently brief to be used feasibly as a screening tool.

The Personality Inventory for Children, Second Edition (PIC-2), and two associated measures are reviewed in Chapter 12 by Lachar and Boyd. The original PIC was designed to provide comprehensive information about problems in child adjustment, with scales to assess disruptive behavior, psychological discomfort, social and family adjustment, cognitive development, and school behaviors. Over the last several years, the original PIC has evolved into the PIC-2 and two companion measures completed by teachers (the Student Behavior Survey, or SBS) and by youths (the Personality Inventory for Youth, or PIY).

The Diagnostic Interview Schedule for Children: Present State Voice (Voice DISC) is reviewed by Wasserman and colleagues in Chapter 13. The Voice DISC assesses more than 30 DSM-IV diagnoses and conditions warranting further evaluation, in self-report modules that correspond to diagnostic groupings (e.g., Major Depression, Generalized Anxiety, Oppositional Defiant). Each youth receives a unique computerized interview, depending upon the pattern of his or her responses. "Voice" refers to the fact that the computer administration "speaks" the items to the youth while they are displayed on the video monitor, reducing the need for the youth to be able to read the items. The DISC family of instruments also includes a parent version (not currently "voiced") that assesses a caretaker's report of a youth's mental health disorder.

The final two instruments included in Part IV are the Minnesota Multiphasic Personality Inventory—Adolescent (MMPI-A), reviewed in Chapter 14 by Archer and Baker, and the Millon Adolescent Clinical Inventory (MACI), reviewed by Salekin and colleagues in Chapter 15. Both instruments are administered only to the youth and address a broad range of psychological, emotional, behavioral, substance use, and peer/family difficulties. They also evaluate aspects of adolescent development (e.g., egocentricity, risk-taking behavior) that are of increasing interest to juvenile justice and forensic mental health examiners.

CHAPTER 11

Achenbach System of Empirically Based Assessment

Thomas Achenbach

PURPOSE

The Achenbach System of Empirically Based Assessment (ASEBA, which sounds like "zebra") was developed to meet the need for practical, low-cost assessment of youths in many contexts. These contexts include juvenile justice, mental health, medical, and educational settings. The ASEBA is designed to assess a broad spectrum of behavioral, emotional, and social problems. Because it is also important to evaluate youths' personal strengths, the ASEBA assesses favorable aspects of functioning, as well as problems. Furthermore, because youths may not be willing or able to provide complete and accurate reports of their own functioning, the ASEBA is designed to obtain multiple perspectives on the youths' functioning. The ASEBA does this by providing forms for completion by parent figures and other caregivers, teachers, clinical interviewers, and psychological examiners. It also provides forms for documenting observations of youths' behavior in group settings, such as classrooms and recreational activities.

Youths' behavior may differ markedly from one context to another. To document the variations in youths' behavior, the ASEBA is designed to compare and coordinate reports by people who see the youths in different contexts. In addition, many youths who enter the juvenile justice system have been or will be evaluated in mental health and/or educational settings. As a consequence, there is a need for juvenile justice, mental health, and education personnel to share their knowledge of the youths. To meet the need for communication among all these different personnel, information obtained from the ASEBA can be readily understood by people who have diverse professional backgrounds.

BASIC DESCRIPTION

Forms in the ASEBA

Youth Self-Report Form

The ASEBA includes the Youth Self-Report for Ages 11 to 18 (YSR), which obtains youths' reports of their competencies and problems in both quantitative and qualitative form. Paper forms and interactive computer entry options are available for self-administration by youths having at least fifth-grade reading skills. For youths who cannot complete forms independently, the YSR can be easily administered in about 15 minutes by an interviewer. An interviewer hands a youth a copy of the YSR to look at while retaining a second copy of the YSR. The interviewer then says, "I'm going to read you the questions on this form, and I'll write down your answers." This procedure maintains standardization while avoiding embarrassment and errors on the part of youths who cannot complete YSRs independently. Because the YSR itself is read to the youth, the interviewer does not need any specialized training. The Adult Self-Report for Ages 18 to 59 (ASR) can be used for emancipated minors and youths who have reached age 18. The ASR includes many of the YSR items, plus other items that are geared toward transitions to adulthood. (Users can decide whether the YSR or ASR is more appropriate for particular 18-year-olds.)

Companion Forms for Multiple Perspectives

Youths are important sources of information about their own functioning. However, they may not always provide accurate reports of their competencies and problems. Consequently, it is essential to obtain other perspectives on youths' functioning whenever possible. To do this economically, the ASEBA includes the following companions to the YSR:

- Child Behavior Checklist for Ages 6 to 18 (CBCL/6–18), which is completed by parents, parent surrogates, and others who play parental roles, such as relatives, foster parents, and staff members of residential facilities.
- Adult Behavior Checklist for Ages 18 to 59 (ABCL), which is completed for emancipated minors and youths who have reached age 18 by people who know them.
- Teacher's Report Form (TRF), which is completed by teachers and other educational personnel.

- Semistructured Clinical Interview for Children and Adolescents (SCICA), which is used to assess youths in clinical interviews.
- Direct Observation Form (DOF), which is used to assess youths' functioning in group settings, such as classrooms and group activities.
- Test Observation Form (TOF), which is completed by examiners who administer ability and achievement tests.

Depending on the perspective that is being tapped, the forms are scored on syndromes of behavioral, emotional, and social problems; scales consisting of problem items that are consistent with categories for psychopathology specified by the *Diagnostic and Statistical Manual of Mental Disorders* fourth edition (DSM-IV; American Psychiatric Association, 1994); and scales for favorable characteristics that reflect competence in activities, relationships, and school. Table 11.1 lists the ASEBA forms, the perspectives they tap, and the kinds of scales they include. Table 11.1 also lists references for details about the forms, their applications, reliability, validity, and norms. Each form

TABLE 11.1. ASEBA Forms for Assessing Youths

Forms	Ages	Completed by:	Scales[e]
Youth Self-Report (YSR)[a]	11–18	Youths	Competence, syndromes, DSM-oriented
Adult Self-Report (ASR)[b]	18–59	Emancipated youths, adults	Adaptive, syndromes, DSM-oriented
Child Behavior Checklist (CBCL)[a]	6–18	Parent figures, residential staff	Competence, syndromes, DSM-oriented
Teacher's Report Form (TRF)[a]	6–18	Educational personnel	Academic, adaptive, syndromes, DSM-oriented
Adult Behavior Checklist (ABCL)[b]	18–59	People who know the subject	Adaptive, syndromes, DSM-oriented
Semistructured Clinical Interview for Children and Adolescents (SCICA)[c]	6–18	Interviewers	Syndromes, DSM-oriented, observational, self-report
Direct Observation Form (DOF)[a]	5–14	Observers	Syndromes, on-task behavior
Test Observation Form (TOF)[d]	6–18	Test administrator	Syndromes, DSM-oriented

Note. Footnotes *a–d* below cite references for details of the forms, their applications, reliability, validity, and norms.
[a]Achenbach and Rescorla (2001).
[b]Achenbach and Rescorla (2003).
[c]McConaughy and Achenbach (2001).
[d]McConaughy and Achenbach (2004).
[e]All forms also include scales for Internalizing, Externalizing, and Total Problems scores. "Internalizing" refers to problems that are mainly within the self, such as anxiety, depression, and physical complaints without apparent medical cause. "Externalizing" refers to problems that involve conflicts with other people and with social mores, such as fighting, stealing, and lying.

takes about 15 minutes to complete. To facilitate multicultural applications, translations are available in 71 languages.

The ASEBA forms tap many characteristics that are important for juvenile justice, mental health, educational, and risk evaluations. These characteristics include aggression, rule-breaking behaviors, substance use, depression, anxiety, withdrawal, somatic problems, social problems, attention-deficit/hyperactivity problems, thought problems, and suicidal thoughts and behavior. Because ASEBA forms can obtain and compare data from multiple respondents in diverse contexts, they enable users to obtain comprehensive pictures of youths' functioning that include, but also extend well beyond, self-reports in juvenile justice contexts. Clerical workers can quickly score the forms by hand or computer. The ASEBA profiles display scores in relation to national norms that are gender-, age-, and respondent-specific. The ASEBA software provides systematic comparisons among problems reported by youths, parent figures, and educational personnel.

Multiple Modes for Obtaining Data

ASEBA forms can be used to obtain data in multiple ways, including classic paper-and-pencil formats, machine-readable forms that include both Teleform and optical mark-reading formats, and interactive self-administration on desktop and laptop computers. In addition, a Web-based application called Web-Link enables a user to transmit forms to any Web-enabled computer to be printed on paper or to be displayed on a monitor for interactive entry, with options for different languages. Data from the completed forms are then transmitted back to the user's computer for scoring and comparisons among respondents. Web-Link thus enables users to obtain data from diverse respondents without requiring them to come to the juvenile justice site or to mail forms.

Some of the items on ASEBA forms ask respondents to provide descriptions and comments, as well as ratings of the youth's behavior. The respondents' descriptions and comments provide individualized, qualitative information that is useful for understanding the respondents' ratings and that provides a basis for subsequent queries. Examples of YSR items that request descriptions in addition to ratings are "I drink alcohol without my parents' approval (describe)," "I can't get my mind off certain thoughts (describe)," "I hear sounds or voices that other people think aren't there (describe)," "I have thoughts that other people would think are strange (describe)," and "I use drugs for nonmedical purposes (describe)." To reflect degrees of intensity and frequency, all the problem items are rated 0 = "not true," 1 = "somewhat or sometimes true," or 2 = "very true or often true," based on the preceding 6 months. Other respondents rate and report on analogous items, plus items that youths are unlikely to report about themselves, such as "Plays with own sex parts in public," "Sexual problems (describe)," and "Stares blankly."

Competence, Adaptive Functioning, Problem, and DSM-Oriented Scales

The YSR and CBCL competence items are scored on scales designated as Activities, Social, School, and Total Competence. The Activities scale assesses the quality and amount of the youth's involvement in sports and in other kinds of activities. The Social scale assesses the youth's interpersonal relationships. The School scale assesses the youth's performance and problems in school. And the Total Competence scale combines scores for the Activities, Social, and School scales. The TRF includes scales for Academic Performance and Adaptive Functioning, which includes the teacher's ratings of favorable characteristics that reflect effective adaptation to the school environment.

The YSR, CBCL, and TRF all have eight scales for scoring "syndromes," which constitute patterns of problems identified in statistical analyses of forms completed by 11,982 respondents. Because the syndromes reflect patterns of problems found in parent, teacher, and self-report ratings, they are called "cross-informant syndromes." The eight syndromes are Anxious/Depressed, Withdrawn/Depressed, Somatic Complaints, Social Problems, Thought Problems, Attention Problems, Rule-Breaking Behavior, and Aggressive Behavior. Problem items are also scored in terms of broader groupings designated as Internalizing (comprising the first three syndromes), Externalizing (comprising the last two syndromes), and Total Problems (comprising all problem items on the form). The term "Internalizing" refers to problems that are primarily within the self, such as anxiety, depression, and physical problems without known medical cause. The term "Externalizing" refers to problems that involve conflict with others and with social mores, such as fighting, stealing, and lying.

To provide links to psychiatric diagnoses, the forms are also scored in terms of the following scales, which comprise items selected by an international panel of experts from 16 cultures as being very consistent with diagnostic categories of the American Psychiatric Association's (1994) DSM-IV: Affective Problems, Anxiety Problems, Somatic Problems, Attention Deficit/Hyperactivity Problems, Oppositional Defiant Problems, and Conduct Problems.

Each scale of problems is scored by summing the 0, 1, and 2 ratings for the items comprising the scale. To help users judge whether a youth's score on each scale is normal or deviant, the scales are displayed on profiles. For each scale, percentiles and standard scores (T-scores) are provided that indicate how a youth's score compares with scores obtained by a national sample of peers of the same gender and age, rated by the same type of respondent (e.g., self, parent figure, educator). A percentile indicates the percentage of youths in the national sample who obtained scores less than or equal to a particular score. For example, if a youth obtains a score on the YSR Aggressive Behavior scale that is at the 98th percentile, this means that 98% of youths in the national normative sample obtained scores lower than or equal to the youth's score. Conversely, only 2% of youths obtained higher scores. In other words, the youth's ratings of aggressive behavior on the YSR are higher than the self-ratings of aggression obtained from most youths in the normative sample. *T*-scores also indicate how high a youth's scale score is in comparison to the scale scores obtained by the normative sample of youths. The *T*-scores provide a standard set of numbers for all the scales that show how deviant a youth's scale score is, even though the distributions of raw scores differ from one scale to another. For example, a *T*-score of 70 on any scale indicates that a youth's score is at the 98th percentile, regardless of how many items are on the scale.

Lines printed on the profiles of scale scores indicate scores that are in the "normal" range, "borderline clinical" range, and "clinical" range on each scale. For example, the clinical range for the DSM-oriented and syndrome scales includes scores that are at or above the 98th percentile (*T*-score = 70). The borderline clinical range includes scores that are at the 93rd through 97th percentiles (*T*-scores = 65–69). And the normal range includes scores that are below the 93rd percentile. When evaluating youths, users can consider the ranges shown on the profile, as well as the precise raw score, percentile, and *T*-score obtained by the youth on each scale.

HISTORY OF THE METHOD'S DEVELOPMENT

Development of the ASEBA forms began in the 1960s with efforts to identify patterns of problems (i.e., syndromes) that had not been recognized by the official diagnostic system of the time, which was the first edition of the American Psychiatric Association's (1952) *Diagnostic and Statistical Manual of Mental Disorders* (DSM-I). Statistical analyses of problems reported in psychiatric case histories revealed considerably more syndromes among youths than had been recognized in the official DSM-I system (Achenbach, 1966).

Development of the YSR, CBCL, and TRF

Based on the initial findings and subsequent testing of successive pilot editions with thousands of youths, the YSR, CBCL, and TRF were published with manuals that included extensive reliability, validity, and normative data (e.g., Achenbach & Edelbrock, 1983). The "reliability" data showed that the forms could be relied upon to produce consistent results if they were repeated on the same youths over periods when the youths' behavior was not likely to change. The "validity" data showed that scores obtained from the forms validly identified youths who needed mental health services. And the normative data consisted of scores for large samples of typical youths that provided "norms" (i.e., yardsticks with which to determine whether scores obtained by particular youths deviate from those obtained by most typical youths). The three forms were scored on profiles of scales. The scales were derived and normed separately for each gender within particular age ranges, as rated by each type of informant. This was done to reflect possible gender, age, and informant differences in the patterning of problems. Because the scales were statistically derived separately for each gender/age group, there were substantial differences between some of the scales on the different profiles.

In 1991, revised profiles were published that included eight "cross-informant syndromes"—that is, patterns of problems identified in ratings by different kinds of informants, including parents, teachers, and youths, for both genders at different ages (Achenbach, 1991). The cross-informant syndromes made it easy to directly compare a youth's scores on each syndrome as seen by the youth, by parent figures, and by educational personnel. Software was published that provided systematic comparisons between item and scale scores obtained from each informant in terms of the eight syndromes, Internalizing, Externalizing, and Total Problems.

In 2001, slightly revised versions of the YSR, CBCL, and TRF and their scoring profiles were published with a new manual that documents their reliability, validity, and norms based on a new national probability sample (Achenbach & Rescorla, 2001). The revised forms included new items for alcohol and tobacco use; for breaking rules at home, school, or elsewhere; for lack of enjoyment (anhedonia); and for attention deficits. Based on extensive analyses that included the new items, the eight cross-informant syndromes were revised somewhat. The name of the Delinquent Behavior syndrome was changed to Rule-Breaking Behavior, to take account of its broad range of problem behaviors that include (but are not limited to) behaviors subject to adjudication as delinquent. Because the correlations between the 2001 syndromes and their 1991 counterparts were very high (Achenbach & Rescorla, 2001), the numerous findings obtained with the earlier versions can be generalized to the 2001 versions of the syndromes.

Profiles of DSM-Oriented Scales

Another important innovation of the 2001 forms was the addition of DSM-oriented scales that indicate deviance in terms of major DSM-IV diagnostic categories. Like the syndrome scales, the DSM-oriented scales display scores on profiles in relation to norms that are specific to boys and girls of particular ages, as reported by parent figures, educational personnel, and the youths themselves. As explained earlier, these scales comprise items that an international panel of experts identified as being very consistent with DSM-IV diagnostic categories. Scores on the DSM-oriented scales are significantly associated with DSM-IV diagnoses (Achenbach & Rescorla, 2001, pp. 129–130). However, neither the DSM-oriented scales nor any other measure should be the sole basis for making diagnostic decisions. Instead, multiple kinds and sources of data need to be integrated as a basis for diagnostic decisions.

Critical Items, Narrative Reports, and Bar Graph Comparisons

The software for scoring the 2001 forms prints scores for critical items that are of particular clinical concern. It also prints narrative reports that verbally summarize findings. These reports can be easily understood by nonclinical personnel (e.g., juvenile justice administrators/staff and court personnel) who are unfamiliar with standardized psychological assessment instruments. An additional important innovation of the software is the display of bar graphs that compare scale scores obtained from up to eight respondents for each youth. These bar graphs enable users to see at a glance the areas in which respondents consistently report problems in the clinical versus borderline clinical versus normal range. The bar graphs also enable users to quickly identify differences among informants' reports. For example, users can quickly identify youths who report high levels of anxiety, depression, or somatic problems that are not reported by other respondents. Conversely, users can identify youths who fail to report problems, such as aggression and rule-breaking behavior, that are reported by other respondents. Both kinds of discrepancies are crucial for identifying mental health issues, for planning appropriate services, and for evaluating change as seen both by the youths and by people who know them.

Forms for Assessing Adults and Emancipated Minors

Youths often remain involved with juvenile justice systems during the transition to adulthood. For example, commitment to the juvenile justice system can be "extended" beyond 18 years of age (usually to age 21) for youths who pose a high recidivism risk, but are not viewed as appropriate subjects for criminal court. To provide continuity of developmentally appropriate, multi-informant assessment, the Young Adult Self-Report (YASR) and Young Adult Behavior Checklist (YABCL) were published as upward extensions of the YSR and CBCL, respectively (Achenbach, 1997). Revised versions of the YASR and YABCL were published in 2003 as the ASR and the ABCL, respectively (Achenbach & Rescorla, 2003).

The ASR and ABCL have many problem items in common with the ASEBA forms for youths. However, they also have problem and adaptive functioning items and scales that are appropriate for adults and emancipated minors. Examples include questions about job performance, relations with spouse or partner, drinking too much alcohol, meeting responsibilities, staying away from job when not sick and not on vacation, failing to pay debts, and doing things that may cause trouble with the law. In addition, the adult forms have scales for assessing the number of times per day the individual used tobacco, the number of days on which the individual was drunk, and the number of days on which drugs were used for nonmedical purposes in the preceding 6 months. Separate norms are provided for each gender at ages 18–35 and 36–59, based on self-reports for the ASR scores and reports by people who know the individual being assessed with the ABCL.

RESEARCH EVIDENCE

Over 5,000 publications report the use of ASEBA forms in 62 cultures (Bérubé & Achenbach, 2005). Norms and research studies provide data for each gender at ages 6–11 and 12–18 on the CBCL and TRF, and 11–18 on the YSR. Adolescent development issues have been taken into account by obtaining self-reports and feedback from 11- to 18-year-olds, their parents, their teachers, and clinicians during the development of each ASEBA form and scoring profile. In addition, ASEBA manuals display the percentage of youths, their parents, and their teachers who endorsed each ASEBA item, separately for clinically referred and nonreferred boys and girls in 2-year age intervals. Because so many studies have been published on hundreds of topics, only a few examples are possible in the space available here.

The ASEBA manuals summarize key research findings and present detailed analyses of ethnic and socioeconomic (SES) differences in national probability samples that are representative of the United States. In brief, when SES is controlled for, ethnic differences for ASEBA scores within the United States are typically found to be negligible (Achenbach & Rescorla, 2001, 2003). In addition, comparisons of ASEBA problem scores across multiple cultures have indicated that the differences in reported problems among most cultures are remarkably small. Furthermore, there is considerable cross-cultural similarity in the problems that are most common versus least common. These findings were obtained from parents' CBCL ratings of 13,697 children and youths from the following 12 cultures: Australia, Belgium, China, Germany, Greece, Israel, Jamaica, The Netherlands, Puerto Rico, Sweden, Thailand, and the United States (Crijnen, Achenbach, & Verhulst, 1997, 1999). Similar findings were obtained on YSRs completed by 7,137 youths from the following seven cultures: Australia, China, Israel, Jamaica, The Netherlands, Turkey, and the United States (Verhulst et al., 2003). The levels of agreement between ratings by youths, parents, and teachers have also been found to be similar in China, Jamaica, The Netherlands, Puerto Rico, and the United States (Verhulst & Achenbach, 1995).

Examples of findings for juvenile justice populations include strong associations between CBCL/YSR scores on the one hand and drug abuse, symptoms of the DSM-IV diagnosis of conduct disorder, and suicidality on the other (Crowley, Mikulich, Ehlers, Whitmore, & MacDonald, 2001; Ruchkin, Schwab-Stone, Koposov, Vermeiren, & King, 2003). Examples of long-term prediction of delinquent behaviors from ASEBA scores include significant prediction of police contacts and substance abuse over 6- and 8-year periods from childhood to adolescence and from adolescence to young adulthood (Achenbach, Howell, McConaughy, & Stanger, 1995, 1998; Ferdinand, Blum, & Verhulst, 2001). Similar significant predictions have also been found over 10-year periods from childhood and adolescence to young adulthood (Hofstra, van der Ende, & Verhulst, 2001). In addition, these studies showed significant prediction of other problems that may be of concern to juvenile justice, such as suicidal behavior, unwed pregnancy, dropping out of school, receipt of mental health services, and being fired from jobs.

To obtain references for reports relating to juvenile justice, ethnic characteristics, particular kinds of problems, outcomes, and other topics, readers can consult the *Bibliography of Published Studies Using the ASEBA Instruments* (Bérubé & Achenbach, 2005), which is updated annually. Examples of juvenile justice topics in the 2005 volume include the following, with the number of references for each topic shown in parentheses: Aggression (276), Alcohol (58), Antisocial Conduct (116), Conduct Disorder (169), Delinquent (Rule-Breaking) Behavior (95), Outcomes (384), Substance Abuse (134), and Violence (108). Reports of findings related to ethnic and cultural factors include the following topics: African American (97), Asian (160), Hispanic/Latino (66), Native American (15), and Cross-Cultural Research (1,420). Numerous findings support the reliability, validity, utility, and generalizability of scores obtained with ASEBA instruments (reviewed by Achenbach & Rescorla, 2001, 2003).

APPLICATION

ASEBA forms, software, manuals, and training videos are available from the Research Center for Children, Youth, and Families, a nonprofit center at the University of Vermont. Information about ordering, practical applications, references, and research updates from around the world can be obtained at *http://www.aseba.org*. As documented in over 5,000 publications by some 8,000 authors, ASEBA instruments are used in many settings for many purposes (Bérubé & Achenbach, 2005). Because the YSR, CBCL, TRF, ASR, and ABCL are self-administered, no special qualifications are needed for administering them. Personnel who give the forms to respondents should explain the purpose for completing the forms and should be available to answer questions. Questions should be answered in a straightforward manner without clinical probing.

Interpretations of ASEBA profiles should be done by people with training in standardized assessment of youths. The level of training is typically commensurate with what can be obtained in master's-degree programs in psychology, special education, social work, counseling, and related fields. The most important preparation for users is to read the relevant ASEBA manual and related documentation.

ASEBA forms can be used in many ways in juvenile justice contexts. For example, initial assessment can include having a youth complete the YSR and having any available parent figures complete the CBCL. If the youth has attended an educational program, all available teachers and other educational personnel can be asked to complete TRFs. To facilitate data collection, Web-Link can be used to send electronic requests and forms to respondents who have access to Web-enabled computers. The data can then be returned electronically or on paper forms to the user's computer for scoring and cross-informant comparisons.

Profiles of syndromes, DSM-oriented scales, and competence scales, as well as cross-informant bar graphs and item comparisons, can be generated by clerical workers. Juvenile justice staffers and mental health professionals can examine comments and open-ended responses made on the completed ASEBA forms. They can also examine computer-scored or hand-scored profiles to identify scores that indicate needs for mental health evaluation. Examples include scores on items and scales concerning suicidal ideation and behavior, depression, anxiety, withdrawal, social problems, attention problems, thought problems, and aggression. Depending on the patterns of cross-informant similarities and differences, as well as other information, it may be decided that a clinical interview is needed. If an interview is needed, the SCICA can be administered and then scored on a profile that is analogous to the profiles scored from the YSR, CBCL, and TRF. It may also be decided that one or more ability or achievement tests should be administered. The examiner who administers the test(s) can use the TOF to record psychopathology observed during testing. If it is decided to observe behavior in group settings, the DOF can be used to record problems and on-task behavior.

As an example, suppose that a youth displays strange behavior or strange ideas. It would then be important to answer questions about whether the youth has a thought disorder, mental retardation, and/or substance use problems that affect the youth's behavior and cognition. ASEBA forms completed by the youth, parent figures, other caregivers, and/or teachers can be compared to determine whether they indicate strange behavior or thoughts. If only one or two informants report strange behavior or thoughts, those informants can be asked to describe the circumstances, in order to determine whether situational factors explain the strange behavior or thoughts. This information can also be used to determine whether clinical problems need to be considered in plans for treatment, diversion programs, probation, or other options. However, psycholegal decisions should always be based on multiple factors, including the youth's offenses, past history, medical examinations, and the availability of suitable options.

In general, youths who consistently obtain high scores for competencies and adaptive functioning, and low scores for problems according to multiple informants, may be especially good candidates for diversion and community service options. Youths who consistently obtain moderate scores for competencies, adaptive functioning, and problems may be appropriate candidates for probation and other forms of close judicial supervision in the community. Youths who consistently obtain low scores for competence and adaptive functioning, but high scores for anxiety, depression, thought problems, and/or attention problems, are apt to need mental health services. And youths who consistently obtain low scores for competencies and adaptive functioning, but high scores mainly for aggressive and rule-breaking behavior, may be the most appropriate for structured correctional settings (if such settings are warranted by their offenses).

In order to measure changes in diverse aspects of youths' functioning, ASEBA forms can be readministered periodically (e.g., at intervals of 3–6 months). Because the YSR, CBCL, TRF, ASR, and ABCL can be self-administered and are scored by clerical workers, they do not require time on the part of juvenile justice or mental health workers. Multi-informant ASEBA forms can be readministered again to evaluate outcomes after youths' complete particular programs. By comparing multirespondent profiles at completion of a program with profiles obtained at the beginning of the program, juvenile justice and mental health staffers can evaluate evidence for improvement or deterioration in individual youths.

If the same forms and profiles are used in more than one program, they can be compared for youths in each program to identify differences in outcomes for the different programs. If randomized procedures are used to assign youths to different programs, statistical comparisons of ASEBA data can be used to test differences in the effectiveness of the programs.

CASE EXAMPLE

Fifteen-year-old Robert L. was brought to a juvenile detention center after he was apprehended in a stolen car. To the intake worker, Robert looked like a scared little boy who was trying to act tough. As part of the center's admission procedure, the worker told Robert about the center, how long he might stay there, and what might happen next. He also told Robert that he wanted to get to know him so that he could contact Robert's family and provide any help that Robert needed for medical and other problems. The worker then asked several standard questions about illnesses, medications, allergies, and special dietary needs. Robert answered mainly in monosyllables. When the worker asked where Robert went to school, he named an alternative high school program. The police report indicated that Robert was living at a group home.

To initiate screening for mental health problems and adaptive functioning, the worker asked Robert what kinds of things he liked to do in his spare time. He learned that Robert especially liked computers and could do programming. Because Robert was clearly very comfortable with computers, the worker told Robert that he would like him to fill out the YSR, and that he could do it on a computer if he preferred. When Robert agreed, the worker took him to the center's computer room and set him up to do the computerized client entry version of the YSR. The worker remained nearby in case there were questions or other issues.

After the 15 minutes needed for Robert to complete the computerized YSR, the worker printed out the protocol of Robert's responses. This included his open-ended responses, plus his YSR profiles for competence, syndromes, and DSM-oriented scales; the list of his scores on critical items; and the narrative report. By looking at Robert's YSR syndrome profile (Figure 11.1), the worker saw that Robert scored in the clinical range on the Anxious/Depressed, Withdrawn/Depressed, and Thought Problems syndromes. On the profile of DSM-oriented scales, the worker saw that Robert scored in the clinical range on the Affective (i.e., depressive) Problems and Anxiety Problems scales. Critical items endorsed by Robert included "I deliberately try to hurt or kill myself," "I hear sounds or voices that other people think aren't there," and "I think about killing myself." Altogether, enough possible mental health problems were evident to place Robert on suicide precautions and to get information from others who knew him.

The intake worker contacted the house parents at Robert's group home to ask them to complete CBCLs and to obtain consent for two of Robert's teachers to complete TRFs. Because both the group home and the school were equipped with computers connected to the Web, it was easy to transmit the forms electronically. The house parents and the two teachers entered their own data and transmitted the data to the detention center via Web-Link, which avoided the need for any key entry by data clerks. The data were scored and cross-informant comparisons were printed out on a computer at the detention center.

Robert had lived with his mother until he entered the group home 4 months earlier. Because she lived in the area and continued to have contact with Robert, it was decided to ask her to complete a CBCL. Although she could not read or write English very well, she was literate in her native language, for which a translation of the CBCL was available. Because the layout of the translation is the same as the layout of the English-language CBCL, a clerical worker at the detention center could easily enter the data into the English-language scoring software.

Profiles and cross-informant comparisons displayed item and scale scores from the YSR completed by Robert, the three CBCLs completed by the group home parents and his mother, and the TRFs completed by the two teachers. The completed ASEBA forms, profiles, and cross-informant comparisons were provided to the detention center's mental health consultant with other information about Robert's case.

By looking at the bar graphs comparing syndrome scores from all six respondents, the mental health consultant quickly saw that, like Robert, most of the adult respondents reported enough problems in the Anxious/Depressed and Withdrawn/Depressed syndromes to place Robert in the clinical range, as shown in Figure 11.2. The bar graphs of the DSM-oriented scales showed that most of the respondents also reported enough problems on the Affective (i.e., depressive) Problems and Anxiety Problems scales to place Robert in either the borderline clinical or the clinical range. As explained earlier, the borderline clinical range spans the 93rd through the 97th percentiles (T-scores of 65–69). Unlike Robert, most of the adult respondents reported enough problems of the Social Problems and Rule-Breaking Behavior syndromes to place him in

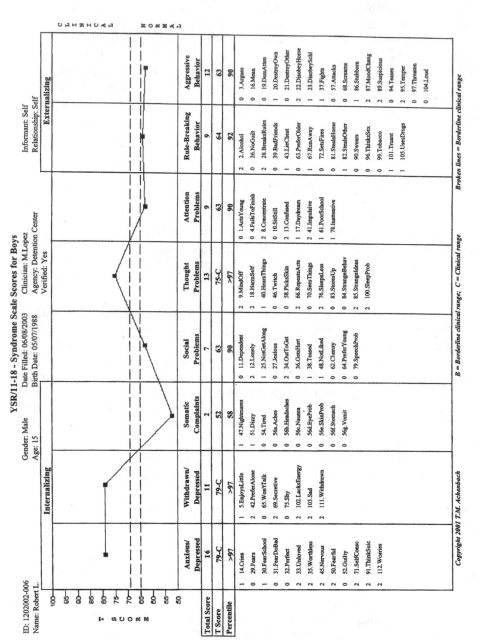

FIGURE 11.1. Profile of syndrome scale scores obtained from the YSR completed by Robert L.

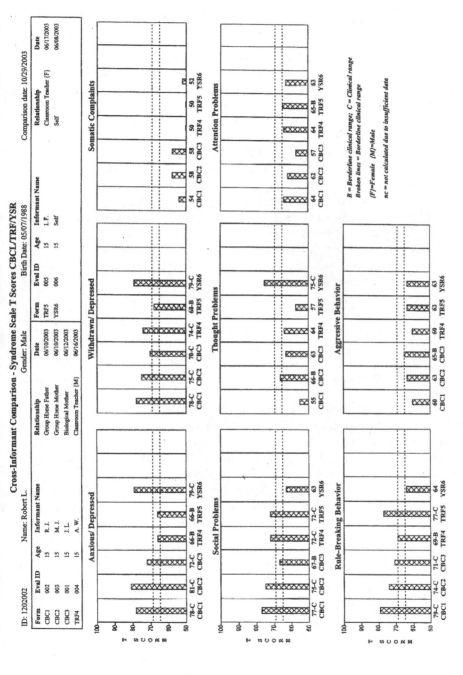

FIGURE 11.2. Cross-informant comparison of syndrome scale scores obtained from the YSR, three CBCL/6–18 forms, and two TRFs completed for Robert L.

the borderline or clinical range. However, only Robert reported suicidal tendencies and enough problems on the Thought Problems scale to reach the clinical range. This last scale includes problems such as "Can't get mind off certain thoughts," "Deliberately tries to hurt or kill self," "Hears sounds or voices that other people think aren't there," and "Strange ideas."

There was thus great consistency among all the respondents in reporting considerably more problems of depression, anxiety, and withdrawal than were reported for national normative samples of adolescent boys. There was also consistency among the adult respondents in reporting elevated rates of social problems and rule-breaking behavior, which were not reported by Robert. This suggested that Robert was unwilling or unable to report these problems, but that they were evident to other people. On the other hand, only Robert reported thought problems and suicidal tendencies, indicating that these were not evident to his mother, his group home parents, or his teachers.

In Robert's case, his own reports of thought problems and suicidal tendencies prompted the detention center staff to take suicide precautions. On the other hand, his failure to report social problems and rule-breaking behaviors that were reported by all the other informants indicated that he could not be relied upon to report all aspects of his problems.

On the competence and adaptive functioning scales, there was consistency in reports that Robert had some important skills and strengths, but that his relations with peers and adults were poor. On open-ended items focused on the best things about Robert, most respondents noted his talent for computers and ability to spend long hours working and playing on them. His interest and ability in information technology provided a potential focus for helping him.

Robert's prior lack of serious delinquency, his problems with anxiety and depression, and the potential for capitalizing on his interest and ability in information technology warranted a recommendation for a court diversion program. The diversion program was designed to include mental health services to treat his depressive and anxiety problems, suicidal tendencies, and alienation; to improve his social skills; and to overcome problems with reality testing. A psychiatrist was to evaluate Robert for antipsychotic and antidepressant medications. A therapist was to work closely with Robert's teachers and group home parents to foster the development of his computer skills in ways that would also enhance his social skills, such as through membership in a computer club. The ASEBA forms were to be completed 6 months later to evaluate Robert's progress, and 12 months later to evaluate the outcome of the 1-year diversion program.

REFERENCES

Achenbach, T. M. (1966). The classification of children's psychiatric symptoms: A factor-analytic study. *Psychological Monographs, 80*(Whole No. 615).

Achenbach, T. M. (1991). *Integrative guide for the 1991 CBCL/4–18, YSR, and TRF Profiles.* Burlington: University of Vermont, Department of Psychiatry.

Achenbach, T. M. (1997). *Manual for the Young Adult Self-Report and Young Adult Behavior Checklist.* Burlington: University of Vermont, Department of Psychiatry.

Achenbach, T. M., & Edelbrock, C. (1983). *Manual for the Child Behavior Checklist and Revised Child Behavior Profile.* Burlington: University of Vermont, Department of Psychiatry.

Achenbach, T. M., Howell, C. T., McConaughy, S. H., & Stanger, C. (1995). Six-year predictors of problems in a national sample of children and youth: II. Signs of disturbance. *Journal of the American Academy of Child and Adolescent Psychiatry, 34,* 488–498.

Achenbach, T. M., Howell, C. T., McConaughy, S. H., & Stanger, C. (1998). Six-year predictors of problems in a national sample: IV. Young adult signs of disturbance. *Journal of the American Academy of Child and Adolescent Psychiatry, 37,* 718–727.

Achenbach, T. M., & Rescorla, L. A. (2001). *Manual for the ASEBA School-Age Forms and Profiles.* Burlington: University of Vermont, Research Center for Children, Youth, and Families.

Achenbach, T. M., & Rescorla, L. A. (2003). *Manual for the ASEBA Adult Forms and Profiles.* Burlington: University of Vermont, Research Center for Children, Youth, and Families.

American Psychiatric Association. (1952). *Diagnostic and statistical manual of mental disorders.* Washington, DC: Author.

American Psychiatric Association. (1994). *Diagnostic and statistical manual of mental disorders* (4th ed.). Washington, DC: Author.

Bérubé, R. L., & Achenbach, T. M. (2005). *Bibliography of published studies using the Achenbach System of Empirically Based Assessment (ASEBA): 2005 edition.* Burlington: University of Vermont, Research Center for Children, Youth, and Families.

Crijnen, A. A. M., Achenbach, T. M., & Verhulst, F. C. (1997). Comparisons of problems reported by parents of children in 12 cultures: Total Problems, Externalizing, and Internalizing. *Journal of the American Academy of Child and Adolescent Psychiatry, 36,* 1269–1277.

Crijnen, A. A. M., Achenbach, T. M., & Verhulst, F. C. (1999). Comparisons of problems reported by parents of children in twelve cultures: The CBCL/4–18 syndrome constructs. *American Journal of Psychiatry, 156,* 569–574.

Crowley, T. J., Mikulich, S. K., Ehlers, K. M., Whitmore, E. A., & MacDonald, M. J. (2001). Validity of structured clinical evaluations in adolescents with conduct and substance problems. *Journal of the American Academy of Child and Adolescent Psychiatry, 36,* 1269–1277.

Ferdinand, R. F., Blüm, M., & Verhulst, F. C. (2001). Psychopathology in adolescence predicts substance use in young adulthood. *Addiction, 96,* 861–870.

Hofstra, M. B., van der Ende, J., & Verhulst, F. C. (2001). Adolescents' self-reported problems as predictors of psychopathology in adulthood: 10-year follow-up study. *British Journal of Psychiatry, 179,* 203–209.

McConaughy, S. H., & Achenbach, T. M. (2001). *Manual for the Semistructured Clinical Interview for Children and Adolescents* (2nd ed.). Burlington: University of Vermont, Research Center for Children, Youth, and Families.

McConaughy, S. H., & Achenbach, T. M. (2004). *Manual for the Test Observation Form for Ages 2 to 18*. Burlington: University of Vermont, Research Center for Children, Youth, and Families.

Ruchkin, V. V., Schwab-Stone, M., Koposov, R. A., Vermeiren, R., & King, R. A. (2003). Suicidal ideations and attempts in juvenile delinquents. *Journal of Child Psychology and Psychiatry, 44*, 1058–1066.

Verhulst, F. C., & Achenbach, T. M. (1995). Empirically based assessment and taxonomy of psychopathology: Cross-cultural applications. *European Child and Adolescent Psychiatry, 4*, 61–76.

Verhulst, F. C., Achenbach, T. M., van der Ende, J., Erol, N., Lambert, M. C., Leung, P. W. L., et al. (2003). Comparisons of problems reported by youths from seven countries. *American Journal of Psychiatry, 160*, 1479–1485.

CHAPTER 12

Personality Inventory for Children, Second Edition; Personality Inventory for Youth; and Student Behavior Survey

David Lachar
Jenine Boyd

PURPOSE

Over 45 years ago, two University of Minnesota psychology professors (Robert D. Wirt and William E. Broen, Jr.)—influenced by the development of a comprehensive objective measure of adult adjustment, the Minnesota Multiphasic Personality Inventory (MMPI)—began to develop a similar measure for children and adolescents. The Personality Inventory for Children (PIC; Wirt, Lachar, Klinedinst, & Seat, 1977) represented one of the first multidimensional questionnaires that was designed to be completed by a parent to provide estimates of child adjustment. It took 25 years of effort to finally publish the PIC. Validity scales were also developed to estimate the accuracy of these adjustment estimates (Wirt et al., 1977).

The PIC was designed to provide comprehensive information about problems in child adjustment, with scales to assess disruptive behavior, psychological discomfort, social and family adjustment, cognitive development, and school behaviors. The PIC efficiently generates the type of information that is valued and most often requested in various assessment settings where parents participate in developing a better understanding of youth adjustment. One example of such an application is a court-ordered evaluation of a detained juvenile. In this application, the judge requests a psychological evaluation to obtain additional information about a juvenile's mental status and emotional needs, in order to assist in determining the necessary services and disposition. In this regard, the development of statistically derived standards that identify problems deemed to be of clinical significance and in need of professional attention was especially valuable in meeting this objective.

Over the last several years, the PIC has evolved into a "family" of similar objective assessment measures completed by parents (the Personality Inventory for Children, Second Edition, or PIC-2); by teachers (the Student Behavior Survey, or SBS); and by youth (the Personality Inventory for Youth, or PIY). These measures can be administered jointly or individually to answer specific questions. For example, when diagnostic standards (e.g., the criteria for a diagnosis of attention-deficit/hyperactivity disorder [ADHD]) require evidence that disruptive behavior is demonstrated in two or more settings, the PIC-2 and SBS may be applied to survey home and classroom adjustment, respectively, by application of indexes that measure relevant problem behavior dimensions. The PIY may also be applied to assess both a student's adjustment problems and his or her willingness to share such problems with concerned professionals. When applied together, the PIC-2, PIY, and SBS provide clinical information that meets contemporary testing standards for the comprehensive assessment of mental health needs in youth (Lachar, 1998, 2003).

BASIC DESCRIPTION

Personality Inventory for Children, Second Edition

The PIC-2 (Lacher & Gruber, 2001), which is also available in Spanish (see Lachar & Gruber, 2001, Appendix D), requires informant reading comprehension skills at the fourth-grade level. The statements are completed by endorsing a response of either "true" or "false." Responses to all 275 statements (completed in 40–60 minutes) generate a profile of 3 validity scales, 9 clinical scales, and 21 subscales (see Figure 12.1 for an example of a computer-generated PIC-2 Standard Form Profile). PIC-2 scales were standardized on two gender-specific student samples collected across all of the school years, kindergarten through 12th grade (ages 5 through 18).

The "scale," an accumulation of statement responses, is the primary element of assessment for the PIC-2, PIY, and SBS. Items were selected for these scales by application of a multiple-stage process. Potential statements were first identified because of dominant content or previous use in another test. Statement performance was then investigated to demonstrate statistical support for scale placement. Scales placed on published versions of these tests evidenced adequate internal consistency, test–retest stability, and concurrent validity (the ability of a scale to predict important clinical behaviors and symptoms). Scales may also be further divided on the basis of statement factor analysis (a form of item analysis) into shorter subscales that are characterized by increased content homogeneity. These subscales facilitate test interpreta-

Personality Inventory for Children, Second Edition (PIC-2)
A WPS TEST REPORT by David Lachar, Ph.D., Christian P. Gruber, Ph.D.
Copyright ©2003 by Western Psychological Services
12031 Wilshire Blvd., Los Angeles, California 90025-1251
Version 1.110

Child Name: Case Study
Birthdate: 10-6-88
Age: 15
Respondent: Not Entered
Date Administered: 11/24/03

Gender: Male
Grade: 8

Date Processed: 11/27/03

Child ID: Not Entered
Ethnicity: White

Relationship to Child: Father
Administered By: Jenine Boyd

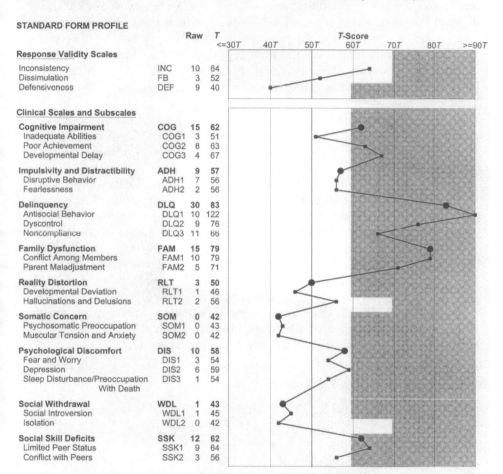

STANDARD FORM PROFILE

		Raw	T				T-Score			

Response Validity Scales

Scale	Code	Raw	T
Inconsistency	INC	10	64
Dissimulation	FB	3	52
Defensiveness	DEF	9	40

Clinical Scales and Subscales

Scale	Code	Raw	T
Cognitive Impairment	**COG**	**15**	**62**
Inadequate Abilities	COG1	3	51
Poor Achievement	COG2	8	63
Developmental Delay	COG3	4	67
Impulsivity and Distractibility	**ADH**	**9**	**57**
Disruptive Behavior	ADH1	7	56
Fearlessness	ADH2	2	56
Delinquency	**DLQ**	**30**	**83**
Antisocial Behavior	DLQ1	10	122
Dyscontrol	DLQ2	9	76
Noncompliance	DLQ3	11	66
Family Dysfunction	**FAM**	**15**	**79**
Conflict Among Members	FAM1	10	79
Parent Maladjustment	FAM2	5	71
Reality Distortion	**RLT**	**3**	**50**
Developmental Deviation	RLT1	1	46
Hallucinations and Delusions	RLT2	2	56
Somatic Concern	**SOM**	**0**	**42**
Psychosomatic Preoccupation	SOM1	0	43
Muscular Tension and Anxiety	SOM2	0	42
Psychological Discomfort	**DIS**	**10**	**58**
Fear and Worry	DIS1	3	54
Depression	DIS2	6	59
Sleep Disturbance/Preoccupation With Death	DIS3	1	54
Social Withdrawal	**WDL**	**1**	**43**
Social Introversion	WDL1	1	45
Isolation	WDL2	0	42
Social Skill Deficits	**SSK**	**12**	**62**
Limited Peer Status	SSK1	9	64
Conflict with Peers	SSK2	3	56

NOTE: Actuarial interpretive guidelines for the scales of the PIC-2 Standard Form Profile are highlighted in chapter 3 (pages 19 - 53) of the 2001 PIC-2 manual.

FIGURE 12.1. Personality Inventory for Children, Second Edition (PIC-2) Standard Form Profile generated from paternal response for case study. The PIC-2 Standard Form Profile copyright (c) 2001, 2003 by Western Psychological Services. Reprinted by permission of the publisher, Western Psychological Services, 12031 Wilshire Boulevard, Los Angeles, CA 90025, U.S.A., *http://www. wpspublish.com*. Not to be reprinted in whole or in part for any additional purpose without the express written permission of the publisher. All rights reserved.

tion. On the other hand, scales may be combined into composite dimensions on the basis of their similarity or frequent correlation to provide summary measures that are sensitive to symptomatic change upon readministration.

The validity scales, as explained in more detail later in this chapter, play a critical role in evaluating the accuracy of the information obtained by estimating the role that defensiveness, exaggeration, or inadequate attention or comprehension contributed to questionnaire response. Scale raw scores are transformed into a standard score, the *T*-score, in which the normative average score is set as a standard of 50 and the distribution or variability of scores is transformed with 1 standard deviation set at 10. In this manner, average *T*-score values most often fall between 40*T* and 60*T*, with mild problems most often designated in the 60s, moderate problems in the 70s, and extreme problems most often designated in excess of 79*T*.

A critical-items list comprises 106 items arranged into nine categories (Cognitive Status and School Adjustment; Developmental Deviation; Inattention and Disruptive Behavior; Depression and Worry; Health Concerns; Reality Distortion; Peer Relations; Dyscontrol and Antisocial Orientation; Family Discord). This list provides a comprehensive evaluation of deficits in adaptation, emotion, and behavior across a wide range of intensity and frequency. Completion of the first 96 items in the PIC-2 administration booklet or a self-scoring form (in 15 minutes or less) provides a standard score display of nine short adjustment scales and four scale composites, entitled the PIC-2 Behavioral Summary Profile. Because of the manner in which the statements of the short scales were selected (see the description later in this chapter), this profile was designed to support the selection of treatment interventions. The scale composites, as summary measures, were designed to quantify change in adjustment through repeated administration (see Figure 12.2 for an example of a computer-generated PIC-2 Behavioral Summary Profile).

Personality Inventory for Youth

The PIY (Lachar & Gruber, 1995), which is also available in Spanish (Negy, Lachar, & Gruber, 1998; Negy, Lachar, Gruber, & Garza, 2001), includes 270 self-report statements primarily derived from PIC statement content. The items require a mid-third-grade to low-fourth-grade reading comprehension level, and are completed by endorsing a response of either "true" or "false." PIY results are presented via a profile of 4 validity scales, 9 clinical scales, and 24 subscales with content dimensions comparable to the PIC-2 (see Figure 12.3 for an example of a computer-generated PIY Profile). In addition, 32 statements from the first 80 items of the PIY form a screening scale intended to provide optimal identification of those regular education students who, when administered the full PIY, produce clinically significant results. Also included are three "scan items" for each clinical scale, selected in such a manner that students who endorse at least two of each set of three items will have

PIC-2: BEHAVIORAL SUMMARY PROFILE

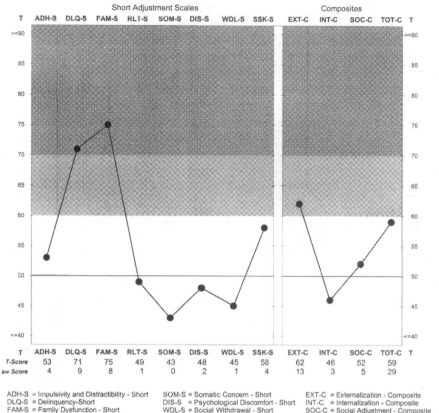

T	ADH-S	DLQ-S	FAM-S	RLT-S	SOM-S	DIS-S	WDL-S	SSK-S	EXT-C	INT-C	SOC-C	TOT-C	T
T-Score	53	71	75	49	43	48	45	58	62	46	52	59	
aw Score	4	9	8	1	0	2	1	4	13	3	5	29	

ADH-S = Impulsivity and Distractibility - Short
DLQ-S = Delinquency-Short
FAM-S = Family Dysfunction - Short
RLT-S = Reality Distortion - Short

SOM-S = Somatic Concern - Short
DIS-S = Psychological Discomfort - Short
WDL-S = Social Withdrawal - Short
SSK-S = Social Skill Deficits-Short

EXT-C = Externalization - Composite
INT-C = Internalization - Composite
SOC-C = Social Adjustment - Composite
TOT-C = Total Score - Composite

NOTE: Actuarial interpretive guidelines for the scales of the PIC-2 Behavioral Summary Profile are highlighted in chapter 4 (pages 55 - 66) of the 2001 PIC-2 manual

FIGURE 12.2. PIC-2 Behavioral Summary Profile generated from paternal response for case study. The PIC-2 Behavioral Summary Profile copyright (c) 2001, 2003 by Western Psychological Services. Reprinted by permission of the publisher, Western Psychological Services, 12031 Wilshire Boulevard, Los Angeles, CA 90025, U.S.A., *http://www.wpspublish.com.* Not to be reprinted in whole or in part for any additional purpose without the express, written permission of the publisher. All rights reserved.

Personality Inventory for Youth (PIY)

A WPS TEST REPORT by David Lachar, Ph.D., Christian P. Gruber, Ph.D.
Copyright ©1997-2003 by Western Psychological Services
12031 Wilshire Blvd., Los Angeles, California 90025-1251
Version 1.110

Youth Name: Case Study
Birthdate: 10-6-88
Age: 15
Date Administered: 11/24/03

Gender: Male
Grade: 8
Date Processed: 11/27/03

Youth ID: Not Entered
Ethnicity: White

Administered By: Jenine Boyd

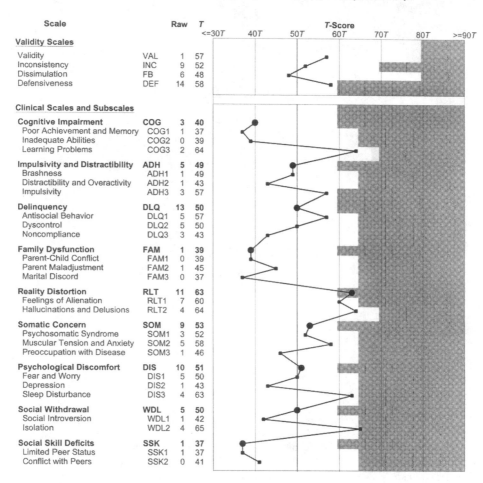

NOTE: Actuarial interpretive guidelines for PIY scales may be found on pages 14 - 21 of the 1995 PIY Administration and Interpretation Guide.

FIGURE 12.3. Personality Inventory for Youth (PIY) Profile generated from youth response for case study. The PIY Profile copyright (c) 1995, 1997, 2003 by Western Psychological Services. Reprinted by permission of the publisher, Western Psychological Services, 12031 Wilshire Boulevard, Los Angeles, CA 90025, U.S.A., *http://www.wpspublish.com*. Not to be reprinted in whole or in part for any additional purpose without the express, written permission of the publisher. All rights reserved.

a high probability of scoring more than *59T* on the corresponding clinical scale. Scales were standardized on two gender-specific samples of 4th- through 12th-grade students (ages 8 through 19). Significant endorsements of an 87-statement critical-items list arranged into nine categories are also available when the PIY is scored by hand or by computer.

Student Behavior Survey

The SBS (Lachar, Wingenfeld, Kline, & Gruber, 2000) includes 102 items that were not derived from the PIC-2 or PIY, but instead are new rating statements that capture content appropriate to teacher observation. Review of the SBS revealed that 58 out of its 102 items specifically refer to in-class or in-school behaviors and to judgments that can only be made by school staff members, such as "Follows the teacher's directions" and "Disrupts class by misbehaving" (Wingenfeld, Lachar, Gruber, & Kline, 1998). SBS items are placed into 14 scales that generate gender-specific standard scores for two age groups, 5–11 years and 12–18 years. SBS statements and their rating options are arrayed on both sides of one sheet of paper. These items are sorted into content-meaningful dimensions and are placed under 11 scale headings to enhance the clarity of item meaning, rather than being presented in a random order.

The SBS administration form consists of three sections. In the first section, the teacher selects one of five rating options ("deficient," "below average," "average," "above average," or "superior") to describe eight areas of academic achievement, such as reading comprehension and mathematics; these ratings are then summed to provide an estimate of current Academic Performance. The remaining 94 SBS items are rated on a 4-point frequency scale: "never," "seldom," "sometimes," or "usually." The second section (Academic Resources) presents positively worded statements that are divided into three scales. The first two of these scales consist of descriptions of positive behaviors that describe the student's adaptive behaviors: Academic Habits and Social Skills. The third scale, Parent Participation, consists of ratings of the student's parents (or other caregivers) that are very school-specific. In these six items, the teacher is asked to rate the degree to which the parents support the student's educational program. The third SBS administration section, Problems in Adjustment, presents seven scales consisting of negatively worded items: Health Concerns, Emotional Distress, Unusual Behavior, Social Problems, Verbal Aggression, Physical Aggression, and Behavior Problems. Three additional 16-item nonoverlapping Disruptive Behavior scales complete the SBS Profile (see Figure 12.4 for an example of a computer-generated SBS Profile). These scale items were drawn from several of the basic 11 scales and were consensually nominated as representing the characteristics associated with youth who obtain one of three *Diagnostic and Statistical Manual of Mental Disorders*, fourth edition (DSM-IV) diagnoses. These scales have been named Attention-Deficit/Hyperactivity, Oppositional Defiant, and Conduct Problems (Pisecco et al., 1990).

Student Behavior Survey (SBS)

A WPS TEST REPORT by David Lachar, Ph.D., Christian P. Gruber, Ph.D.
Copyright ©2003 by Western Psychological Services
12031 Wilshire Blvd., Los Angeles, California 90025-1251
Version 1.110

Student Name: Case Study
Birthdate: 10-6-88
Age: 15
Rater: Spec Education
Date Administered: 11/26/03

Gender: Male
Grade: 8
Role of Rater: Teacher
Date Processed: 12/04/03

Student ID: Not Entered
Ethnicity: White

Months Observing Child: 4
Administered By: Jenine Boyd

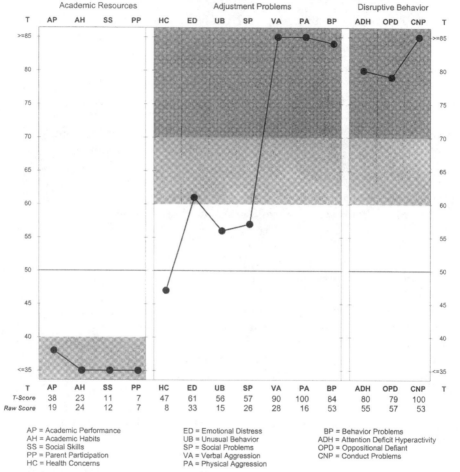

	AP	AH	SS	PP	HC	ED	UB	SP	VA	PA	BP	ADH	OPD	CNP
T-Score	38	23	11	7	47	61	56	57	90	100	84	80	79	100
Raw Score	19	24	12	7	8	33	15	26	28	16	53	55	57	53

AP = Academic Performance
AH = Academic Habits
SS = Social Skills
PP = Parent Participation
HC = Health Concerns

ED = Emotional Distress
UB = Unusual Behavior
SP = Social Problems
VA = Verbal Aggression
PA = Physical Aggression

BP = Behavior Problems
ADH = Attention Deficit Hyperactivity
OPD = Oppositional Defiant
CNP = Conduct Problems

NOTE: Actuarial interpretive guidelines for SBS scales may be found on pages 13 - 17 of the 2000 SBS manual.

FIGURE 12.4. Student Behavior Survey (SBS) Profile generated from teacher response for case study. The SBS Profile copyright (c) 2000, 2003 by Western Psychological Services. Reprinted by permission of the publisher, Western Psychological Services, 12031 Wilshire Boulevard, Los Angeles, CA 90025, U.S.A., *http://www.wpspublish.com*. Not to be reprinted in whole or in part for any additional purpose without the express, written permission of the publisher. All rights reserved.

The PIC-2, PIY, and SBS manuals present scale content and empirically derived interpretive guidelines; describe scale construction procedures that provide evidence of scale accuracy; give estimates of psychometric performance; and provide various examples of test application. Readers interested in learning more about these measures may also consult a number of relatively detailed chapters available in contemporary reference works (see Lachar, 2003, 2004a, 2004b; Lachar & Gruber, 2003).

HISTORY OF THE METHOD'S DEVELOPMENT

For all three informant-specific measures, items were assigned to scales based on their manifest elements, and each statement was retained for a questionnaire based on the most substantial correlation to its assigned scale (vs. all remaining scales). The application of consistent methods of development for the scales within a profile facilitates the subsequent application of the same interpretive standards to these scales. For the nine basic scales of the standard PIY and PIC-2, interpretation has been further enhanced by the development of subscales through factor analysis of scale items. This divides the scales into subscales of smaller sets of items with greater homogeneity. For example, the disruptive behavior scale Delinquency (DLQ) of both the PIC-2 and PIY has been further divided into three subscales reflecting specific acts (Antisocial Behavior), poorly modulated anger (Dyscontrol), or disobedience to the requests of authority figures (Noncompliance).

In the majority of instances, each descriptive statement contributes to only one scale, as in the case of the 11 basic SBS and 9 clinical PIY scales. In the PIC-2, only 16 items (6% of 264 placed items) appear in more than one clinical scale, because these 16 statements obtained substantial and equivalent correlations with more than one subscale. For example, "Others often say that my child is moody" is in the Depression subscale of the Psychological Discomfort scale, reflecting "moody" as a measure of dysphoria, and on the Dyscontrol subscale of the DLQ scale, reflecting "moody" as a measure of anger and irritability.

The historical evolution of PIC scales may be demonstrated by the examination of the DLQ scale. The 1977 "empirically keyed" version of DLQ was constructed by the identification of questionnaire items with endorsement rates that statistically separated samples of normative and adjudicated delinquents, regardless of statement content. The resulting 47 items (40 items retained in the 280-statement PIC-R; Lachar, 1982) correctly identified 95% of independent normative and adjudicated delinquent samples reserved for repeated scale application (Lachar, Abato, & Wirt, 1975, cited in Wirt et al., 1977). Lachar and Gdowski (1979) obtained numerous scale correlates for DLQ in a large child guidance/child psychiatry sample, and developed interpretive narratives for four T-score ranges: 80–89, 90–99, >99, and >109. McAuliffe and Handal (1984) demonstrated that DLQ could identify antisocial acting-out tendencies in high school students, in that this scale was moderately related to self-reported delinquency. Rothermel (1985) demonstrated the diagnostic potential of the PIC, especially DLQ, when compared to a self-report questionnaire in a large sample of adolescents recruited from a juvenile court population. Although scale construction methods differed in the comparable PIC-2 and PIY scales, more than half of the original DLQ items were retained in these revisions. The PIC-R and PIC-2 versions have been found to be highly correlated (r = .93), although correlations across informants for the PIC-R and PIY versions were lower (r = .52 for males, .60 for females). The comparability of the self-report PIY and parent report PIC-2 versions of DLQ was demonstrated, in that the content dimensions of each scale informant version generated three identically labeled subscales, and review of scale statements revealed an 85% item overlap between versions. Although these three DLQ subscales obtained the most robust self-report to parent report correlations in a referred sample, the correlations only achieved values in the low to middle .40s.

Specialized scales for the PIC-2, PIY, and SBS were constructed by using different methods selected to achieve each scale's purpose. The three SBS Disruptive Behavior scales each consist of 16 nonoverlapping items from the standard 11 profile scales consensually nominated to reflect the behaviors expected of students who obtain a specific clinical diagnosis. The eight short scales of the PIC-2 Behavioral Summary each consist of the 12 statements that best matched multiple specific criteria: use of present tense versus historical context, frequent endorsement in samples referred for clinical assessment, description of phenomena that are often the focus of contemporary short-term therapeutic intervention, and selection of statements incorporating the most varied scale content. The Behavioral Summary composites consist of more items than the short scales in order to more accurately measure increments of behavioral change obtained in PIC-2 repeated administration. Composite scales are combinations of short scales and reflect three behavior/symptom dimensions achieved by the statistical analysis of statement relations in factor analysis; in addition, a total score summarizes all 96 Behavioral Summary items. "Externalization" (a label commonly given to behaviors and symptoms characterized by poor self-control and overt or disruptive behaviors) is a composite that includes the 24 items from the DLQ and the Impulsivity and Distractibility short scales. The "Internalization" (a label commonly assigned to symptoms and behaviors characterized by behavioral overcontrol and feelings of discomfort) composite includes the 36 items from the Reality Distortion, Somatic Concern, and Psychological Distress short scales. The "Social Adjustment" composite consists of the 24 items of the Social Withdrawal and Social Skill Deficits short scales.

The PIC-2 and PIY validity scales were developed to identify inconsistency and defensiveness in self-report, given that many referred youths may be inadequately motivated or insufficiently educated to meet the demands of many of these questionnaires. There are three types of validity scales: Inconsistency, Defensiveness, and Dissimulation.

The Inconsistency scales of the PIY and PIC-2 were developed through the identification of highly correlated questionnaire item pairs. Elevated Inconsistency scale scores reflect substantial inconsistent responses between items with highly similar content, suggesting that the youth or parent informant did not pay adequate attention to, or could not understand, the questionnaire statements. The Defensiveness scales identify possible minimization or denial of current problems. These statements were for the most part specifically designed to represent either denial of common problems ("Sometimes I put off doing a chore [false]," "My child almost never argues [true]") or attribution of improbable positive adjustment ("My child always does his/her homework on time [true]," "I am always on time and remember what I am supposed to do [true]"). The Dissimulation scales were constructed to identify distortion of description through item analyses of three samples: the accurate description of nonreferred students; a second description of the same students, following direction to portray these students as in need of mental health services; and test protocols obtained in routine clinical assessment. These scored items reflect either the exaggeration of current problems or a malingered pattern of atypical or infrequent symptoms. Additional study of PIY validity scale performance has been provided by Wrobel and colleagues (1999).

RESEARCH EVIDENCE

Demographic Influence on Normative Scale Performance

Standardization samples for development of the instruments were large (PIC-2, $N = 2,306$; PIY, $N = 2,327$; SBS, $N = 2,612$), and each test manual demonstrates the relative minimal effect of age upon scale score. Only the SBS required the application of two age ranges to avoid age-related errors. This will be of little concern to juvenile justice personnel, however, as the majority of youths will fall within the older age norms (ages 12–18 years).

In contrast to the influence of age, gender has been found to have a robust influence on scales of all three measures. In the normative samples, boys obtained descriptions equivalent to more than 4 T-score points higher than the ones for girls on the SBS dimensions Academic Habits, Behavior Problems, and Attention-Deficit/Hyperactivity. Similarly, boys were described by their parents as demonstrating more problems than girls on the PIC-2 subscales Poor Achievement, Disruptive Behavior, and Fearlessness. Gender effects on PIY scales suggest that boys describe themselves as more problematic on DLQ and on Impulsivity and Distractibility, while girls describe themselves as more problematic on Psychological Discomfort.

Internal Consistency and Reliability

Scale item lengths and their median alpha coefficients (in parentheses) are as follows. For the PIC-2: scales, average 31 items (.89); subscales, average 13 items (.89); Behavioral Summary short scales, 12 items (.82); composite scales

(.94); total score (.95). For the PIY: scales, average 26 items (.85); subscales, average 10 items (.73). For the SBS: scales, average 11 items (.90).

Median short-term test–retest reliability estimates (r_{tt}) are as follows. For the PIC-2: scales (.90); subscales (.88); Behavioral Summary short scales (.87); and each of the four composites (.89). For the PIY: scales (.83); subscales (.73). For the SBS: scales (.88). The PIC-2 manual provides comparisons of parent descriptions. These interrater correlation values were calculated for both referred and nonreferred children. The median interrater correlation value for PIC-2 scales was .73 (.80); comparable values were .71 (.80) for subscales and .68 (.72) for PIC-2 Behavioral Summary short scales; and comparable values for the four composite scores ranged from .68 to .78 (.71 to .86). These values are consistently above a comparable mean value of .61 reported in a meta-analysis of parent agreement (Duhig, Renk, Epstein, & Phares, 2000). Comparable values for SBS scales were obtained by analyzing a sample of paired student descriptions obtained from fourth- and fifth-grade teachers working in teams, and from teachers and their teacher assistants in elementary-grade self-contained classrooms. The median interrater correlation for this sample was .73.

Validity

When normative (nonclinical) and clinic-referred youth were compared, the differences obtained on the PIC-2 clinical scales represented a large effect (a difference of approximately 8 T-score points) for six scales and a moderate effect (a difference of approximately 5 T-score points) for the remaining three scales. For PIC-2 subscales, these differences represented at least a moderate effect for 19 of these 21 subscales. Comparable analysis for the PIC-2 Behavioral Summary demonstrated that these differences were similarly robust for all of its 12 dimensions (10 obtained a difference equal to a large effect, 2 a moderate effect). Factor analysis of the PIC-2 subscales resulted in five dimensions that accounted for 71% of the variability among these dimensions. Comparable analysis of the eight short scales of the PIC-2 Behavioral Summary extracted the same two scale dimensions or groupings in both referred and normative protocols, representing commonly derived patterns of youth symptoms and problem behaviors: Externalizing Problems and Internalizing Problems. Independent evidence of scale meaning (i.e., criterion validity) was demonstrated by correlations between PIC-2 dimensions and 6 clinician rating dimensions, 14 SBS scales, and 24 PIY subscales. In addition, the PIC-2 demonstrated its ability to differentiate among 11 DSM-IV-diagnosis-based samples (discriminant validity). Our current examination of subscale score elevation differences among these samples suggests that youths diagnosed with conduct disorder may be identified by DLQ subscale elevations (DLQ1 greater than 79T, DLQ2 greater than 79T, DLQ3 greater than 69T), Fearlessness subscale elevations (ADH2 greater than 69T), and reports of poor academic achievement (COG2 greater than 69T). The PIC-2 manual also provides a bibliography of over 350 relevant publications that study or apply PIC scales.

Several estimates of the PIY's validity are presented in its manual (Lachar & Gruber, 1995). PIY dimensions were correlated with profile and content scales of the Minnesota Multiphasic Personality Inventory. The scales of PIY protocols obtained in clinical evaluation were correlated with scores on several self-report scales and questionnaires: the Social Support Scale, the Adolescent Hassles Scale, the State–Trait Anxiety Inventory, the Reynolds Adolescent Depression Scale, the Sensation Seeking Scale, the State–Trait Anger Inventory, and the Personal Experience Inventory. PIY scores were also correlated with adjective checklist items in college freshmen, and with chart-derived symptom dimensions in adolescents hospitalized for psychiatric evaluation and treatment.

Additional evidence of validity was obtained from the comparison of valid PIY profiles of adolescents diagnosed with major depression to the PIY profiles of adolescents diagnosed with conduct disorder who were hospitalized at the same facility (Lachar, Harper, Green, Morgan, & Wheeler, 1996). This comparison revealed that adolescents with conduct disorder obtained disproportionately more elevations on the DLQ scale and its three subscales, while adolescents diagnosed with major depression obtained disproportionately more elevations on the Psychological Discomfort and Social Withdrawal scales and on the Depression and Social Introversion subscales. Another study compared two samples of Spanish- or English-speaking male adolescents from south Texas: regular education high school students and students incarcerated in a state juvenile justice facility (Negy et al., 2001). Although language-related differences resulted in Spanish-speaking adolescents' scoring approximately 1 T-score point higher, incarcerated youths scored an average of 8.6 and 7.5 T-score points higher on scales and subscales. Among a variety of scale and subscale elevations, DLQ1 (Antisocial Behavior) demonstrated the greatest group difference (73.1T vs. 49.5T) and obtained a significant elevation in 77% of the incarcerated sample.

The SBS manual provides considerable evidence of scale validity (Lachar et al., 2000). As similarly considered for the PIC-2 and PIY, SBS scale comparisons of normative and referred samples resulted in large-effect differences for 10 scales and medium-effect differences for an additional 3 scales (leaving only Parent Participation to represent a small-effect group difference). The 11 nonoverlapping SBS scales formed three clearly interpretable factors that represented 71% of the variability among these measures: Externalization, Internalization, and Academic Performance. SBS scales were correlated with six clinical rating dimensions and with the scales and subscales of the PIC-2 and the PIY obtained in referred samples. The rating dimension Disruptive Behavior obtained substantial correlations with several SBS scales (Oppositional Defiant, $r = .70$; Verbal Aggression, $r = .64$; Behavior Problems, $r = .64$; Academic Habits, $r = -.63$). The rating dimension Antisocial Behavior correlated .58 with Behavior Problems and .54 with Conduct Problems, while the rating dimension Psychological Discomfort obtained substantial correlations with Emotional Distress ($r = .55$), Oppositional Defiant ($r = .48$), Social Problems ($r = .47$), and Social Skills ($r = -.44$).

The SBS scales were also correlated with the four scales of the Conners Teacher Rating Scale, Short Form, in students with learning disabilities and in students nominated by their elementary school teachers as having most challenged their teaching skills over the previous school year. SBS scale discriminant validity was also demonstrated by comparison of samples defined by the Conners Hyperactivity Index. Similar comparisons were conducted across samples of special education students who had been classified with intellectual impairments, emotional impairments, or learning disabilites.

The Actuarial Process

Comprehensive data analyses have provided actuarial, or empirically based, scale interpretations for the PIC-2, PIY, and SBS. These analyses first identified the fine detail of the significant correlations between a specific scale and nonscale clinical information, and then determined the range of scale T-scores for which this detail was the most descriptive. This process first defined a normal range and a range of clinically meaningful scale standard scores, and then assigned correlated clinical information to score ranges within this clinical range. The content of scale correlates has been integrated directly into narrative text that is provided in the test manuals and used in computer-generated interpretive systems.

APPLICATION

The PIC-2, PIY, and SBS manuals and test materials are available from the test publisher (Western Psychological Services, 12031 Wilshire Boulevard, Los Angeles, CA 90025). These measures include the structure necessary for scoring and assignment of standard scores, or they may be scored by hand with templates or by using a computer scoring program that may also provide narrative scale interpretations. Parents and youth find PIC-2 and PIY content, respectively, reasonable and appropriate. These informants should be encouraged to be open and respond sincerely to questionnaire statements. Youth may benefit from a discussion of PIY validity scales, and PIY statements may be presented with the use of the standardized audiotape presentation if a youth has difficulty with reading comprehension or limited attention or motivation. When school adjustment and classroom behavior are of interest, or community placement is a possibility, an effort should be made to administer the SBS.

The challenge inherent in interpretation of the 96 scores generated by administration of the PIC-2, PIY, and SBS can be simplified somewhat by the addition of some structure to the scales and subscales that achieve a clinical elevation. The various scales generated by these three measures may be efficiently considered by their classification under one of the following five headings: Academic and Cognitive Status, Undercontrolled Behavior, Overcontrolled Behavior, Social Adjustment, and Family and Parent Status (see Lachar & Gruber, 2001, Table 10, p. 79, for this classification system). These headings have been applied to the following case example.

CASE EXAMPLE

The PIC-2, PIY, and SBS were administered as part of a court-ordered evaluation of John, a 15-year-old European American adolescent. John was detained consequent to being charged with burglary of a building. His prior legal history included criminal mischief and runaway behavior. A judge requested a psychological evaluation to provide diagnostic impressions and treatment considerations that might assist in the disposition phase of his proceedings. John had a history of accessing special education services and maintained only minimal contact with his biological mother; he lived with his biological father. Prior to being detained, John was enrolled in a self-contained classroom for children who exhibited extremely disruptive school behavior. John had a history of psychiatric outpatient treatment. He was prescribed Ritalin for treatment of ADHD at the age of 9, but discontinued treatment at the age of 13, despite his perception that the medication helped him "concentrate in school."

John reported a history of auditory and visual hallucinations, as well as the use of marijuana several times a week. John's father participated in a parent interview. He reported that John bullied, threatened, and intimidated others; had engaged in burglary and stealing; lied excessively; and ignored the household curfew almost daily. The results presented in Figures 12.1 through 12.4 are discussed under the five headings and scale assignments referred to above. In addition, relevant observations and other test results are discussed in light of these inventory results.

Academic and Cognitive Status

As part of the evaluation, John was administered tests measuring intellectual functioning and academic achievement. John's intellectual ability was estimated to be in the borderline range, and his reading, spelling, and arithmetic skills were all 3 or more years below the skills expected for a youth his age. The pattern obtained suggested the presence of a specific arithmetic disability.

John's custodial parent, his biological father, completed the 275-item version of the PIC-2. These results suggested the presence of a poor academic adjustment and poor language skills (Poor Achievement = 63T, Developmental Delay = 67T). His father endorsed the following critical items: "Reading has been a problem for my child," "My child has failed a grade (repeated a year) in school," and "My child first talked before he was 2 years old [false]."

John was administered the PIY by having him listen to the standardized audiocassette of PIY statements while he read these statements in the administration booklet, given his extremely limited reading skills. The PIY provided limited indication of problematic academic achievement (Learning Problems = 64T). John's responses indicated that he was aware of his academic limitations. John endorsed these critical items: "Because of my learning problems, I get extra help or am in a special class at school," and "Reading has been hard for me."

John's academic history and psychological assessment supported his teacher's SBS-derived description of a very problematic school adjustment, even given his placement in a self-contained classroom that focused on behavior management. (Note that scores below 40T on the following scales reflect a problem status: Academic Performance = 38T, Academic Habits = 23T.) Representative teacher observations included "Demonstrates a logical and organized approach to learning [never]," "Follows the teacher's directions [never]," and "Performance consistent with ability [never])." These inventory descriptions supported a consistent focus on the need for a detailed learning disability assessment as well as academic remediation.

Undercontrolled Behavior

The PIC-2 profile for John was substantially defined by considerable elevations of the Antisocial Behavior (122T) and Dyscontrol (76T) subscales. His teacher endorsed similar behavior in SBS scale elevations on Verbal Aggression (90T), Physical Aggression (100T), and Behavior Problems (84T), with the three Disruptive Behavior scales similarly elevated. The PIC-2 Behavioral Summary Profile suggested that noncompliance and undercontrolled behaviors should be the focus of therapeutic intervention, and that the Behavioral Summary should be readministered following intervention to document treatment effectiveness. The father's Disruptive Behavior value (56T), in contrast to the teacher's response on Academic Habits (23T) and Attention-Deficit/ Hyperactivity (80T), provided inconsistent evidence of the value of psychostimulant treatment in this case (although the total pattern on the SBS was consistent with a diagnosis of conduct disorder). This diagnostic issue might be resolved through a neuropsychological assessment to evaluate the presence of problematic inattention.

Considering the documented value of the PIY to describe problem behaviors (Lachar et al., 1996; Negy et al., 2001), the absence of similar elevations on the PIY appeared to be a curious anomaly, although a careful look at the PIY Defensiveness scale (58T) suggested that John might have minimized or underreported some of his problems. Additional support for problem minimization was derived from an interview. John had admitted to being expelled from three schools for fighting with peers, cursing, and fighting with teachers. John said, "When somebody tells me to do something and I don't like it, I go off on them." He also endorsed items on the Suicide Ideation scale of the Massachusetts Youth Screening Instrument—Version 2 (see Chapter 5) during the detention intake process, and further stated during the intake process that he was experiencing current suicidal ideation, with the mistaken belief that he would be released from detention sooner if he articulated thoughts of self-harm. This theme of "return to home" had been repeated throughout his sentence completion form (e.g., "I hate being here," "I suffer in the juvenile detention center," "I miss my Dad," "I am best when I am with my Dad," "I can't go home," "My greatest worry is getting out of here").

Overcontrolled Behavior

Little evidence of problematic overcontrolled behavior was elicited by these three questionnaires. On the PIC-2 dimensions of Psychological Discomfort, Somatic Concern, and Reality Distortion, John obtained scores within the average range, suggesting no problems with depression, anxiety, or psychosis. However, John's marginal elevation on the Reality Distortion scale suggested that he might feel different from his peers. His teacher's responses on the SBS resulted in an elevation on Emotional Distress that was only 1 point into the clinical range ($61T$). A Children's Depression Inventory (Kovacs, 1992) total score within the normal range ($46T$) was consistent with these findings.

Social Adjustment

Marginal evidence of poorly developed social skills, limited social interest, and little social influence was suggested across these three inventories (PIC-2: Limited Peer Status, $64T$; PIY: Isolation, $65T$; SBS: Social Skills, $11T$).

Family and Parent Status

PIC-2 elevations suggested that family interactions and the adjustment of other family members were important clinical considerations for John (Conflict Among Members = $79T$, Parent Maladjustment = $71T$, Family Dysfunction—Short = $71T$). His teacher expressed similar concern in describing parent interaction with the school program (Parent Participation = $7T$; "Parent expectations of school resources and responsibilities are realistic [never]," "Parent(s) meet with school staff when asked [never]," "Parent(s) cooperate with school efforts to improve class behavior and achievement [never]," "Parent's expectations concerning child's potential for achievement are realistic [never]," "Parent(s) facilitate completion of homework when necessary [never]").

Considering this youth's desire to return home, his extreme denial of all but 1 of 29 items would be expected ($39T$, when the normative expectation is at least 7 or 8 items, with the clinical range starting at 13 items endorsed = $60T$), indicating an intense avoidance of portraying family and parent adjustment in a negative light. Indeed, family members had exerted and continued to exert an important negative influence on this youth's life. His biological mother had left the family when he was a toddler; he had been neglected by his stepmother (there were allegations that she had fed him dog food); and he had received inadequate attention from his father.

John was given a DSM-IV diagnosis of conduct disorder, adolescent-onset type, moderate, based on probation records, school records, parent interview, and PIC-2 and SBS test results. A diagnosis of cannabis abuse was also rendered, based on John's report that he smoked marijuana several times a week and on a current urinalysis. Mathematics disorder (provisional) was indicated as well. The following recommendations were made in order to decrease the likelihood that John would engage in future delinquent behavior: drug counseling; anger management; further testing by the school district to determine whether John met the criteria for a specific learning disability, given his limited math skills; a behavior modification program that was consistent in the home and school; psychiatric outpatient services; and intense probation supervision. However, John's father was insufficiently involved in his child's education, did not cooperate with recommended psychiatric interventions or requests of the juvenile probation department, and admitted that he was incapable of managing his son. At a subsequent hearing, the judge ordered John to a residential treatment facility, given his father's lack of interest in his son. Upon release, John became a ward of the state.

REFERENCES

Duhig, A. M., Renk, K., Epstein, M. K., & Phares, V. (2000). Interparental agreement on internalizing, externalizing, and total behavior problems: A meta-analysis. *Clinical Psychology: Science and Practice, 7,* 435–453.

Kovacs, M. (1992). *Children's Depression Inventory (CDI): Manual.* North Tonawanda, NY: Multi-Health Systems.

Lachar, D. (1982). *Personality Inventory for Children (PIC): Revised format manual supplement.* Los Angeles: Western Psychological Services.

Lachar, D. (1998). Observations of parents, teachers, and children: Contributions to the objective multidimensional assessment of youth. In A.S. Bellack & M. Hersen (Series Eds.) & C. R. Reynolds (Vol. Ed.), *Comprehensive clinical psychology: Vol. 4. Assessment* (pp. 371–401). New York: Pegamon.

Lachar, D. (2003). Psychological assessment in child mental health settings. In I. B. Weiner (Series Ed.) & J. R. Graham & J. A. Naglieri (Vol. Eds.), *Handbook of psychology: Vol. 10. Assessment psychology* (pp. 235–260). New York: Wiley.

Lachar, D. (2004a). The Personality Inventory for Children, Second Edition (PIC-2), Personality Inventory for Youth (PIY), and Student Behavior Survey (SBS). In M. Hersen (Series Ed.) & M. J. Hilsenroth & D. L. Segal (Vol. Eds.), *Comprehensive handbook of psychological assessment: Vol. 2. Personality assessment* (pp. 192–212). New York: Wiley.

Lachar, D. (2004b). Personality Inventory for Children, Second Edition (PIC-2), Personality Inventory for Youth (PIY), and Student Behavior Survey (SBS). In M. Maruish (Ed.) *The use of psychological testing for treatment planning and outcome assessment* (3rd ed.). Vol. 2. *Instruments for children and adolescents* (pp. 141–178). Mahwah, NJ: Erlbaum.

Lachar, D., & Gdowski, C. L. (1979). *Actuarial assessment of child and adolescent personality: An interpretive guide for the Personality Inventory for Children profile.* Los Angeles: Western Psychological Services.

Lachar, D., & Gruber, C. P. (1995). *Personality Inventory for Youth (PIY): Manual; administration and interpretation guide; technical guide.* Los Angeles: Western Psychological Services.

Lachar, D., & Gruber, C. P. (2001). *Personality Inventory for Children, Second Edition (PIC-2): Standard form and behavioral summary manual.* Los Angeles: Western Psychological Services.

Lachar, D., & Gruber, C. P. (2003). Multisource and multidimensional objective assessment of adjustment: The Personality Inventory for Children, Second Edition; Personality Inventory for Youth; and Student Behavior Survey. In C. R. Reynolds & R. W. Kamphaus (Eds.), *Handbook of psychological and educational assessment of children: Personality, behavior, and context* (2nd ed., pp. 337–367). New York: Guilford Press.

Lachar, D., Harper, R. A., Green, B. A., Morgan, S. T., & Wheeler, A. C. (1996, August). *The Personality Inventory for Youth: Contribution to diagnosis.* Paper presented at the 104th annual meeting of the American Psychological Association, Toronto.

Lachar, D., Wingenfeld, S. A., Kline, R. B., & Gruber, C. P. (2000). *Student Behavior Survey: Manual.* Los Angeles: Western Psychological Services.

McAuliffe, T. M., & Handal, P. J. (1984). PIC Delinquency scale: Validity in relation to self-reported delinquent acts and a socialization scale. *Criminal Justice and Behavior, 11,* 35–46.

Negy, C., Lachar, D., & Gruber, C. P. (1998). The Personality Inventory for Youth (PIY)—Spanish Version: Reliability and equivalence to the English version. *Hispanic Journal of Behavioral Sciences, 20,* 391–404.

Negy, C., Lachar, D., Gruber, C. P., & Garza, N. D. (2001). The Personality Inventory for Youth (PIY): Validity and comparability of English and Spanish versions for regular education and juvenile justice samples. *Journal of Personality Assessment, 76,* 250–263.

Pisecco, S., Lachar, D., Gruber, C. P., Gallen R. T., Kline, R. B., & Huzinec, C. (1999). Development and validation of disruptive behavior scales for the Student Behavior Survey (SBS). *Journal of Psychoeducational Assessment, 17,* 314–331.

Rothermel, R. D., Jr. (1985). A comparison of the utility of the Personality Inventory for Children and the Jesness Inventory in assessing juvenile delinquents (Unpublished doctoral dissertation, Wayne State University, 1985). *Dissertation Abstracts International, 46*(5), 1740B.

Wingenfeld, S. A., Lachar, D., Gruber, C. P., & Kline, R. B. (1998). Development of the teacher-informant Student Behavior Survey. *Journal of Psychoeducational Assessment, 16,* 226–249.

Wirt, R. D., Lachar, D., Klinedinst, J. K., & Seat, P. D. (1977). *Multidimensional description of child personality: A manual for the Personality Inventory for Children.* Los Angeles: Western Psychological Services.

Wrobel, T. A., Lachar, D., Wrobel, N. H., Morgan, S. T., Gruber, C. P., & Neher, J. A. (1999). Performance of the Personality Inventory for Youth validity scales. *Assessment, 6,* 367–376.

CHAPTER 13

Diagnostic Interview Schedule for Children: Present State Voice Version

Gail A. Wasserman
Larkin S. McReynolds
Prudence Fisher
Christopher P. Lucas

PURPOSE

The Present State Voice version of the Diagnostic Interview Schedule for Children (Voice DISC) is one of a family of instruments developed to provide an accurate and efficient assessment of child and adolescent mental health problems. Developed for epidemiological purposes (Shaffer, Fisher, Lucas, Dulcan, & Schwab-Stone, 2000; Shaffer, Restifo, Garfinkel, Enhrensaft, & Munfah, 1998), the DISC's most recent format renders it particularly useful for typically low-resource justice settings (Wasserman, McReynolds, Lucas, Fisher, & Santos, 2002). Based on the fourth edition of the *Diagnostic and Statistical Manual of Mental Disorders* (DSM-IV; American Psychiatric Association, 1994), scoring algorithms generate provisional diagnoses that can inform clinicians in justice settings about youths' individual service needs, and can provide justice administrators with information about program needs in their facilities.

Justice agencies typically have limited resources in terms not only of trained and available staff but of updated evaluation materials, and both types of limitations can hinder identification of youths' mental health concerns. Nonetheless, agencies are faced with increased pressure to assess youths' mental health status. Although the DISC-IV is not a screen, the self-administered, computerized format of the Voice DISC lends itself to this use, providing one important assessment component (youth interview) in a timely, cost-effective manner. Because it electronically stores data in computer files, the Voice DISC allows aggregation of collected data for institutional reporting and grant development purposes. Recent reviews of mental health assessment methods for youths in the juvenile justice system have recommended adopting only validated instruments (LeBlanc, 1998; Wiebush, Baird, Krisberg, & Onek, 1995). Among available tools for developing DSM-IV diagnoses with children and adolescents, the DISC is the most thoroughly researched.

Recently, the fields of psychology and psychiatry have moved dramatically to establish treatment guidelines based on empirical evidence (Chambless et al., 1996; Grisso & Barnum, 2003; Kim, Fendrich, & Wislar, 2000; Task Force on Promotion and Dissemination of Psychological Procedures, 1995). Beyond its efficiency and the wealth of research data available on the DISC, a major advantage is that it provides provisional diagnoses. Obtaining diagnoses is central to the assessment and referral process, because treatment recommendations should vary according to diagnosis. Most evidence-based treatments map onto specific disorders, with efficacy only demonstrated for youths with those disorders. At a recent consensus conference, experts in mental health assessment and in juvenile justice policy and practice agreed that assessment of diagnostic status is essential to service planning for youths in the justice population (Wasserman, Jensen, Ko, Trupin, & Cocozza, 2003).

A 1992 monograph reviewing mental health needs and services for youths in the juvenile justice system (Otto, Greenstein, Johnson, & Friedman, 1992) pointed to high levels of disorders among these youths, compared to the general population. That review cautioned that our understanding is often limited by use of inappropriate instruments (with inadequate psychometrics), lack of specification of the time frame for diagnosis, and the failure to consider comorbidity. Rates of "comorbidity," or the co-occurrence of more than one disorder (or type of disorder) in an individual, are also elevated among youths in justice settings. Comorbidity also complicates treatment decisions, as clinicians must understand which conditions to treat first, and how different mental health conditions interrelate with each other. These clinical concerns are well addressed by the DISC's ability to assess a range of disorders.

BASIC DESCRIPTION

A Measure of Diagnostic Status and Impairment

The Voice DISC assesses more than 30 current (past-month) DSM-IV diagnoses and conditions warranting further evaluation, in modules that correspond to diagnostic groupings (see Table 13.1). Each youth gets a unique interview, depending upon the pattern of his or her responses. Because the Voice DISC is based on the DSM-IV, obtaining a diagnosis requires more than tallying symptoms. Specific criteria must be met regarding the types of symptoms; their onset, frequency, and duration; and the degree of impairment for the particular disorder. Each module has "gate questions" that determine whether to continue questioning about that disorder. Most gate questions inquire about presence–absence of symptoms, and follow-up questions determine symptoms' severity, frequency, and duration (see Table 13.1).

For youths who meet diagnostic criteria (as defined above) or who meet at least half of the defined (American Psychiatric Association, 1994) criteria for a given disorder, the Voice DISC includes a detailed assessment of impairment attributed to symptoms in that disorder. Six questions at the conclusion of each diagnostic module address impairment in relationships with parents/caretakers, participating in family activities, participating in activities with peers, relationships with teachers (employers), academic (occupational) functioning, and being distressed about the endorsed symptoms. Each question utilizes the same two-part structure—first asking about problems in that area, and then inquiring further about frequency and severity of those problems (see Table 13.2).

The self-report nature of the Voice DISC forces reliance on youths' awareness of the social and personal consequences of their disorders when impairment is being determined. Relying on the self-judgments of youths in the justice system, who are likely to have difficulties in insight, remorse, and empathy, probably results in substantial underreporting of impairment (Ko, Wasserman, McReynolds, & Katz, 2004). For example, in an earlier study of incarcerated youths (Wasserman et al., 2002), among 59 youths with substance use disorders who denied impairment, 19 (32%) were currently incarcerated for substance-related offenses.

TABLE 13.1. Voice DISC Disorder Modules and Sample Questions

Introduction (i.e., demographics and timeline)	
Module A: Anxiety	Module C: Mood
Social Phobia	Major Depression
Separation Anxiety	Dysthymia
Specific Phobia	Mania
Panic	Hypomania
Agoraphobia	
Generalized Anxiety	Module E: Disruptive Behavior
Selective Mutism[a]	Attention-Deficit/Hyperactivity
Obsessive–Compulsive	Oppositional Defiant
Posttraumatic Stress	Conduct
Module B: Miscellaneous[a]	Module F: Substance Use
Eating (Anorexia/Bulimia)	Alcohol Abuse/Dependence
Elimination Disorders	Nicotine Abuse/Dependence[a]
Tic Disorders	Marijuana Abuse/Dependence
Pica	Other Substance Abuse/Dependence
Trichotillomania	

[a]Many juvenile justice facilities do not include these modules as part of the Voice DISC interview.

TABLE 13.2. Sample Questions and Impairment Questions from the Voice DISC

Sample questions

Obsessive–Compulsive: "In the last four weeks, have you often worried over and over again that things you touch are dirty or have germs?"

Major Depression: "In the last four weeks, have you often felt self sad or depressed?"

Suicide: "Now thinking about the last four weeks, have you tried to kill yourself?"

Conduct: "In the last year, have you ever threatened someone in order to steal from them?"

Marijuana Abuse/Dependence: "In the last year, did you miss [school/work] to use marijuana or because you were too high on marijuana to go to [school/work]?"

Impairment questions (appearing at the end of each disorder module)

"When the problems were worst, did feeling sad or depressed make it difficult for you to do your schoolwork or cause problems with your grades?"

If yes: "How bad were the problems you had with your schoolwork because you felt this way? Would you say: very bad, bad, or not too bad?"

In considering impairment for the purpose of making a diagnosis, a clinician should rely on multiple informants and various pieces of information. Alternative "impairment algorithms" for each DISC diagnosis are undergoing testing. Currently, we recommend that juvenile justice agencies and clinicians rely on multiple sources of information for determining impairment in youths.

Procedure and Materials

Administration

The Voice DISC presents prerecorded questions via headphones, while the same questions appear on the computer screen. Youths use the keyboard or mouse to enter responses, completing the instrument at their own pace. Most questions have a "yes–no" format. The Voice DISC requires no special clinical expertise to administer and is readily scored by computer. Support staffers can administer the instrument; it requires 5 minutes to initialize (i.e., to enter a youth's identifying information), and 5 minutes to orient the youth (or youths, in group administration) to the computer and the DISC interview. Questions can be replayed if not understood or heard properly at first. The program stores responses as they are entered, and answers cannot be changed once a module is completed. The interview can be stopped at any time without losing any information. Justice staff members can immediately review completed interview results on the screen, save them to a diskette, and/or print a report for later review.

Length of Administration Time

Because of the gated-format questions, administration time can vary; a commonly used protocol (18 diagnoses) takes approximately an hour for youths in the juvenile justice system to complete (Wasserman et al., 2002), with expectably longer completion times for youths endorsing more symptoms. Administration time can be shortened by reconfiguring computer software to skip certain disorders if other reliable and valid instruments are in use for their assessment.

Scoring and Reporting

The Voice DISC provides four different reports. The "Diagnostic Report" is most widely used by justice staff, and lists youths' diagnoses, diagnostic criteria met, and symptoms endorsed. The briefer "Clinical Report" lists positive, subthreshold, and negative diagnoses; "impairment" and "symptom" scores by diagnosis; and a preset list of "clinically significant symptoms." The "Reconstruction Report" includes the text of all questions asked and the corresponding answers. The "Symptom Report" (in preparation) lists all endorsed symptoms.

Materials Required

The Voice DISC requires a personal computer with a 486 processor, 1 gigabyte of free space on the hard drive, a Windows 2000 or XP operating system, a Windows sound card, a CD-ROM drive, a pointing device, at least 570K free conventional DOS memory, and headphones. A quiet location reduces distraction.

The DISC family of instruments also includes a parent version (not currently "voiced"), available in both English and Spanish, that assesses a caretaker's report of a youth's disorder in the past year. Other versions currently under psychometric testing are the Quick DISC (shorter administration time) and the Young Adult DISC (suitable for 18- to 25-year-olds).

Language Requirements

The Voice DISC requires minimal reading ability because of its audio presentation. The questions are written to be understood by individuals with at least a third-grade oral English-language comprehension ability. Most juveniles will be able to meet this requirement; in a recent Texas probation intake sample, only 6 of 1,244 approached youths (<1%) were unable to complete the Voice DISC because of language limitations (Wasserman, McReynolds, Ko, Katz, & Carpenter, in press). Although the instrument is suitable for individuals as young as 9 years old, the verbal limitations common among youths in the justice system lead us to caution against use with very young or cognitively limited juveniles. Interviewer-assisted adaptations are appropriate alternatives.

The Spanish-language version of the DISC (not voiced, but computerized) will also need interviewer assistance.

Special Features

Increased Accuracy in Recall of Time-Based Events

Timing of symptom history is essential for diagnosis, but most individuals find it difficult to date past events accurately. A unique feature of the Voice DISC allows the derivation of an individual timeline that assists respondents in answering questions about timing. Youths identify salient events (e.g., past birthdays) that occurred at designated past reference points (2 weeks, 4 weeks, 3 months, 6 months, and 1 year), producing an individual timeline. Throughout the interview, the timeline appears whenever a question relates to the timing of symptoms, as an anchor to help increase accuracy in reporting of time frames.

Enhanced Disclosure

The computer administration of the Voice DISC has an advantage over interview methods, because interviewer-administered instruments may result in underreporting of sensitive information by youths. For example, adolescent boys are more forthcoming about stigmatizing behavior, such as drug and alcohol use and suicidal behavior, on self-administered surveys than when they are interviewed (Turner et al., 2004).

Privacy Concerns

The Voice DISC offers confidentiality in administration, even in group presentation. Because the interview occurs over headphones, and responses are entered via keyboard, others cannot hear either questions or answers. Given the individualized branching format, respondents are generally on different "pages" of the interview after a few minutes. Use of privacy screens or computers oriented in different directions enhances confidentiality. We recommend that some staff members be available in the room to troubleshoot and ensure that juveniles remain focused. They should remain at a sufficiently removed distance to allow privacy, however.

HISTORY OF THE METHOD'S DEVELOPMENT

Work on the DISC began in 1979, when the National Institute of Mental Health (NIMH) convened an expert advisory panel to study the feasibility of structured psychiatric interviews for children. After reviewing the initial version's field trials, colleagues at Columbia University/New York State Psychiatric Institute took the lead in further development. Since then, there have been three major revisions (DISC-R, DISC-2 [2.1 and 2.3], and DISC-IV), each extensively field-tested. Revisions have been based upon consultation with DISC users and diagnostic experts about the best wording and formatting of questions. As the DSM criteria have evolved, necessary changes have been incorporated into the DISC structure. For example, the DISC-2.1 was field-tested in the Methods for Epidemiology of Child and Adolescent Mental Disorders (MECA) study (Lahey et al., 1996) with 9- to 17-year-olds from both clinical and community settings (Jensen et al., 1995).

The DISC-2.3 (Shaffer et al., 1996), appearing in 1991, included algorithms for "diagnosis-specific" impairment and was computerized. After the MECA trials, the NIMH appointed the DISC Editorial Board (DEB) to oversee development of the DISC-IV, based on review of the reliability and validity data collected in the DISC-2 field studies, expert consultation, user feedback, and adherence to the newly released criteria of the DSM-IV and the *International Classification of Diseases*, 10th revision. The DEB was responsible for reviewing and approving all scoring algorithms for the DISC. They also approved all "official" versions of the instrument and scoring algorithms to ensure standard presentation and use. Since the dissolution of the DEB in 2000, the DISC Development Group at Columbia University has continued with further DISC-related development and testing.

The computerized Voice DISC was created in 1990. The first report of its use in a juvenile justice sample examined approximately 300 males newly admitted to reception centers in New Jersey and Illinois (Wasserman et al., 2002). Following this initial "feasibility" study, the Center for the Promotion of Mental Health in Juvenile Justice at Columbia University/New York State Psychiatric Institute has collaborated with juvenile justice facilities in over 38 sites in 16 states. This has resulted in assessment of over 7,000 youths with the Voice DISC since 2002.

RESEARCH EVIDENCE

This section describes evidence for the reliability and validity of various earlier versions of the DISC (the "DISC family of instruments," as described above in "History of the Method's Development") from which the Voice DISC was derived, as well as research examining the Voice DISC itself. A separate subsection focuses specifically on DISC family and Voice DISC results with youths in juvenile justice samples.

Reliability of the DISC Family of Instruments

A complete report on DISC-IV test–retest reliability (administered twice a few weeks apart) in clinical and community samples is in preparation. Partial results (Shaffer et al., 2000) demonstrate acceptable reliability for most diagnoses. Changing a single answer can change a diagnosis from negative to positive (or vice versa), so it tends to be better to base reliability on a count of symptoms or criteria than on a categorical determination of diagnostic status, regardless of informant. Every symptom scale had good reliability.

Parent-reported DISC diagnoses showed moderate to good test–retest reliability on the earlier DISC-2.3 in a community sample (Schwab-Stone et al., 1996), as did diagnoses using combined parent and child report. Youth report was less reliable than parent report, except for conduct disorder. Reliabilities for the symptom and criterion counts were considerably better than for diagnostic status (Shaffer et al., 1996). There are no significant differences in 1-month reliability of diagnoses between self- and interviewer-administered versions of the Voice DISC, with agreement comparable to, or better than, that of earlier versions (Lucas, 2003). Test–retest reliability of the Voice DISC is as good as or better than that of prior versions (Shaffer et al., 2000).

Validity of the DISC Family of Instruments

Methodology varies greatly for studies comparing DISC-generated diagnoses with other indicators of diagnostic status, and this variation complicates conclusions regarding validity. Concordance between other structured interviews and clinician diagnosis is also generally moderate to poor (Aronen, Noam, & Weinstein, 1993; Ezpeleta et al., 1997; Steiner, Tebes, Sledge, & Walker, 1995; Vitiello, Malone, Bushcle, Delanyey, & Behar, 1990; Weinstein, Stone, Noam, Grimes, & Schwab-Stone, 1989). Although the primary source of these discrepancies remains unknown, studies show that clinician diagnoses are subject to biases (relying on contextual and demographic factors, prematurely determining diagnosis before collecting all relevant information, assigning familiar diagnoses, and selectively collecting information to confirm rather than disconfirm suspected diagnoses) (Angold & Fisher, 1999; Lewczyk, Garland, Hurlburt, Gearity, & Hough, 2003). Structured interviews such as the DISC improve reliability and eliminate such biases by standardizing information gathering and decision making. Further research is needed to determine more clearly how structured diagnostic interviews and clinician diagnoses compare to a "gold standard," although there is little consensus in the field regarding what the "gold standard" for diagnosis might be. Given all these factors, evidence relating DISC-generated diagnoses to other indicators of diagnostic status is mixed.

A useful construct for describing an instrument's psychometric properties is "sensitivity" (see Chapter 4—i.e., how well a screen correctly identifies individuals who are "truly disordered," as determined by some second assessment). The sensitivity of the DISC-2.1 in identifying certain disorders has been measured on samples from centers specializing in treatment of particular diagnoses, with those centers' "standard-practices" diagnoses as criterion measures (Fisher et al., 1993). The sensitivity of the DISC-2.1 in identifying such disorders was good to excellent.

In a study of 245 youths from clinical settings, clinician diagnosis (DSM-III-R) was compared to the DISC-2.3; agreement was low (Jensen & Weisz, 2002). The DISC identified higher rates of anxiety disorders and comorbidity, but was also more likely to designate youths as disorder-free. In contrast, another study (Lahey et al., 1996) found overall moderate to very good agreement between DISC-2.3 and clinician diagnoses (Schwab-Stone et al., 1996). For 240 youths receiving mental health services, there was a low rate of agreement between DISC-IV diagnosis and community clinician diagnosis (Lewczyk et al., 2003). Clinicians diagnosed higher rates of mood disorders, while youths reported higher rates of attention-deficit/hyperactivity disorder (ADHD), disruptive behavior disorders, anxiety disorders, and comorbidity on the DISC-IV. Again, the DISC-IV identified more youths as disorder-free than did clinicians.

Research in Juvenile Justice Samples

In studies using the DISC to investigate prevalence of mental disorder among youths in justice settings (Atkins, Pumariega, & Rogers, 1999; Duclos et al., 1998; Garland et al., 2001; Randall, Henggeler, Pickrel, & Brondino, 1999; Teplin, Abram, McClelland, Dulcan, & Mericle, 2002; Wasserman et al., 2002), Voice DISC prevalence rates are comparable to those reported based on earlier computerized versions of the DISC administered by interviewers. Rates of approximately 15% anxiety, 10% mood, 32% disruptive, and 50% substance use disorders are generally reported (Wasserman et al., 2002), and comorbidity is high (Teplin et al., 2002; Wasserman et al., 2002). Studies of incarcerated youths generally agree that approximately 65% show some diagnosable disorder, as measured on the DISC (given high comorbidity, this estimate is not based upon adding across disorder categories). Above and beyond expectably high rates of disruptive behavior and substance use disorders, approximately 20% of juveniles in the justice system meet criteria for either a mood or an anxiety disorder. Juveniles entering secure care are likely to report elevated rates of separation anxiety symptoms, which may be more a contextual response to pending removal from family rather than a mark of enduring disorder (Ko et al., 2004; Wasserman, Ko, & McReynolds, 2004; Wasserman et al., in press). Rates of most disorders appear similar across secure detention (Teplin et al., 2002) and postadjudication corrections (Wasserman et al., 2002) settings. Rates are closer to community samples (i.e., generally lower) for youths at earlier processing points, such as probation intake, perhaps because less seriously delinquent youths are included (Wasserman et al., in press).

Preventing suicide and suicide attempts is very important to juvenile justice agencies, especially as many risk factors for suicide attempts are elevated among youths in this population (e.g., mood and substance use disorders, access to weapons, and stressful life events ("Practice parameters," 2001). Those with histories of past attempts are at continuing risk. While inquiring about major depressive disorder, the DISC-IV queries about suicidal ideation, past attempts, and current plans. Importantly, past-month rates of self-reported suicide attempts in incarcerated youths (Wasserman et al., 2002; Wasserman & McReynolds, 2004) correspond closely (i.e., 2–3% per month) to rates reported by facility directors in the Office of Juvenile Justice and Delinquency Prevention's (1994) *Conditions of Confinement* report, and both sources appear considerably higher than the benchmark of approximately 9% of high school students attempting suicide per year (Centers for Disease Control and Prevention, 2001).

Validity data are available for some diagnostic conditions among youths in the juvenile justice system. In a sample of mostly male juvenile offenders, those diagnosed with disruptive behavior disorders on the DISC had more disciplinary problems during residential stay than did nondisordered youths (Friman et al., 2000). Incarcerated youths who reported a substance use disorder on the Voice DISC were more likely to have been charged with a substance-related offense than were nondisordered youths or those with no substance use disorder (37.3%, 23.2%, and 13.5%, respectively) (Wasserman et al., 2002).

Gender comparisons on the DISC within justice samples concur in documenting increased rates of comorbidity and of mood and anxiety disorders in girls relative to boys (Teplin et al., 2002; Wasserman et al., in press)—findings consistent with community studies (Ferdinand, Stijnen, Verhulst, & Van der Reijden, 1996; Overbeck, Vollebergh, Meeus, Engels, & Luijpers, 2002). Some information is available regarding ethnic differences in rates of disorder in justice samples (Teplin et al., 2002; Wasserman et al., 2002). By design, there are no differences in the questions or diagnostic algorithms as they are presented to different subgroups of youths, since the same pattern of behaviors should underlie a given disorder, regardless of the gender or ethnicity of the person answering the questions. Disorders appropriate only to very young children or to youths over 18 are not included in the DISC-IV or the Voice DISC.

APPLICATION

The Value of Diagnostic Information

A recent consensus conference of expert mental health assessment researchers and juvenile justice practitioners made six recommendations regarding mental health assessment for youths in the justice system. Participants distinguished two separate purposes for which mental health information should be examined (Wasserman et al., 2003). The first evaluates emergent risk of harm to self or others at intake; the second considers mental health service needs. Practitioners have not consistently differentiated these two purposes, for which different sets of instruments and procedures are useful. Consensus conference participants agreed that mental health service needs should be assessed for all youths prior to disposition and for those who remain in secure care or supervision. Having available information on diagnostic status allows appropriate incorporation of mental health services into treatment plans for youths in both community and secure care settings. Ongoing research at our center is evaluating the degree to which access to accurate information about diagnostic status better informs treatment planning, and whether appropriate receipt of such services in turn reduces recidivism.

The Voice DISC provides information on mental health service need. Consensus conference participants identified a youth's self-report as one component in a comprehensive approach to case identification. Other components included service use history, a caretaker's report, mental status evaluation, and family history of disorder. There are few guidelines for integrating information across multiple sources to decide who needs services (Ko et al., 2004).

For most juvenile justice agencies, offering a comprehensive mental health assessment for every youth in their care is a daunting task. Efficiency demands might lead agencies to streamline identification of either emergent risk or mental health service need by using two-stage screening procedures (Shrout, Skodel, & Dohrenwend, 1986). Although the Massachusetts Youth Screening Instrument—Version 2 (MAYSI-2) was not developed to identify diagnostic status (Grisso & Barnum, 2003), many facilities use it as a first-stage screen for identifying service needs (see Chapter 5). We recently examined the utility of this procedure by comparing youths' responses on the MAYSI-2 and the Voice DISC (Wasserman et al., 2004). Although the MAYSI-2 could quickly determine the likely presence of *some* psychiatric disorder, we found that it might be more challenging to use it as a screen for service needs, as it was less able to identify the *particular* disorder a youth reported. Knowing that some mental health problem exists, a clinical staff member would need to conduct a direct interview with the youth to determine diagnostic status before commencing treatment. The DISC allows a clinical staffer to conduct a more efficient subsequent direct interview, focusing on reported symptoms.

When and by Whom the Voice DISC Should Be Administered

Having information about mental health service needs early in processing helps inform decisions about which programs and settings might best address a youth's problems. On the other hand, concerns may exist regarding the ease with which a youth newly entering the justice system may be able to focus on a diagnostic assessment. A comparison of DISCs administered on the date of probation or reception center intake to those occurring in the first 2 weeks after intake revealed few differences in rates of disorder or in administration time (McReynolds & Wasserman, 2004). This suggest that even newly admitted youths can efficiently report on their mental health status.

The Voice DISC was designed to be administered by lay staff members. Individuals with basic computer skills are able to administer the software. No professional training is required, although standardized training is essential. Columbia University provides such training in a variety of formats (see below). Alternatively, since clinical skills are required for interpretation, a mental health clinician (e.g., a psychologist, social worker, or psychiatrist) should review the DISC report for youths endorsing a disorder and conduct a clinical interview before proceeding to treatment. In settings where a positive diagnosis triggers only a referral to another agency or provider, no additional clinical training is required.

Decision Making about Mental Health Referral

Since a high level of mental health service need is likely to be uncovered by the Voice DISC, agencies may need to prioritize which conditions they can undertake to treat. Most agencies have existing programs targeting disruptive behavior and substance use. Addressing youths' internalizing (mood and anxiety) disorders may be more of a departure for clinical practice in justice settings. Internalizing disorders may contribute to considerable difficulty in youths' management, and effective psychosocial and psychopharmacological treatments exist for most (Columbia University Division of Child and Adolescent Psychiatry, 2003).

In particular, youths' increased willingness to disclose sensitive information to a computer makes the Voice DISC particularly useful for evaluating suicide risk. The DISC provides information on recent (4-week) and lifetime suicide attempts, as well as reported ideation and suicide planning over the past 4 weeks. Clearly, all youths endorsing current ideation as well as a plan or a recent attempt should be referred for immediate emergency clinical care. Even those with current ideation alone should be referred for a clinical evaluation within 24 hours. Other considerations in identifying youths' treatment needs include length of stay, as well as availability of trained staff members and of collaborating mental health providers. Although these factors should be considered proactively, it is beyond the scope of this chapter to make specific recommendations.

Requests for more information regarding the Voice DISC or other formats can be obtained online (*http://www.promotementalhealth.org*), or by a phone call to our center (212-543-5298) or the DISC Development Group (888-814-3472). As noted, our center has developed training materials for use in juvenile justice settings.

CASE EXAMPLE

At age 17, Charles was convicted of felony burglary in adult court and admitted to a juvenile detention center before he was to be transferred to an adult prison on his 18th birthday to complete a 10-year sentence. He had previously been cited for several offenses, including assault with a deadly weapon, shoplifting, driving under the influence, larceny, and assault and battery. Following a history of early problems in school (misbehavior in the classroom, excessive absences, assaultive behavior), Charles dropped out early in the 9th grade. His home life was chaotic and unstructured; his father had alcoholism, and his mother was disabled, homebound, and heavily medicated for chronic pain. Charles had run away on several occasions. He began abusing marijuana and alcohol by age 13, using more serious drugs as he became older. Many of his delinquent acts occurred while he was drinking or using drugs; he supported his drug addiction by theft.

Charles completed the Voice DISC while in detention for his burglary charge; he endorsed ADHD and multiple substance use disorders (i.e., alcohol, marijuana, and other substance use). A forensic psychiatrist later incorporated the Voice DISC results into other data sources to inform a dispositional evaluation requested by the court. As a result of this evaluation, Charles's attorney argued for an alternative sentence to adult prison, and he applied to a residential substance abuse treatment program. The rehabilitation plan offered by the forensic psychiatrist also included a trial of medication to address the ADHD symptoms. Charles completed his general equivalency diploma while he was detained awaiting treatment.

Various systems had missed several earlier opportunities to identify and address Charles's problems. Had underlying mental health issues been addressed when he first came to the attention of school or juvenile justice authorities, intervention might have responded to his needs before they became exacerbated. Instead, he was already awaiting sentencing on an adult felony charge by the time his mental health and substance use needs were well identified.

REFERENCES

American Psychiatric Association. (1994). *Diagnostic and statistical manual of mental disorders* (4th ed.) Washington, DC: Author.

Angold, A., & Fisher, P. W. (2000). Interviewer based interviews. In D., Shaffer, C. P. Lucas, & J. E. Richters (Eds.), *Diagnostic assessment in child and adolescent psychopathology* (pp. 34–65). New York: Guilford Press.

Aronen, E. T., Noam, G. G., & Weinstein, S. R. (1993). Structured diagnostic interviews and clinicians' discharge diagnoses in hospitalized adolescents. *Journal of the American Academy of Child and Adolescent Psychiatry, 32,* 674–681.

Atkins, D. L., Pumariega, A. J., & Rogers, K. (1999). Mental health and incarcerated youth: I. Prevalence and nature of psychopathology. *Journal of Child and Family Studies, 8,* 193–204.

Centers for Disease Control and Prevention, Division of Adolescent and School Health. (2001). *National Youth Risk Behavior Surveillance System: Trends in the prevalence of suicide ideation and attempts.* Retrieved from *http://www.cdc.gov/YRBSS*

Chambless, D. L., Shoham, V., Sanderson, W. C., Johnson, S. B., Pope, K. S., Cris-Christoph, P., et al. (1996). An update on empirically validated therapies. *The Clinical Psychologist, 49,* 5–18.

Columbia University Division of Child and Adolescent Psychiatry. (2003). *Columbia University guidelines for child and adolescent mental health referral* (2nd ed.). New York: Author.

Duclos, C. W., Belas, J., Novins, D. K., Martin, C., Jewett, C. S., & Manson, S. M. (1998). Prevalence of common psychiatric disorders among American Indian adolescent detainees. *Journal of the American Academy of Child and Adolescent Psychiatry, 37,* 866–873.

Ezpeleta, L., De la Osa, N., Domenech, J. M., Navarro, J. B., Losillo, J. M., & Judez, J. (1997). Diagnostic agreement between clinicians and the Diagnostic Interview for Children and Adolescents (DICA-R) in an outpatient sample. *Journal of Child Psychology and Psychiatry, 38,* 431–440.

Ferdinand, R. F., Stijnen, T., Verhulst, F. C., & Van der Reijden, M. (1996). The prevalence of self-reported problems in young adults from the general population. *Social and Psychiatric Epidemiology, 31,* 10–20.

Fisher, P. W., Shaffer, D. M., Piacentini, J. C., Lapkin, J., Kafantaris, V., Leonard, H., et al. (1993). Sensitivity of the Diagnostic Interview Schedule for Children, 2nd edition (DISC-2.1) for specific diagnoses of children and adolescents. *Journal of the American Academy of Child and Adolescent Psychiatry, 32,* 666–673.

Friman, P. C., Handwerk, M. L., Smith, G. L., Larzelere, R. E., Lucas, C. P., & Shaffer, D. M. (2000). External validity of conduct and oppositional defiant disorders determined by the NIMH Diagnostic Interview Schedule for Children. *Journal of Abnormal Child Psychology, 28,* 277–286.

Garland, A. F., Hough, R. L., McCabe, K. M., Yeh, M., Wood, P. A., & Aarons, G. A. (2001). Prevalence of psychiatric disorders in youths across five sectors of care. *Journal of the American Academy of Child and Adolescent Psychiatry, 40,* 409–418.

Grisso, T., & Barnum, R. (2003). *Massachusetts Youth Screening Instrument— Version 2 (MAYSI-2): User's manual and technical report.* Sarasota, FL: Professional Resource Press.

Jensen, A. L., & Weisz, J. R. (2002). Assessing match and mismatch between practitioner-generated and standardized interview-generated diagnoses for clinic-referred children and adolescents. *Journal of Consulting and Clinical Psychology, 70,* 158–168.

Jensen, P. S., Roper, M., Fisher, P. W., Piacentini, J. C., Canino, G. J., Richters, J. E., et al. (1995). Test–retest reliability of the Diagnostic Interview Schedule for Children (DISC 2.1): Parent, child, and combined algorithms. *Archives of General Psychiatry, 52,* 61–71.

Kim, J. Y. S., Fendrich, M., & Wislar, J. S. (2000). The validity of juvenile arrestees' drug use reporting: A gender comparison. *Journal of Research in Crime and Delinquency, 37,* 419–432.

Ko, S. J., Wasserman, G. A., McReynolds, L. S., & Katz, L. M. (2004). Contribution of parent report to Voice DISC-IV diagnosis among incarcerated youths. *Journal of the American Academy of Child and Adolescent Psychiatry, 43,* 868–877.

Lahey, B. B., Flagg, E. W., Bird, H. R., Schwab-Stone, M. E., Canino, G. J., Dulcan, M. K., et al. (1996). The NIMH Methods for the Epidemiology of Child and Adolescent Mental Disorders (MECA) study: Background and methodology. *Journal of the American Academy of Child and Adolescent Psychiatry, 35,* 855–864.

LeBlanc, M. (1998). Screening of serious and violent juvenile offenders: Identification, classification, and prediction. In R. Loeber & D. P. Farrington (Eds.), *Serious and violent juvenile offenders: Risk factors and successful interventions* (pp. 167–193). Thousand Oaks, CA: Sage.

Lewczyk, C. M., Garland, A., Hurlburt, M. S., Gearity, J., & Hough, R. L. (2003). Comparing DISC-IV and clinician diagnoses among youths receiving public mental health services. *Journal of the American Academy of Child and Adolescent Psychiatry, 42,* 349–356.

Lucas, C. P. (2003). The use of structured diagnostic interviews in clinical child psychiatric practice. *Review of Psychiatry, 22,* 75–102).

McReynolds, L. S., & Wasserman, G. A. (2004). *The timing of DISC administration in juvenile justice settings.* Manuscript in preparation.

Office of Juvenile Justice and Delinquency Prevention. (1994). *Conditions of confinement: Juvenile detention and corrections facilities* (Report No. 145793). Washington, DC: Author.

Otto, R. K., Greenstein, J. J., Johnson, M. K., & Friedman, R. M. (1992). Prevalence of mental disorders among youth in the juvenile justice system. In J. J. Cocozza (Ed.), *Responding to the mental health needs among youth in the juvenile justice system* (pp. 7–48). Seattle, WA: National Coalition for the Mentally Ill in the Criminal Justice System.

Overbeck, G., Vollebergh, W., Meeus, W., Engels, R., & Luijpers, E. (2002). Course, co-occurrence, and longitudinal associations of emotional disturbance and delinquency from adolescence to young adulthood: A six-year three-wave study. *Journal of Youth and Adolescence, 30,* 401–426.

Practice parameters for the assessment and treatment of children and adolescents with suicidal behavior. (2001). *Journal of the American Academy of Child and Adolescent Psychiatry, 40,* 24S–51S.

Randall, J., Henggeler, S. W., Pickrel, S. G., & Brondino, M. J. (1999). Psychiatric comorbidity and the 16-month trajectory of substance-abusing and substance-dependent juvenile offenders. *Journal of the American Academy of Child and Adolescent Psychiatry, 38,* 1118–1124.

Schwab-Stone, M. E., Shaffer, D. M., Dulcan, M. K., Jensen, P. S., Fisher, P. W., Bird, H. R., et al. (1996). Criterion validity of the NIMH Diagnostic Interview Schedule for Children Version 2.3 (DISC 2.3). *Journal of the American Academy of Child and Adolescent Psychiatry, 35,* 878–888.

Shaffer, D. M., Fisher, P. W., Dulcan, M. K., Davies, M., Piacentini, J. C., Schwab-Stone, M. E., et al. (1996). The NIMH Diagnostic Interview Schedule for Children (DISC-2.3): Description, acceptability, prevalence and performance in the MECA study. *Journal of the American Academy of Child and Adolescent Psychiatry, 35,* 865–877.

Shaffer, D. M., Fisher, P. W., Lucas, C., Dulcan, M. K., & Schwab-Stone, M. E. (2000). NIMH Diagnostic Interview Schedule for Children Version IV (NIMH DISC-IV): Description, differences from previous versions, and reliability of some common diagnoses. *Journal of the American Academy of Child and Adolescent Psychiatry, 39,* 28–38.

Shaffer, D. M., Restifo, R., Garfinkel, W. H., Enhrensaft, M., & Munfah, J. (1998, October–November). *Screening for young-adult suicidality and mood disorders in high school: The cost benefits of one- and two-stage strategies.* Poster presented at the 45th annual meeting of the American Academy of Child and Adolescent Psychiatry, Anaheim, CA.

Shrout, P. E., Skodel, A. E., & Dohrenwend, B. P. (1986). A two-stage approach for case identification and diagnosis: First-stage instruments. In J. E. Barrett & R. M. Rose (Eds.), *Mental disorders in the community: Progress and challenge* (pp. 286–303). New York: Guilford Press.

Steiner, J. L., Tebes, J. K., Sledge, W. H., & Walker, M. L. (1995). A comparison of the Structured Clinical Interview for DSM-III-R and clinical diagnoses. *Journal of Nervous and Mental Disease, 183*, 365–369.

Task Force on Promotion and Dissemination of Psychological Procedures. (1995). Training in and dissemination of empirically-validated psychosocial treatments: Report and recommendations. *The Clinical Psychologist, 48*, 3–23.

Teplin, L. A., Abram, K. M., McClelland, G. M., Dulcan, M. K., & Mericle, A. (2002). Psychiatric disorders in youth in juvenile detention. *Archives of General Psychiatry, 59*, 1133–1143.

Turner, C. F., Ku, L., Rogers, S. M., Lindberg, L. D., Pleck, J. H., & Sonenstein, F. L. (2004). Adolescent sexual behavior, drug use, and violence: Increased reporting with computer survey technology. *Science, 280*, 867–873.

Vitiello, B., Malone, R., Bushcle, P. R., Delanyey, M. A., & Behar, D. (1990). Reliability of DSM-III diagnoses of hospitalized children. *Hospital and Community Psychiatry, 41*, 63–67.

Wasserman, G. A., Jensen, P. J., Ko, S. J., Trupin, E. W., & Cocozza, J. J. (2003). Mental health assessments in juvenile justice settings: Report of the consensus conference. *Journal of the American Academy of Child and Adolescent Psychiatry, 42*, 752–761.

Wasserman, G. A., Ko, S. J., & McReynolds, L. S. (2004). Assessing the mental health status of youth in juvenile justice settings. *OJJDP Juvenile Justice Bulletin*. Retrieved from *http://ojjdp.ncjrs.org/publications/PubAbstract.asp?pubi=11733*

Wasserman, G. A., McReynolds, L., Lucas, C., Fisher, P. W., & Santos, L. (2002). The Voice DISC-IV with incarcerated male youth: Prevalence of disorder. *Journal of the American Academy of Child and Adolescent Psychiatry, 41*, 314–321.

Wasserman, G. A., & McReynolds, L. S. (2004). *Suicide risk at juvenile probation intake*. Manuscript under review.

Wasserman, G. A., McReynolds, L. S., Ko, S. J., Katz, L. M., & Carpenter, J. R. (in press). Gender differences in psychiatric disorders at juvenile probation intake. *American Journal of Public Health*.

Wasserman, G. A., McReynolds, L. S., Ko, S. J., Katz, L. M., Cauffman, E., Haxton, W., & Lucas, C. P. (2004). Screening for emergent risk and service needs among incarcerated youth: Comparing MAYSI-2 and Voice DISC-IV. *Journal of the American Academy of Child and Adolescent Psychiatry, 43*, 629–639.

Weinstein, S. R., Stone, K., Noam, G. G., Grimes, K., & Schwab-Stone, M. (1989). Comparison of DISC with clinicians' DSM-III diagnoses in psychiatric inpatients. *Journal of the American Academy of Child and Adolescent Psychiatry, 28*, 53–60.

Wiebush, R. G., Baird, C., Krisberg, B., & Onek, D. (1995). Risk assessment and classification for serious, violent, and chronic juvenile offenders. In J. C. Howell, B. Krisberg, J. D. Hawkins, & J. J. Wilson (Eds.), *Serious, violent, and chronic juvenile offenders: A sourcebook* (pp. 171–212). Thousand Oaks, CA: Sage.

CHAPTER 14

Minnesota Multiphasic Personality Inventory— Adolescent

Robert P. Archer
Emily M. Baker

PURPOSE

Within a few years of its original publication in 1943, the Minnesota Multiphasic Personality Inventory (MMPI) became the most widely used and studied objective personality assessment instrument (Archer, 1997). Although the MMPI was primarily intended for evaluating adults, it was also used with adolescent populations as early as the 1940s. There were some marked areas of ambiguity for clinicians and researchers, however, in extending the original MMPI to assess teenagers. For example, there were concerns that many test items were not relevant to adolescent development and experiences. Others observed that the MMPI was too long (566 items) to use effectively with many adolescents, and that specific test items were often written at too demanding a reading level for adolescent populations. Criticism was also aimed at limitations of the various sets of adolescent norms developed for the original MMPI (e.g., Archer, 1987; Butcher & Williams, 2000). For example, Marks and Briggs (1972) developed adolescent norms for the original MMPI that were based on samples of predominantly white adolescents collected between the 1940s and 1960s. Their normative data set lacked ethnic diversity and became increasingly outdated, underscoring the need for new norms that represented contemporary American teenagers (e.g., Pancoast & Archer, 1988).

Butcher and colleagues (1992) created the Minnesota Multiphasic Personality Inventory—Adolescent (MMPI-A) in response to these growing concerns. A major aim in the development of the MMPI-A was to obtain contemporary norms based on a nationally representative sample of 1,620 adolescents. Many test items were revised to simplify or modernize wording, and items were eliminated as inappropriate for adolescents. The test length was reduced from 566 to 478 items, and several new content and supplementary scales were created to assess adolescent problem areas. Throughout these revisions, Butcher and colleagues sought to improve the test while also maintaining, as much as possible, the integrity of the original MMPI's basic validity and clinical scales. Their goal was to develop a form of the MMPI, including a contemporary set of adolescent norms, that would help to standardize assessment practices for adolescents.

BASIC DESCRIPTION

The MMPI-A is designed to assess psychopathology for adolescents ages 14 through 18. Eighteen-year-olds may be evaluated with this instrument if they are living with their parents in a dependent environment, but should be administered the adult version (the MMPI-2) if they are living independently (Butcher et al., 1992).

Scales of the MMPI-A

The MMPI-A consists of 478 items that contribute to a number of scales. These include 7 validity scales and 10 clinical scales in the Profile for Basic Scales, 15 content scales and 6 supplementary scales in the Profile for Content and Supplementary Scales, and 28 Harris–Lingoes and 3 *Si* subscales in the Profile for Harris–Lingoes and *Si* Subscales. Table 14.1 provides an overview of the MMPI-A's scale and subscale structure.

Among the MMPI-A validity scales, there are two measures of defensiveness (*L* and *K*), three infrequency scales and subscales (*F, F1,* and *F2*), and two measures of response consistency (*VRIN* and *TRIN*). Defensiveness scales assess the test taker's tendency to consciously or unconsciously underreport symptoms, whereas the infrequency scales measure the tendency to overreport or exaggerate symptoms. The consistency scales measure the extent to which the adolescent responds to items in a reliable or consistent manner. Eight of the MMPI-A basic scales measure dimensions of psychopathology, such as depression, anxiety, and antisocial behaviors and attitudes. The remaining two basic clinical scales, *Mf* and *Si,* are unique in containing "nonclinical" dimensions and are often seen as significantly different from the remaining eight basic scales in terms of *T*-score distributions and nonclinical correlate patterns. There are 15 content scales, including a number of scales that are related to acting-out or externalizing behaviors: the *A-ang, A-cyn,* and *A-con* scales. Elevations on these scales are generally related to behaviors that place adolescents in conflict with others and result in rule violations and behavioral difficulties (Williams, Butcher, Ben-Porath, & Graham, 1992).

TABLE 14.1. MMPI-A Scale Structure

Basic validity and clinical scales

Variable Response Inconsistency (*VRIN*)	Scale 1	Hypochondriasis (*Hs*)
True Response Inconsistency (*TRIN*)	Scale 2	Depression (*D*)
Infrequency 1 (*F1*)	Scale 3	Hysteria (*Hy*)
Infrequency 2 (*F2*)	Scale 4	Psychopathic Deviate (*Pd*)
Infrequency (*F*)	Scale 5	Masculinity–Femininity (*Mf*)
Lie (*L*)	Scale 6	Paranoia (*Pa*)
Defensiveness (*K*)	Scale 7	Psychasthenia (*Pt*)
	Scale 8	Schizophrenia (*Sc*)
	Scale 9	Hypomania (*Ma*)
	Scale 0	Social Introversion (*Si*)

Content and supplementary scales

Anxiety (*A-anx*)	Anxiety (*A*)
Obsessiveness (*A-obs*)	Repression (*R*)
Depression (*A-dep*)	MacAndrew Alcoholism (*MAC-R*)
Health Concerns (*A-hea*)	Alcohol/Drug Problem Proneness (*PRO*)
Bizarre Mentation (*A-biz*)	Alcohol/Drug Problem Acknowledgment
Anger (*A-ang*)	(*ACK*)
Cynicism (*A-cyn*)	Immaturity (*IMM*)
Alienation (*A-aln*)	
Conduct Problems (*A-con*)	
Low Self-Esteem (*A-lse*)	
Low Aspirations (*A-las*)	
Social Discomfort (*A-sod*)	
Family Problems (*A-fam*)	
School Problems (*A-sch*)	
Negative Treatment Indicators (*A-trt*)	

Harris–Lingoes and *Si* subscales

D_1	Subjective Depression	Sc_1	Social Alienation
D_2	Psychomotor Retardation	Sc_2	Emotional Alienation
D_3	Physical Malfunctioning	Sc_3	Lack of Ego Mastery, Cognitive
D_4	Mental Dullness	Sc_4	Lack of Ego Mastery, Conative
D_5	Brooding	Sc_5	Lack of Ego Mastery, Defective
Hy_1	Denial of Social Anxiety	Sc_6	Inhibition
Hy_2	Need for Affection	Ma_1	Bizarre Sensory Experiences
Hy_3	Lassitude–Malaise	Ma_2	Amorality
Hy_4	Somatic Complaints	Ma_3	Psychomotor Acceleration
Hy_5	Inhibition of Aggression	Ma_4	Imperturbability
Pd_1	Familial Discord	Si_1	Ego Inflation
Pd_2	Authority Problems	Si_2	Shyness/Self-Consciousness
Pd_3	Social Imperturbability	Si_3	Social Avoidance
Pd_4	Social Alienation		Self/Other Alienation
Pd_5	Self-Alienation		
Pa_1	Persecutory Ideas		
Pa_2	Poignancy		
Pa_3	Naiveté		

Two of the supplementary scales (A and R) were developed by Welsh (1956) to measure major factor dimensions in the MMPI item pool. The two major stylistic influences that run through the MMPI-A item pool are emotional distress (Anxiety) and the tendency to repress or deny the occurrence of unpleasant or threatening feelings or events (Repression). The Immaturity (IMM) scale, developed by Archer, Pancoast, and Gordon (1994), measures an adolescent's maturation based on the developmental model of Loevinger (1976). Higher IMM scores are related to functioning within Loevinger's preconformist stage, as reflected in concrete thinking, egocentric self-occupation, and the inability to empathize with others or develop group loyalties. The remaining three content scales (ACK, PRO, and MAC-R) are measures of attitudes and behaviors related to alcohol and other substance abuse (Weed, Butcher, & Williams, 1994). Finally, the Harris–Lingoes and Si subscales provide information useful for refining our interpretation of the MMPI-A basic scale results, by providing a more detailed perspective on the specific areas endorsed to produce a basic scale elevation. Harris–Lingoes subscale information is not available for MMPI-A basic scales Hs, Mf, Pt, and Si.

Scoring and Interpretation

Individual MMPI-A results are compared, through the conversion of raw scores to T-scores, to adolescents' psychological functioning as reported by the 805 boys and 815 girls in the MMPI-A normative sample. T-scores are generated separately for females and males, because females generally report more symptomatology than males on the MMPI-A (as well as most other self-report measures). Because systematic age differences in test responses were not identified by the authors of the MMPI-A, specific age norms were not developed. Therefore, one set of norms was created that included all adolescents between the ages of 14 and 18.

T-scores above 64 are considered to be "clinically elevated," while T-scores between 60 and 64 are classified as "marginally elevated." It is expected that adolescents in this marginal elevation range will show some of the less extreme clinical symptoms associated with a particular scale (e.g., Archer, 1997). T-scores below 60 are within normal ranges, similar to response patterns produced by typical adolescents. T-scores on the MMPI-A are generated so that the mean for the normative population on each scale is 50 and the standard deviation is 10 T-score points. Therefore, a T-score of 60 is at approximately the 84th percentile, and a T-score of 70 is roughly at the 98th percentile for the normative sample.

Behavioral/clinical descriptions of T-score elevations have been developed for the MMPI-A scales on the basis of empirical research, and are critical for understanding and communicating test results. For example, T-scores greater than 64 on the Depression (D) basic scale have been associated with adolescents who are described as sad, dissatisfied, apathetic, guilty, and socially isolated (e.g., Archer & Krishnamurthy, 2002). When basic scale profiles are classified based on the most elevated single scale with T greater than or equal to 60, this is referred to as a "one-point codetype" or "single-scale high-point codetype." A "two-point codetype" is based on the two clinical scales most elevated in the basic scale profile, as long as the elevation of each scale is above a T-score of 60. Behaviors or traits that correlate with the one-point and two-point codetypes provide the basis for most MMPI-A interpretive statements.

The MMPI-A can be repeated or readministered to examine possible changes in adolescents' psychopathology across time. Adolescence is a developmental period marked by significant and rapid changes, including modifications in personality and psychopathology. Repeated administration of the MMPI-A during adolescence is therefore particularly valuable for gauging changes both in psychological dysfunction (as a result of treatment effects) and in developmental maturity (e.g., Archer, 1997; Archer & Krishnamurthy, 2002).

Administration and Materials

Administering the MMPI-A is relatively simple, and responses may be scored by a variety of methods. A typical MMPI-A administration requires approximately 1 hour to complete, depending on the adolescent's reading speed and level of concentration. The test is available in both softcover and hardcover test booklets. Multiple versions of the answer sheet are available, and the appropriate choice is dependent on the scoring option to be used by the evaluator (i.e., hand, mail-in, or optical scoring). In addition to the traditional paper-and-pencil administration, two other administration alternatives are offered by Pearson Assessments: (1) an audiotape version, with a running time of 100 minutes, which is useful with adolescents who have reading or visual difficulties; and (2) computer administration with the purchase of software. Two MMPI-A interpretive software programs are available for guidance in interpreting MMPI-A profiles. These are The Minnesota Report: Adolescent System Interpretive Report, distributed by Pearson Assessments and developed by Butcher and Williams; and the MMPI-A Interpretive System (Version 3), distributed by Psychological Assessment Resources and created by Archer. Both of these interpretive programs have report content that is specific for adolescents evaluated in juvenile justice settings.

It is important to establish rapport with an adolescent prior to administration of any psychological test, but it is particularly relevant for the MMPI-A because of its length. Engaging in nonthreatening dialogue with the adolescent prior to testing may help increase his or her involvement, motivation, and interest in the testing process. The adolescent can be encouraged to use this pretest interview to identify questions or concerns about him- or herself that might be clarified by the testing results (Archer & Krishnamurthy, 2002). The evaluation should occur in a noise-free testing environment that is comfortable and free from distraction. The adolescent should be monitored by the evaluator throughout the testing to ensure accuracy and compliance, and to provide assistance when needed. The MMPI-A testing should be completed in one session if possible, but may be broken into separate sessions if necessary. The MMPI-A cannot be sent home with the teenager for completion or administered in any other nonsupervised setting.

Reading level and comprehension are essential considerations when an evaluator is determining an adolescent's ability to complete the MMPI-A. The MMPI-A requires a seventh-grade reading level to comprehend test items at a level consistent with an interpretable and valid test protocol (Dahlstrom, Archer, Hopkins, Jackson, & Dahlstrom, 1994). This is especially important in juvenile justice settings, because many offenders have prior histories of learning difficulties in school (e.g., specific reading/language disabilities). The audiotape version of the test may help produce valid results for those adolescents who struggle with reading comprehension. Finally, several foreign-language translations are available for the MMPI-A. For example, the test is currently available in Dutch/Flemish, French, Italian, Spanish for Mexico, and Spanish for the United States. It is expected that MMPI-A researchers will follow in the path of the MMPI-2 by developing many more foreign-language adaptations in the future.

HISTORY OF THE METHOD'S DEVELOPMENT

The process of developing the MMPI-A began with the creation of an experimental test booklet (MMPI Form TX) that contained 704 items. This version of the MMPI was administered to 805 boys and 815 girls in the MMPI-A normative sample in many of the same geographic locations used as data collection sites used for the MMPI-2. Form TX was also used in the collection of test data from various clinical samples. The first section of the TX booklet contained the 550 items from the original form of the MMPI, followed by 154 experimental items that covered a variety of content areas believed potentially relevant to youths' developmental experiences; these areas included familial and peer relationships, eating disorders, identity problems, and abuse of alcohol or drugs (Archer, 1997). Approximately 13% of the 550 original items in the Form TX booklet were reworded to improve reading clarity for adolescents. Items related to childhood or adolescent experiences, for example, were generally worded in the past tense in the original test booklet because it was primarily developed for adult respondents, but were changed to the present tense in Form TX.

The MMPI-A manual provides information on test–retest reliability on the basic, content, and supplementary scales (Butcher et al., 1992). Based on these reliability data, the typical standard error of measurement (the degree to which scores can fluctuate by chance) for the basic scales is 4–6 *T*-score points. Consequently, one can assume that if an adolescent retakes the MMPI-

A within a relatively short time span, without significant change in his or her psychological functioning, the adolescent's basic scale scores will fall in the range of approximately 4–6 T-score points about 50% of the time. These data are important in evaluating the practical significance of any T-score differences obtained by readministering the test (to measure possible changes in functioning over time).

RESEARCH EVIDENCE

The MMPI has a considerable literature base with adolescents, which can be extended to the MMPI-A because of the substantial similarities between these instruments (Archer, 1997). Archer (1987) noted that there were roughly 100 studies using the original form of the MMPI in adolescent populations between its release in 1943 and the mid-1980s. Moreover, Forbey (2003) recently reviewed the literature on the MMPI-A and identified approximately 112 books, chapters, and research articles published in just the few years since its release in 1992.

Forbey observed that the content areas addressed in the MMPI-A literature had been fairly broad, so that it was helpful to group the articles and chapters into several categories. One category focused on general methodological issues, including articles describing the validity scale and basic clinical scale construction, and research evaluating the usefulness of the validity scales in detecting various forms of invalid responding. A second general content area included use of the MMPI-A with specific diagnostic groups (e.g., depressed adolescents). A third major grouping of MMPI-A articles addressed cultural or language issues. Finally, Forbey identified several books and book chapters as instructional guides for the use of the MMPI-A. Notably, Pope, Butcher, and Seelen (2000) have provided a guide to using the MMPI-2 and MMPI-A in courtroom settings, and Archer (2005) has provided a chapter in his MMPI-A text on forensic applications of the MMPI-A. Overall, research with the MMPI-A is progressing at a faster pace than that shown in adolescent research investigations of the original form of the MMPI.

MMPI research specific to juvenile delinquents began with Capwell (1945) and Hathaway and Monachesi (e.g., 1952, 1963). Capwell demonstrated the ability of scale 4 (Pd) to discriminate between groups of delinquent and nondelinquent girls. Hathaway and Monachesi (1963) collected data in the Minnesota school system to identify MMPI characteristics of adolescents who would later engage in delinquent behaviors. They found that scales 4 and 9 were especially valuable in predicting delinquency. Early studies such as theirs demonstrated the usefulness of the original MMPI in identifying and predicting youths' delinquent behaviors.

Subsequent research with the MMPI-A has continued to support the findings that scales 4, 8, and 9 are predictive of higher delinquency rates, as evidenced by their frequent elevations among delinquent youths. Hathaway and

Monachesi labeled this triad the "excitatory scales," to describe their relationship to acting-out behavior. More recently, studies have examined the use of the MMPI-A to identify patterns of juvenile offenders. Archer, Bolinskey, Morton, and Farris (2003) found that the 4-9 and 4-6 two-point codetypes are particularly frequent in male young offender populations. Adolescents who produce these codetypes, reflecting their two most elevated basic clinical scales, are more likely to report family discord, foster care placements, adoption, and involvement with law enforcement. These adolescents are described as defiant, disobedient, and primarily using acting out as their defense mechanism. Adolescents with a 2-4 codetype are often described as having difficulty with impulse control and oppositional behaviors. The impulsivity and conduct-disordered behaviors of these adolescents often lead to legal problems and substance abuse.

The content and supplementary scales are an additional source of information for evaluating delinquent youths. Their profiles often display elevations on scales related to substance abuse (*MAC-R, ACK, PRO*) and scales related to impulsive and acting-out behaviors (*IMM, A-ang, A-cyn, A-sch*, and *A-con*). Information on these particular dimensions can inform the clinician that a more intensive and comprehensive substance abuse evaluation or treatment program is necessary.

APPLICATION

A survey of clinical psychologists (Archer & Newsom, 2000) found that the MMPI-A is the most widely used objective personality assessment instrument with adolescents. Multiple factors contribute to the popularity of this test, including ease of administration and scoring, ability to assess adolescent psychopathology accurately, and usefulness in evaluating change over time. Consistent with the requirements for utilizing any test, the MMPI-A test user should have a comprehensive understanding of the test, as well as a general appreciation of test theory and construction issues. Butcher and colleagues (1992) and Archer and Krishnamurthy (2002) recommend that at a minimum, the interpreter should have completed graduate-level coursework in psychological testing, adolescent development, personality, psychopathology, and psychodiagnosis. The MMPI-A manual (Butcher et al., 1992) does allow for administration by carefully trained support staffers under close supervision of a clinician.

It may be helpful to provide examples of the ways the MMPI-A can be of use to professionals who use it in juvenile justice settings. MMPI-A validity scale results can be combined with findings from the basic, content, and supplementary scales in order to evaluate an adolescent's willingness to engage in psychotherapy, need for structure and consistently applied limits, and capacity to exercise appropriate impulse control. Using this information, a psychologist is better able to design treatment and rehabilitative planning for an adolescent in juvenile justice settings. For example, adolescents with a 4-9 two-point codetype, and elevated scores on *A-con* and *A-ang*, are likely to have trouble with impulse control and anger, to engage in conduct-disordered behaviors, and to "test limits." These adolescents may benefit from greater levels of structure (e.g., clearly defined consequences for rule breaking). In contrast, adolescents with a 6-8 two-point codetype are likely to be more passive, socially isolated, and prone to victimization in a detention setting. Supplementary safety measures may be developed in order to ensure their protection, because they are often recognized as odd and are preyed on by others, and may eventually be driven into unpredictable, aggressive behavior.

Specific areas of conflict in the adolescent's life, such as family and peer relationships (*A-fam* and *A-sod*), feelings of self-esteem/self-worth (*A-lse*), and/or social discomfort (*A-sod*) can be identified and understood more fully from review of their MMPI-A results. In addition, adolescents who are experiencing substantial emotional distress (e.g., anxiety and depression) may obtain elevations on basic clinical scales 2 and 7; the Anxiety (*A*) supplementary scale; and various content scales (*A-dep, A-anx, A-obs, A-lse*). Adolescents reporting high levels of distress in detention settings may benefit from psychological services and may potentially require monitoring for suicide risk. Moreover, a significant subset of adolescents involved in the juvenile justice system may qualify for dual diagnoses (e.g., psychiatric and substance abuse diagnoses), and several MMPI-A scales (*ACK, PRO,* and *MAC-R*) may assist in identifying those with substance abuse problems. Accurate identification of substance abuse problems can aid parents and law enforcement agents (e.g., probation officers) in monitoring substance use through random urine drug screens when such adolescents are released to an outpatient setting. Finally, reevaluating an adolescent with the MMPI-A during a course of detention or treatment offers the opportunity to examine the extent to which changes in underlying personality and psychopathological features have occurred, and whether any changes in the treatment or rehabilitation plan are indicated or required.

The MMPI-A, like the MMPI-2, is best viewed as an assessment instrument that provides a description of the individual's psychological functioning "at a moment in time." It is limited in its ability to make long-term behavioral or diagnostic predictions. This is a limitation not only of the MMPI-A, but of all psychological assessment instruments, because affective and behavioral instability is characteristic of adolescent development (Archer, 1997). This fluidity in personality structure is a major reason why the *Diagnostic and Statistical Manual of Mental Disorders*, fourth edition (DSM-IV; American Psychiatric Association, 1994) and its text revision (DSM-IV-TR; American Psychiatric Association, 2000) strongly discourage the application of personality disorder diagnoses to adolescents and specifically prohibit the use of the antisocial personality disorder diagnosis for individuals under the age of 18.

The MMPI-A has also been inadequately researched in terms of its ability to assess the risk of violent recidivism in adolescent offenders. The MMPI-A scales related to disinhibition or impulsivity may clearly be relevant to this task (e.g., basic scales 4 and 9, content scales A-*ang* and A-*con*, supplementary scales *IMM* and *MAC-R*), but the extent to which MMPI-A results can accurately identify adolescents at different levels of violence risk has yet to be established. Nonetheless, there are some promising results. For example, in a study by Hicks, Rogers, and Cashel (2000), the MMPI-A was found to be a more effective predictor of behavioral infractions among male residential adolescent offenders than the Hare Psychopathy Checklist: Screening Version (PCL:SV). More specifically, scores from MMPI-A basic scales 6 and 9 were more useful than PCL:SV scores in predicting both violent infractions and self-injurious behaviors.

CASE EXAMPLE

Jared, a 14-year-old African American male, was administered the MMPI-A as part of a psychological evaluation at a community mental health center. He was court-referred for evaluation following charges of burglary and auto theft. The court sought information about either his ability to remain on probation successfully or his need for placement in a secure environment. Jared's prior court history included charges of disorderly conduct, assault, abusive language, and possession of marijuana. He had been on probation for the past 8 months and had spent time in juvenile detention during the previous year. Throughout his evaluation, Jared was defiant and rebellious, impulsively and haphazardly responding to questions.

Jared was the younger of two children, and his older sibling lived away from home. Jared's mother had provided inconsistent living conditions and substandard food and clothing throughout much of his childhood. Jared had lived with his father for a short period, but was removed from his father's care following a physical altercation between them. Jared was then placed in a group home for delinquent boys, and while living there, he was arrested for physically threatening a female staff member. Jared eventually returned to his mother's home, but they continued to have a tumultuous and hostile relationship.

Jared's grades suffered because of frequent school suspensions for disruptive behavior. His peer group included youths also involved with the court system for delinquent behavior. Since age 12, Jared had smoked marijuana and drunk beer with his friends whenever either was available, but he had not received any substance abuse treatment.

Jared was administered the MMPI-A and other test instruments for a comprehensive forensic evaluation that focused on his emotional and behavioral functioning. Jared omitted only four items, and T-scores on measures of response consistency (VRIN = 57, TRIN = 51) were clearly within acceptable ranges. These latter scores indicated that Jared tended to respond consistently to items that were similar in content. His validity scale configuration on L, F, and K also fell below T-scores of 65, suggesting that Jared responded in a reasonably forthright and candid manner. Therefore, the overall validity scale results indicated that the MMPI-A clinical scale scores were valid, accurate, and interpretable.

The following is part of a Configural Clinical Scale Interpretation for Jared produced by the most recent edition of the MMPI-A Interpretive System (Archer, 2003):

> This MMPI-A codetype is classified as a 4-6/6-4 codetype. This codetype is fairly frequent among adolescents and occurs in more than 5% of adolescent assessments in clinical settings. These teenagers are often described as angry, resentful, and argumentative. In addition, an elevation on the A-ang content scale underscores the possibility that this adolescent experiences significant problems in anger control. Such adolescents are usually referred for presenting symptoms involving defiance, disobedience, and negativism. Their treatment referrals are often initiated by court agencies. Adolescents with a 4-6/6-4 codetype typically place excessive demands on others for attention, affection, and sympathy, but are resentful of minor demands that may be placed on them in interpersonal relationships. They are generally suspicious and distrustful of the motives of others and characteristically avoid deep emotional attachments. They display little insight into their psychological problems, and their behaviors often result in rejection and anger by others. In addition, IMM scores indicate that this adolescent might be described as immature, easily frustrated, impatient, defiant, egocentric, and concrete. . . . These adolescents are often referred for psychotherapy as a result of repeated conflicts with parents, which may take the form of chronic intense struggles. . . . The 4-6/6-4 adolescent typically undercontrols his or her impulses and acts without sufficient thought or deliberation. Problems with authority figures are also prevalent for these teenagers, and they are described as provocative by others. Histories of drug abuse are frequently found for these adolescents. . . .
>
> These teenagers tend to avoid responsibility for their behavior. They are difficult to motivate in psychotherapy and are slow to develop a therapeutic relationship. These characteristics may greatly complicate [this teen's] adjustment to life in a detention facility, and he may be more likely than others to have conflicts with staff and other residents. At times, his tendency to be angry and argumentative may result in violent altercations.

There were many points of agreement between the results of this computerized interpretive report and Jared's psychosocial history. Thus a computerized interpretive report based solely on the actuarial features associated with Jared's MMPI-A profile produced a description that accurately reflected the history obtained from Jared's mother. For example, Jared's mother complained of her son's defiant and disobedient behaviors, which are commonly found for adolescents with the 4-6 codetype. Also consistent with the 4-6/6-4 codetype, Jared repeatedly displayed angry behaviors that were not tempered by rules or consequences. He also had multiple encounters with the courts without improvement in his behavior. Typical of adolescents with elevations on scale 6, Jared did not accept responsibility for his problem behaviors. Jared's substance abuse history was also accurately reflected in his elevations on the MMPI-A substance abuse scales.

On the basis of this integration of MMPI-A and psychosocial history data, the forensic psychologist in this case opined that Jared's recidivism risk was moderate to high, and that his intense rehabilitation needs would be best addressed in a structured, secure setting. It was therefore recommended to the court that Jared be placed in a locked residential treatment center under the auspices of the state juvenile justice system. Jared's mother was unable to place the behavioral controls on him that were necessary to prevent future delinquent behavior. A rehabilitation plan was developed from the MMPI-A and other data sources. It included (1) group substance abuse therapy that employed relapse prevention concepts; (2) family therapy that focused on healthy communication between Jared and his mother, as well as his mother's capacity to manage Jared's behavioral issues at home; (3) individual and group counseling to address anger management problems and Jared's tendency to seek out delinquent peers; and (4) milieu therapy to improve Jared's problems with impulse control and relations with authority figures.

REFERENCES

American Psychiatric Association. (1994). *Diagnostic and statistical manual of mental disorders* (4th ed.). Washington, DC: Author.

American Psychiatric Association. (2000). *Diagnostic and statistical manual of mental disorders* (4th ed., text rev.). Washington, DC: Author.

Archer, R. P. (1987). *Using the MMPI with adolescents.* Hillsdale, NJ: Erlbaum.

Archer, R. P. (1997). *MMPI-A: Assessing adolescent psychopathology* (2nd ed.). Mahwah, NJ: Erlbaum.

Archer, R. P. (2003). *MMPI-A Interpretive System (Version 3)* [Computer software]. Lutz, FL: Psychological Assessment Resources.

Archer, R. P. (2005). *MMPI-A: Assessing adolescent psychopathology* (3rd ed.). Mahwah, NJ: Erlbaum.

Archer, R. P., Bolinskey, P. K., Morton, T. L., & Farris, K. L. (2003). MMPI-A characteristics of male adolescents in juvenile justice and clinical treatment settings. *Assessment, 10,* 400–410.

Archer, R. P., & Krishnamurthy, R. (2002). *Essentials of MMPI-A assessment.* New York: Wiley.

Archer, R. P., & Newsom, C. R. (2000). Psychological test usage with adolescent clients: Survey update. *Assessment, 7,* 227–235.

Archer, R. P., Pancoast, D. L., & Gordon, R. A. (1994). The development of the MMPI-A Immaturity (*IMM*) scale: Findings for normal and clinical samples. *Journal of Personality Assessment, 62,* 145–156.

Butcher, J. N., & Williams, C. L. (2000). *Essentials of the MMPI-2 and MMPI-A interpretation* (2nd ed.). Minneapolis: University of Minnesota Press.

Butcher, J. N., Williams, C. L., Graham, J. R., Archer, R. P., Tellegen, A., Ben-Porath, Y. S., et al. (1992). *Minnesota Multiphasic Personality Inventory—Adolescent (MMPI-A): Manual for administration, scoring, and interpretation.* Minneapolis: University of Minnesota Press.

Capwell, D. F. (1945). Personality patterns of adolescent girls: II. Delinquents and non-delinquents. *Journal of Applied Psychology, 29,* 284–297.

Dahlstrom, W. G., Archer, R. P., Hopkins, D. G., Jackson, E., & Dahlstrom, L. E. (1994). *Assessing the readability of the Minnesota Multiphasic Personality Inventory Instruments: The MMPI, MMPI-2, MMPI-A* (MMPI-2/MMPI-A Test Report No.2). Minneapolis: University of Minnesota Press.

Forbey, J. D. (2003, June). *A review of the MMPI-A research literature.* Paper presented at the 38th Annual Symposium on Recent Developments in the Use of the MMPI-2 and MMPI-A, Minneapolis, MN.

Hathaway, S. R., & Monachesi, E. D. (1952). The Minnesota Multiphasic Personality Inventory in the study of juvenile delinquents. *American Sociological Review, 17,* 704–710.

Hathaway, S. R., & Monachesi, E. D. (1963). *Adolescent personality and behavior: MMPI patterns of normal, delinquent, dropout, and other outcomes.* Minneapolis: University of Minnesota Press.

Hicks, M. M., Rogers, R., & Cashel, M. (2000). Prediction of violent and total infractions institutionalized male juvenile offenders. *Journal of the American Academy of Psychiatry and Law, 28,* 183–190.

Loevinger, J. (1976). *Ego development: Conceptions and theories.* San Francisco: Jossey-Bass.

Marks, P. A., & Briggs, P. F. (1972). Adolescent norm tables for the MMPI. In W. G. Dahlstrom, G. S. Welsh, & L. E. Dahlstrom, *An MMPI handbook: Vol. 1. Clinical interpretation* (rev. ed., pp. 388–399). Minneapolis: University of Minnesota Press.

Pancoast, D. L., & Archer, R. P. (1988). MMPI adolescent norms: Patterns and trends across four decades. *Journal of Personality Assessment, 52,* 691–706.

Pope, H. S., Butcher, J. N., & Seelen, J. (2000). *The MMPI, MMPI-2, MMPI-A in court: A practice guide for expert witnesses and attorneys* (2nd ed.). Washington, DC: American Psychological Association.

Weed, N. C., Butcher, J. N., & Williams, C. L. (1994). Development of the MMPI-A alcohol/drug problem scales. *Journal of Studies on Alcohol, 55,* 296–302.

Welsh, G. S. (1956). Factor dimensions *A* and *R.* In G. S. Welsh & W. G. Dahlstrom (Eds.), *Basic reading on the MMPI in psychology and medicine* (pp. 264–281). Minneapolis: University of Minnesota Press.

Williams, C. L., Butcher, J. N., Ben-Porath, Y. S., & Graham, J. R. (1992). *MMPI-A content scales: Assessing psychopathology in adolescents.* Minneapolis: University of Minnesota Press.

CHAPTER 15

Millon Adolescent Clinical Inventory

Randall T. Salekin
Anne-Marie R. Leistico
Crystal L. Schrum
Jana Mullins

PURPOSE

The prevalence of mental disorders is high among youths in juvenile justice settings (Teplin, Abram, McClelland, Dulcan, & Mericle, 2002; Wasserman, McReynolds, Lucas, Fisher, & Santos, 2002). A growing recognition of adolescent mental health problems in juvenile justice settings, and the development of assessment tools specifically tailored to address adolescent psychopathology, have put clinicians in a better position to accurately assess and treat youths who come into contact with the law. One measure designed specifically for use with adolescents is the Millon Adolescent Clinical Inventory (MACI; Millon, 1993). The MACI has gained considerable acceptance because it (1) provides clinicians with information on a wide variety of psychological problems, and (2) has a shorter administration time than some other comprehensive measures of child disorders.

The MACI was designed to assist mental health professionals in assessing and understanding a broad range of psychological problems experienced by adolescents, including general psychopathology, peer difficulties, confusion about self, and family problems. The MACI also assists clinicians in determining which clients are likely to exhibit oppositional and acting-out behavior, anxious feelings, and suicidal tendencies. Notably, the MACI is intended to assess both strengths and weaknesses, and to assist a clinician in maximizing a youth's potential by building on a full scope of personality attributes. The items and norms for the MACI were established by using samples of 13- to 19-year-old youths in a variety of clinical settings. Because the MACI addresses a wide range of problems, the instrument is frequently used in the juvenile justice system to inform decisions about the management and treatment of troubled adolescents.

BASIC DESCRIPTION

The MACI (Millon, 1993) is a brief self-report psychological measure designed to be consistent with the framework of child disorders defined in the *Diagnostic and Statistical Manual of Mental Disorders*, fourth edition (DSM-IV; American Psychiatric Association, 1994), although it does not provide DSM-IV diagnoses. Millon (1993) has also claimed that the MACI contributes to the assessment of developmental issues specific to adolescence. It consists of 3 validity scales, a Reliability scale, 7 Clinical Syndromes scales, 12 Personality Patterns scales, and 8 Expressed Concerns scales. The various scales for the MACI are described in Table 15.1. The measure is appropriate for boys and girls ages 13–18 years, and administration and scoring require approximately 60–80 minutes.

The MACI materials consist of two paper-and-pencil formats, one of which is appropriate for hand scoring and one for computer scoring. Hand-scoring materials include a reusable test booklet and a separate answer sheet. Computer-scoring forms include a combination test booklet and answer sheet and an online format. Audiocassette recordings of the MACI are available for use with both English- and Spanish-speaking clients. All versions are composed of 160 items, to which adolescents respond "true" or "false." Scoring options for the MACI include hand scoring, mail-in scoring, and on-site computer scoring.

Among the MACI's most desirable features is its inclusion of scales assessing three important areas of adolescent psychological functioning: (1) Clinical Syndromes, (2) Personality Patterns, and (3) Expressed Concerns. Clinical Syndromes pertain to major mental illnesses that are thought to be acute, such as depression and anxiety. Personality Patterns represent enduring maladaptive patterns of experiencing oneself and of interacting with others, as opposed to acute clinical syndromes. Expressed Concerns pertain to a youth's perceptions of his or her psychological development and actualization.

The MACI's three validity scales are intended to determine whether or not the profile on the Clinical Syndromes and Personality Patterns scales can be accurately interpreted. More specifically, these three scales assess various ways a youth may misinterpret his or her problems and history: (1) socially desirable responding (Desirability), (2) defensiveness in admitting to common shortcomings (Disclosure); and (3) exaggeration or overreporting of difficulties (Debasement). A fourth scale (Reliability) assesses whether the youth paid attention to or comprehended the MACI items. It should be noted that pathol-

TABLE 15.1. Scales and Scale Descriptions for the MACI

Scale	Name	Description and number of items
Modifying Indices		
X	Disclosure	Assesses how candid and self-revealing or reticent and secretive a client was in responding to MACI items. The scale is based on the overall raw score for the test; that is, totaling all the symptoms across scales results in a total score. Scores between 275 and 400 are considered normal (160 items).
Y	Desirability	Adolescents who present as overly desirable (17 items).
Z	Debasement	Adolescents who have a number of psychological problems that seem excessive or perhaps exaggerated (16 items).
VV	Reliability	This scale is used to test for random responding and the general reliability of the examinee's responses (2 items).
Personality Patterns		
1	Introversive	Adolescents who are indifferent and lack the capacity to experience life as pleasurable or painful (44 items).
2A	Inhibited	Adolescents who are shy or ill at ease with others. Such youths would like to be close to others, but have learned that it is better to keep their distance (37 items).
2B	Doleful	Adolescents who exhibit dejected and/or gloomy moods and have a pessimistic outlook on life (24 items).
3	Submissive	Adolescents who are not very assertive, but may be "soft-hearted," sentimental, and kind. Unlikely to assume a leadership role (48 items).
4	Dramatizing	Adolescents who are talkative, charming, and emotionally expressive (41 items).
5	Egotistic	Adolescents who are seen by others as self-centered, confident, and narcissistic (39 items).
6A	Unruly	Adolescents who act out in an antisocial manner, and often resist efforts by others to help them comply with prosocially acceptable standards (39 items).
6B	Forceful	Adolescents who are strong-willed, "tough-minded," and domineering (22 items).
7	Conforming	Adolescents who are conforming, respectful, and rule-conscious individuals (39 items).
8A	Oppositional	Adolescents who are irritable, unhappy, and passive–aggressive (43 items).
8B	Self-Demeaning	Adolescents who may seem content to suffer and may undermine the efforts of others to help (44 items).
9	Borderline Tendencies	Adolescents who exhibit marked instability in affect, relationships, and self-concept. They may fear abandonment and may engage in self-destructive behaviors (21 items).

(continued)

TABLE 15.1. (continued)

Scale	Name	Description and number of items

Expressed Concerns

A	Identity Diffusion	Adolescents who are confused about who they are and what their personal goals might be (32 items).
B	Self-Devaluation	Adolescents who are dissatisfied with their self-image. These youths may also have low self-esteem (38 items).
C	Body Disapproval	Adolescents who are dissatisfied with their bodies (17 items).
D	Sexual Discomfort	Adolescents who express concern or confusion about sexual thoughts or feelings (37 items).
E	Peer Insecurity	Adolescents who report sadness or concern about being rejected by their peers (19 items).
F	Social Insensitivity	Adolescents who are unconcerned about the welfare of others and override the rights of others for personal gain (39 items).
G	Family Discord	Adolescents who report that their families are tense of conflictual. These youths also have little support from family members and feel as though their parents are detached (28 items).
H	Childhood Abuse	Adolescents who report shame or disgust about receiving verbal, physical, or sexual abuse from parents, other relatives, or friends (24 items).

Clinical Syndromes

AA	Eating Dysfunctions	Adolescents who may have anorexia nervosa or bulimia nervosa (20 items).
BB	Substance Abuse	Adolescents who frequently use or abuse alcohol or other drugs (35 items).
CC	Delinquent Predisposition	Adolescents who have an inclination to break the law or violate the rights of others (34 items).
DD	Impulsive Propensity	Adolescents who have poor control over their impulses including sexual and aggressive impulses (24 items).
EE	Anxious Feelings	Adolescents who are apprehensive and anxious in general. These adolescents are nervous and fretful (42 items).
FF	Depressive Affect	Adolescents who are less energetic, experience fatigue, have a loss of confidence, and feelings of inadequacy (33 items).
GG	Suicidal Tendency	Adolescents who admit to having suicidal thoughts and plans. These adolescents may also believe that others think the world would be better off without them (25 items).

Note. Because there exists some heterogeneity in item context, it is recommended that individual items be examined when there is an elevation on a given scale.

ogy and scores on the Debasement scale are not mutually exclusive; adolescents can obtain elevations on the Debasement scale and also be experiencing severe psychopathology. Because of this, elevations on the Debasement scale may be indicative of severe psychopathology, exaggeration, or both.

The MACI uses base rate scores (called "BR scores"). This means that during the development of the measure the author obtained "base rates," or prevalence rates, for each disorder, problem, or characteristic. This provides important information about how common a problem may be in our communities, clinics, or juvenile justice settings. The raw scale scores were transformed into BR scores by specifying the population prevalence rate for the characteristics represented by each of the MACI Personality Patterns, Expressed Concerns, and Clinical Syndromes scales.

BR scores are anchored at 75 and 85. This means that BR scores of 75 and 85 were assigned to the raw scores that corresponded to the percentile points represented by the target prevalence rates for each psychological problem. For example, suppose the Depressive Affect scale (Scale FF) was estimated to be remarkable (the most characteristic symptom) for 14% of the population and estimated to be present, but not remarkable, in 8% of the population. This would then mean that the raw score on Scale FF that corresponded to the 86th percentile (i.e., 100% minus 14%) was defined to have a base rate of 85. Therefore, those scoring above a BR score of 85 would fit with the base rate group for the disorder. Similarly, the raw score on Scale FF that corresponded to the 78th percentile for the sample (100% minus [14% plus 8%]) was defined to have a base rate of 75. Base rate anchor points were defined in this way so that the proportion of adolescents in the population with BR scores greater than 85 for a particular characteristic would match the target proportion of adolescents for whom the characteristic was *most prominent*. T-scores are different from BR scores because they do not explicitly take base rates into account.

To interpret the MACI, a mental health professional starts by examining the validity scales to determine whether the profile is valid and reliable. Following an examination of the validity scales, the clinician then examines the profile of the Personality Patterns, Expressed Concerns, and Clinical Syndromes scales, typically looking for elevated BR scores (those above 74).

HISTORY OF THE METHOD'S DEVELOPMENT

The MACI has had several forerunners. Specifically, the MACI is a replacement test for an earlier one entitled the Millon Adolescent Personality Inventory (MAPI), which itself was a replacement for the Millon Adolescent Inventory (MAI). The MAI was developed in 1974, and the MAPI was first published by National Computer Systems in 1982 (Millon, Green, & Meagher, 1982). The MACI and its forerunners were developed in consultation with psychiatrists, psychologists, and other mental health professionals working with adolescents. The MAI and MAPI were identical in item content but used different norms (Millon, 1993).

The MAPI was subsequently divided into two forms, one of which was designed to aid mental health workers in assessing teenagers who exhibited emotional or behavioral disorders and who were in a diagnostic or treatment setting at the time of testing. This form was called the MAPI-Clinical (MAPI-C). The second form, the MAPI-Guidance (MAPI-G), was designed for school settings in order to help counselors better understand adolescent personalities and identify students who might benefit from further psychological assessment. According to Millon, the mixed clinical and nonclinical norms for the MAPI led to a loss of precision. Also, clinicians over a 10-year period recommended ways to enhance the instrument by adding scales for important syndromes such as depression and anxiety, which were not assessed by earlier versions of the MACI. Because of these problems, Millon decided to develop a purely clinical reference group with appropriate comparison norms and more relevant scales for the MACI. Millon reported that he took steps to broaden the scope of the MACI, and to maximize the MACI's concordance with its underlying theory of personality and the official DSM classification system. The MACI, as noted earlier, was published in 1993.

RESEARCH EVIDENCE

Reliability

The MACI has been shown to have good internal-consistency and test–retest reliability. As stated in the manual, alpha coefficients range from .73 (Desirability) to .87 (Debasement) for the validity scales. Alphas range from .74 to .90 for Personality Patterns, .75 to .89 for Clinical Syndromes, and .73 to .91 for Expressed Concerns scales. Test–retest data were based on administrations 3–7 days apart. These correlations ranged from .57 to .92, and the median temporal stability coefficient was .82. Given that stability across time was tested with a rather short interval, clinicians may want to limit their statements regarding the longer-term stability of the measure.

Validity

Several studies, primarily in nonforensic samples, have found that the MAPI and MACI have promising concurrent and predictive validity (e.g., Hart, 1993; Hiatt & Cornell, 1999; Millon, 1993; Millon et al., 1982). For example, Hiatt and Cornell (1999), using the Children's Depression Inventory (CDI; Kovacs, 1992) and clinical ratings of depression, found moderate concurrent validity for the MACI. Hart (1993) reported concurrent validity between the MAPI and CDI diagnoses of depression. Johnson, Archer, Sheaffer, and Miller (1992) investigated the validity of the MAPI more broadly by examining the relation between all Minnesota Multiphasic Personality Inventory (MMPI) and MAPI scales. They found that the MAPI scales showed moderate concurrent validity with the MMPI scales.

Some research suggests that the MACI can provide psychologists with relevant information regarding youths' treatment, especially evaluation of its effects. For example, Pantle, Barger, Hamilton, Thornton, and Piersma (1994) found that youths with high scores on the Forceful scale tended to make less gains in psychotherapy. In another study, Piersma, Pantle, Smith, Boes, and Kubiak (1993) found that in a sample of adolescents on an inpatient unit, administering the MAPI at admission and then again at discharge demonstrated significant differences on the Expressed Concerns and Personality Patterns scales in directions suggesting improvement as a consequence of treatment.

The MACI may also assist clinicians in making important treatment distinctions between substance-abusing and non-substance-abusing adolescents. Grilo, Fehon, Walker, and Martino (1995) examined the differences between MACI profiles of adolescent inpatients with and without substance use disorders. They found that the three-dimensional structure of the MACI (i.e., Clinical Syndromes, Personality Patterns, and Expressed Concerns) effectively distinguished between the two groups. The most salient finding was that the substance-abusing group showed significantly higher levels of delinquent predisposition and lower levels of anxiety.

A psychopathy scale (MC-P; Murrie & Cornell, 2000) was recently developed from items of the MACI. The concept of "psychopathy" is important, because in adults it identifies a particularly virulent subset of the criminal population. For example, relative to nonpsychopathic offenders, adult psychopathic offenders engage in more serious and persistent offending, recidivate more quickly after release from prison, and begin their offending at a much earlier age (Salekin, Rogers, & Sewell, 1996). Psychopathy has been described as a disorder with interpersonal, affective, and behavioral features. Interpersonally, those with this disorder are described as superficially charming, manipulative, and deceptive; affectively, as lacking in empathy and remorse; and, behaviorally, as irresponsible sensation seekers (Salekin, Neumann, Leistico, DiCicco, & Duros, 2004).

Murrie and Cornell (2000) found that the MACI MC-P scale was related to the Psychopathy Checklist—Revised (PCL-R; Hare, 1991). Salekin, Ziegler, Larrea, Anthony, and Bennett (2003) investigated the ability of this MACI psychopathy scale to predict recidivism with 55 adolescent offenders 2 years after they had been evaluated at a court evaluation unit. Salekin and colleagues also devised a separate psychopathy scale (P-16) from MACI items that aligned more closely with recommendations by Cooke and Michie (2001) and Frick, Bodin, and Barry (2001) for the refinement of the concept of psychopathy. Results indicated that both the MC-P and the P-16 scales were related to general and violent recidivism. However, especially the interpersonal and affective components of the P-16 scale were stronger predictors of violent recidivism.

The MACI scales that purportedly measure psychopathic traits in youths are relatively new and require more research before they can be used clinically. As Seagrave and Grisso (2002) point out, when youths show behaviors or attitudes that have been called "psychopathic," these may very well be time-limited and not necessarily indicative of budding long-term psychopathy. Measurement of these characteristics could be obscured by typical adolescent developmental issues or by symptoms of treatable mental disorders. In other words, we are not yet certain that measures of adolescent psychopathy are really measuring psychopathy per se (see Hart, Watt, & Vincent, 2002). Finally, it is also important to note that little empirical evidence shows that the disorder is completely resistant to treatment (see Salekin, 2002b).

Although the studies described above suggest the validity of some MACI scales for some purposes, the validation studies described in the MACI manual were not particularly rigorous or supportive regarding the construct validity of the measure. For example, Millon used clinical judgment as the sole basis for establishing the initial validity of the MACI scales, yet found that the MACI was not highly related to clinical judgment. Only two of the three studies in the manual provide criterion-related validity. In one of these studies (n = 139), almost half (13 of the 27) of the MACI scales did not evidence significant correlations with clinical judgment (mean r = .19; range = .00 to .43). On a second sample (n = 194), the validity in relation to clinical judgment was improved, but seven of the scales did not evidence adequate validity, and the average magnitude of the correlation coefficients was still in the low to moderate range. Finally, in regard to juvenile justice settings, much more research is required on race, gender, and age span differences for the MACI in order to maximize its effectiveness in those settings.

Factor-Analytic Work

As described in Chapter 4, "factor analysis" is a method for examining relations between items on a test, to determine whether those relations can be used to create groupings of items that can be labeled as a scale. Similarly, one can examine how the many scale scores in the MACI are related to each other, creating possible groupings of scales to represent overarching concepts. This could be useful to examiners, if it provided more meaningful and simpler ways to summarize youths' MACI results than merely listing all 30 scale scores. It also could lead to research on whether the various factors (groupings of scales) might be helpful in predicting behavior or responsiveness to various treatment interventions.

Romm, Brockian, and Harvey (1999) examined the factor structure of the MACI with 251 adolescents who were consecutively referred to a residential treatment facility. Referrals to this treatment facility did not come specifically from juvenile justice programs, but from a wide range of community services (hospitals, schools, outpatient therapists, and social service agencies). A principal-components factor analysis produced five factors (clusters of MACI scale scores) suggesting the following types of MACI cases: (1) Defiant Externalizers, (2) Intrapunitive Ambivalent Types, (3) Inadequate Avoidants, (4) Self-Deprecating Depressives, and (5) Reactive Abused. Research is needed to determine whether these case types would be useful for purposes of treatment planning or prediction of behavior, and whether they would be useful when employed specifically in juvenile justice facilities or programs.

Salekin (2002a) factor-analyzed MACI scale scores for a sample of 250 adolescent offenders. Findings from the study revealed a two-factor structure for the 7 Clinical Syndromes scales, which he labeled Depressed Mood and Psychopathic Precursors. A two-factor solution was also obtained for the 12 Personality Patterns scales: Factor I (Introversive, Inhibited, and Doleful; 6 scales) and Factor II (Forceful, Unruly, and Dominant; 3 scales). Finally, a two-factor solution was obtained for the Expressed Concerns scales: Factor I (Identity Confusion) and Factor II (Social Sensitivity). MACI users should wait for replication of these results, however, before attempting to apply them in clinical work.

APPLICATION

The MACI is available commercially from Pearson Assessments (formerly National Computer Systems). Because the MACI requires no special conditions or instructions beyond the printed instructions on the test itself, administration can be readily and routinely handled by properly trained assistants in juvenile justice settings. As such, it might serve well as a follow-up assessment for youths who are initially screened as requiring further evaluation. However, once scores are obtained, professional experience is required in order to interpret MACI scores.

Although the MACI has a number of positive features, it also has drawbacks for clinical use. First, one of the most commonly reported concerns is that many items "overlap"; that is, they contribute to more than one scale. This means that the same item can be used to elevate scores on two or more scales in some cases. For example, if a youth endorses an item that is meant to be related to being oppositional (the Oppositional scale), it could very well also elevate the Delinquent Predisposition scale. Thus the youth could be described as oppositional and delinquent, even though the scales measuring these constructs have items in common.

Second, the validity scales may not provide the best estimates of distorted responding, such as exaggerated psychopathology and random responding (reliability). Specifically, adolescents can have bona fide disorders (e.g., depression) and also score high on the Debasement scale. As mentioned, the Debasement scale has items such as "I often feel sad and uninvolved" that are related to psychopathology (e.g., depression). Thus, youths scoring high on the Debasement scale could very well suffer from a disorder. In addition, the Reliability scale consists of only two items and may not always represent the level of agreement or reliability (or unreliability) across the entire test. Youths may be inconsistent on one item pair, and this could invalidate the test, even though they answered questions to the MACI consistently throughout the test with the exception of this one item pair.

Third, further validation data (e.g., testing the MACI scales' level of agreement with clinical judgment and other psychological measures, as well as clinical outcomes) would help clinicians make decisions with greater confidence. Moreover, much more research is needed to determine specifically whether the MACI has clinical utility within the juvenile justice system. For example, the MACI has a Delinquency Predisposition scale, but we have no idea whether this scale actually predicts further delinquency, especially when used in a population in which almost all youths have engaged in past delinquent behaviors. Moreover, there has been almost no research to determine whether MACI scores have similar meanings for youths belonging to various ethnic groups.

CASE EXAMPLE

Courtney, a 16-year-old white female, was brought by the police to a detention center in a Southeastern state. She was charged with harassment because she allegedly pushed and assaulted her stepfather. According to Courtney, the incident occurred because she had used drugs prior to coming home from school, and as a result, her parents wanted to bring her to a hospital for drug testing. This detention center did not use an initial systematic screening process for all youths, and Courtney's initial behavior did not suggest any psychological difficulties at intake; however, after several days in detention, she was noted to be distraught. Specifically, she was observed by the detention staff to be tearful and withdrawn, and had reported feelings of hopelessness to another adolescent in the detention center. The policy at the detention center was to call in a mental health worker for a psychological evaluation if staff members were concerned that a youth had psychological problems and was at risk for suicide.

The mental health professional asked Courtney a wide range of questions about psychiatric symptoms and suicidal thoughts. She denied feeling suicidal, but said that she was "upset" because she wished she had not done the things that had resulted in her being detained. When pressed about being "upset," she said that she was mostly angry about having been detained.

Courtney reported that she had a long history of drug use and had been expelled from school because of it. The clinician was able to obtain some background information on Courtney by consulting court records, talking briefly with her mother by telephone, and (through her mother) obtaining permission to talk with a psychologist who knew and had been treating Courtney. These sources confirmed Courtney's report about her drug use. They also indicated that she had previously been arrested and charged with a variety of offenses, including petit larceny, destruction of property, possession of a controlled substance, and driving under the influence. Courtney's psychologist said that she had been diagnosed with depression at the age of 15 years, and that she had been receiving psychotropic medication and psychotherapy for more than a year to address her depression. Her mother also reported that last year she had tried to commit suicide with an overdose.

In order to address the detention center's concerns about Courtney, data from the MACI, clinical interview, and records provided by Courtney's therapist were integrated by the mental health professional. The MACI validity scales all were within normal limits, suggesting that Courtney responded to the test items in a reasonably forthright manner, neither exaggerating nor minimizing potential problems. The MACI Clinical Syndromes scales indicated elevations beyond a BR score of 85 on Depressive Affect, Suicidal Tendency, and Substance Abuse. Elevations beyond a BR score of 75 were also noted on four other scales: Doleful, Self-Devaluation, Body Disapproval, and Identity Diffusion. These suggested the possibility of a thought disorder related to her depression.

The results of the evaluation were used to make decisions regarding Courtney's treatment and placement. The results suggested the presence of current depressive symptoms, including the need for at least moderate precautions against suicide or other self-harm (despite her hesitance to say this directly during the interview). It was not clear why Courtney admitted to suicidal thoughts on the MACI while failing to report them to the mental health professional in the interview, but some youths will do so because they find it more difficult to admit to some thoughts or behaviors in direct conversation than in paper-and-pencil responding.

Based on the results of the psychological evaluation and MACI data, the recommendation was that Courtney be transferred to an inpatient facility for brief observation and possible intervention with a psychoactive medication that would reduce her depressive symptoms. Courtney was kept under close observation at the detention center, pending her transfer to a local hospital. Later, when the probation staff requested information that might assist in determining a disposition for Courtney's case, the MACI results were used together with other data to help formulate a community-based treatment plan to address her substance use and depression.

REFERENCES

American Psychiatric Association. (1994). *Diagnostic and statistical manual of mental disorders* (4th ed.). Washington, DC: Author.

Cooke, D. J., & Michie, C. (2001). Refining the construct of psychopathy: Towards a hierachical model. *Psychological Assessment, 13,* 171–188.

Frick, P. J., Bodin, D., & Barry, C. (2000). Psychopathic traits and conduct problems in community and clinic-referred samples of children: Further development of the Psychopathy Screening Device. *Psychological Assessment, 12,* 382–393.

Grilo, C. M., Fehon, D. C., Walker, M., & Martino, S. (1995). A comparison of adolescent inpatients with and without substance abuse using the Millon Adolescent Clinical Inventory. *Journal of Youth and Adolescence, 25,* 379–388.

Hare, R. D. (1991). *The Hare Psychopathy Checklist—Revised.* Toronto: Multi-Health Systems.

Hart, R. L. (1993). Diagnosis of disruptive behavior disorders using the Millon Adolescent Personality Inventory. *Psychological Reports, 73,* 895–914.

Hart, S. D., Watt, K. A., & Vincent, G. M. (2002). Commentary on Seagrave and

Grisso: Impressions of the state of the art. *Law and Human Behavior, 26*, 241–245.

Hiatt, M. D., & Cornell, D. G. (1999). Concurrent validity of the Millon Adolescent Clinical Inventory. *Journal of Personality Assessment, 73*, 64–79.

Johnson, C., Archer, R. P., Sheaffer, C. I., & Miller, D. (1992). Relationships between the MAPI and the MMPI in the assessment of adolescent psychopathology. *Journal of Personality Assessment, 58*, 277–286.

Kovacs, M. (1992). *Children's Depression Inventory manual*. North Tonawanda, NY: Multi-Health Systems.

Millon, T. (1993). *Millon Adolescent Clinical Inventory*. Minneapolis, MN: National Computer Systems.

Millon, T., Green, C. J., & Meagher, R. B. (1982). *Millon Adolescent Personality Inventory manual*. Minneapolis, MN: National Computer Systems.

Murrie, D. C., & Cornell, D. G. (2000). The Millon Adolescent Clinical Inventory and psychopathy. *Journal of Personality Assessment, 75*, 110–125.

Pantle, M. L., Barger, C. G., Hamilton, M. C., Thornton, S. S., & Piersma, H. L. (1994). Persistent MAPI scale 6 elevations after inpatient treatment. *Journal of Personality Assessment, 63*, 327–337.

Piersma, H. L., Pantle, M. L., Smith, A., Boes, J., & Kubiak, J. (1993). The MAPI as a treatment outcome measure for adolescent inpatients. *Journal of Clinical Psychology, 49*, 709–714.

Romm, S., Brockian, N., & Harvey, M. (1999). Factor based prototypes of the Millon Adolescent Clinical Inventory in adolescents referred for residential treatment. *Journal of Personality Assessment, 72*, 125–143.

Salekin, R. T. (2002a). Factor-analysis of the Millon Adolescent Clinical Inventory in a juvenile offender population: Implications for treatment. *Journal of Offender Rehabilitation, 34*, 15–29.

Salekin, R. T. (2002b). Psychopathy and therapeutic pessimism: Clinical lore or clinical reality? *Clinical Psychology Review, 22*, 79–112.

Salekin, R. T., Neumann, C. S., Leistico, A. R., DiCicco, T. M., & Duros, R. L. (2004). Psychopathy and comorbidity in a young offender sample: Taking a closer look at psychopathy's potential importance over disruptive behavior disorders. *Journal of Abnormal Psychology, 113*, 416–427.

Salekin, R. T., Rogers, R., & Sewell, K. W. (1996). A review and meta-analysis of the Psychopathy Checklist—Revised: Predictive validity of dangerousness. *Clinical Psychology: Science and Practice, 3*, 203–215.

Salekin, R. T., Ziegler, T. A., Larrea, M. A., Anthony, V. L., & Bennett, A. D. (2003). Predicting dangerousness with two Millon Adolescent Clinical Inventory Psychopathy scales: The importance of egocentric and callous traits. *Journal of Personality Assessment, 80*, 154–163.

Seagrave, D., & Grisso, T. (2002). Adolescent development and the measurement of juvenile psychopathy. *Law and Human Behavior, 26*, 219–239.

Teplin, L., Abram, K., McClelland, G., Dulcan, M., & Mericle, A. (2002). Psychiatric disorders in youth in juvenile detention. *Archives of General Psychiatry, 59*, 1133–1143.

Wasserman, G., McReynolds, L., Lucas, C., Fisher, P., & Santos, L. (2002). The Voice DISC-IV with incarcerated male youths: Prevalence of disorder. *Journal of the American Academy of Child and Adolescent Psychiatry, 41*, 314–321.

PART V

Risk for Violence and Recidivism Assessment Tools

Research has demonstrated that a number of factors put children and youths at risk for involvement in future violence and serious offending. This research thus far has not produced an absolute consensus about the most salient risk factors for youth violence or the most direct pathways to involvement in violent offending among adolescents. Nevertheless, recent literature reviews and analytic summaries (Hawkins et al., 1998; Lipsey & Derzon, 1998; Reppucci, Fried, & Schmidt, 2002; U.S. Department of Health and Human Services, 2001), as well as longitudinal studies (e.g., Farrington & West, 1993; Moffitt & Caspi, 2001), have made valuable contributions to our knowledge of childhood correlates of serious antisocial behavior. A systematic translation of this body of research into practice is still in progress. But taken as a whole, research suggests that (1) in order "to find the antisocial adult of tomorrow, one must look among the antisocial children of today" (Lynam, 1996, p. 210); and (2) a small proportion of males with early-onset delinquency become chronically antisocial in adolescence and adulthood, proceeding to commit over 50% of all crimes (e.g., Farrington, 1995; Loeber & Stouthamer-Loeber, 1998; Moffitt, 1993).

In the last decade, we have seen the advent of case management and risk assessment tools that integrate much of this research. Their aim is to guide early intervention efforts that might prevent later violence and chronic antisocial behavior, and to reduce the current risk of future harm among youths who have recently engaged in harmful aggressive behavior. Part V of this book describes assessment tools developed for this purpose—to evaluate youths' risk of future violence and/or recidivism.

In order to make an informed decision about the selection and use of risk assessment tools for youths, familiarity with the prominent issues in this area is critical. The first issue regards approaches to decision making—namely, clinical or actuarial judgment. "Clinical judgment" generally refers to unstructured assessments where risk variables are not necessarily explicit, may not be empirically validated, and demonstrate little value in the prediction of recidivism (Grisso & Tomkins, 1996; Monahan, 1996). By contrast, "actuarial assessments" generally contain items that are selected empirically, on the basis of a known association with a given outcome (recurrence of violence), and are scored according to some algorithm to produce a judgment about the likelihood of violence.

The second issue pertains to the nature of "risk factors"—circumstances or life events that increase the likelihood of engaging in criminal activity. Risk factors (and, consequently, items in risk assessment tools) are either "static" or "dynamic." Dynamic factors (e.g., current school performance) are variables that can change for a person over time. Thus they can be used to guide rehabilitative efforts by targeting influences on antisocial behavior and guiding interventions aimed at changing those factors. Static factors, on the other hand, are generally historical and difficult if not impossible to change (e.g., age at first arrest). They may be helpful as predictors, but they do not provide any guidance for assessing change as a result of rehabilitative interventions. Some assessment tools also include "protective factors"—positive circumstances or life events that are generally dynamic and reduce the likelihood of a youth's committing crimes.

A crucial third issue for assessments of risk for violence and serious offending among youths is the impact of developmental factors on the time frame for which predictions remain accurate. A significant limitation with the early identification of chronic and violent offenders is the inevitable high false-positive rate. Because youths are in the process of development, many of them who engage in violent behavior at one stage of development do not continue to do so as their development proceeds. Indeed, at least 50% of children who suffer pervasive and serious antisocial behavior prior to age 10 do not develop into violent adolescents (Patterson, Forgatch, Yoerger, & Stoolmiller, 1998; Robins, 1978), and an even greater portion of adolescents with serious offenses do not develop into antisocial adults (Moffitt & Caspi, 2001). Therefore, if we simply use their current violent behavior as a predictor of violence in the future, we will often be wrong (i.e., we will have made a "false-positive" error).

The goal of risk assessments with young people is often to target those in greatest need of rehabilitation efforts and risk monitoring. Generally, mental health examiners will want to use tools with known predictive validity that are capable of guiding treatment planning and capturing changes in risk. Though actuarial judgments have demonstrated predictive validity superior to that of unstructured clinical judgments (Grove & Meehl, 1996), critics have documented the danger of overreliance on actuarial decisions (Berlin, Galbreath, Geary, & McGlone, 2003; Dvoskin & Heilbrun, 2001; Grisso, 2000; Hart, 2003). First, actuarial tools have limited clinical utility, because sometimes empirical methods of constructing tests will identify risk factors that make little sense either theoretically or clinically. For example, imagine that research tells us that a youth's height or shoe size is related to violent behavior. Such things can be measured and may even be used in prediction, but they offer us little guidance for prescribing intervention strategies to reduce violence. Second, actuarial measures are also of little value when it comes to understanding the etiology of antisocial behavior and violence, due to overemphasis on the "effect" of variables rather than the "meaning" of variables (Grubin & Wingate, 1996). Finally, some actuarial tools make exclusive use of static variables, which by definition cannot measure changes in risk and provide little guidance in risk management.

We have already noted two approaches to assessing risk of violence—clinical judgment and actuarial assessment. Recently a third approach has arisen, called "structured professional judgment," to deal with limits of the other two approaches. This is an effort to improve clinical judgment by adding structure for those judgments, while also improving actuarial decision making by adding clinical discretion (Borum, 1996). Such instruments emphasize "prevention" as opposed to "prediction." They typically include both static and dynamic risk factors, because they assume that risk is not entirely stable and can change as a result of various factors (e.g., treatment quality and quantity, developmental factors, protective factors, and context). Assessment tools involving structured professional judgment are designed to guide clinicians to determine what level of risk management is needed, in which contexts, and at what points in time.

Part V comprises five chapters describing different procedures developed for assessing adolescent offenders' risk of violence or recidivism. These instruments are most commonly used for disposition or community reentry decisions to protect public safety, and for intervention and case management planning to guide effective allocation of resources for rehabilitation practices. Due to the nature of these tools, examiners who use them need some training in the specific administration procedures at a minimum, and a professional degree and/or specialized experience in some cases. Furthermore, proper scoring of each of these assessment instruments requires some degree of information from collateral sources (e.g., past records, parents), in addition to interviews with examinees. As such, these assessments can be relatively time-consuming and are often administered on a referral basis or in specific settings. Some have short versions, but most are assessment instruments that would not be feasible for screening of every youth entering a pretrial detention facility.

The first two chapters describe instruments that primarily employ an actuarial approach. In Chapter 16, Barnoski and Markussen describe the Washington State Juvenile Court Assessment (WSJCA) procedure, designed to evaluate youths' risk for reoffending and to guide rehabilitation efforts accordingly. The WSJCA instruments contain empirically selected items and employ algorithms for risk determinations and treatment recommendations. A benefit of the WSJCA is that it incorporates dynamic and protective factors that permit reassessments of risk. The Youth Level of Service/Case Management Inventory (YLS/CMI), reviewed by Hoge in Chapter 17, evaluates risk of recidivism in order to assist with case management and disposition decisions. Most items were derived empirically, and a scoring algorithm is available for decision making; however, the YLS/CMI includes an "override feature" to ensure that final decisions about risk incorporate clinical judgment.

The following two chapters describe instruments employing the structured professional judgment approach. Augimeri and colleagues review the Early Assessment Risk List for Boys (EARL-20B) and the Early Assessment Risk List for Girls (EARL-21G) in Chapter 18. These tools were designed to evaluate the likelihood of future violence and antisocial behavior, and to guide risk management plans, for children under age 12 with disruptive behavior problems. In Chapter 19, Borum, Bartel, and Forth discuss the Structured Assessment of Violence Risk in Youth (SAVRY), an adolescent tool for evaluating the likelihood of future violent acts and assisting with risk management. The two EARLs and the SAVRY produce structured clinical determinations of level of risk (low, medium, or high), while also containing items that inform treatment and management decisions and measure decreases in risk.

Finally, Forth's description in Chapter 20 of the Hare Psychopathy Checklist: Youth Version (PCL:YV) illustrates a minor departure from the other tools included in this section, because the PCL:YV was not originally intended for risk assessment per se. It is a downward extension of the major diagnostic tool for psychopathic personality disorder in adults, and as such, it is designed to assess psychopathic traits in adolescents. As Forth notes, information obtained from this assessment in juvenile justice settings may identify adolescents who are likely to pose serious institutional management problems, and to require intensive interventions and additional resources for management in the community. The PCL:YV is a clinical rating scale and does not prescribe actuarial decision making.

REFERENCES

Berlin, F. S., Galbreath, N. W., Geary, B., & McGlone, G. (2003). The use of actuarials at civil commitment hearings to predict the likelihood of future sexual violence. *Sexual Abuse: A Journal of Research and Treatment, 15*(4), 377–382.

Borum, R. (1996). Improving the clinical practice of violence risk assessment: Technology, guidelines, and training. *American Psychologist, 51*, 945–956.

Dvoskin, J. A., & Heilbrun, K. (2001). Risk assessment and release decision-making: Toward resolving the great debate. *Journal of the American Academy of Psychiatry and the Law, 29*, 6–10.

Farrington, D. P. (1995). The Twelfth Jack Tizard Memorial Lecture: The development of offending and antisocial behavior from childhood: Key findings from the Cambridge Study in Delinquent Development. *Journal of Child Psychology and Psychiatry, 36*, 929–964.

Farrington, D., & West, D. (1993). Criminal, penal and life histories of chronic offenders: Risk and protective factors and early identification. *Criminal Behavior and Mental Health, 3*, 492–523.

Grisso, T. (2000, March). *Ethical issues in evaluations for sex offender re-offending.* Paper presented at the Sex Offender Re-Offence Risk Prediction Training, Sinclair Seminars, Madison, WI.

Grisso, T., & Tomkins, A. J. (1996). Communicating violence risk assessments. *American Psychologist, 51*, 928–930.

Grove, W., & Meehl, P. (1996). Comparative efficiency of informal (subjective, impressionistic) and formal (mechanical, algorithmic) prediction procedures: The clinical-statistical controversy. *Psychology, Public Policy, and Law, 2*, 293–323.

Grubin, D., & Wingate, S. (1996). Sexual offence recidivism: Prediction versus understanding. *Criminal Behavior and Mental Health, 6*, 349–359.

Hart, S. D. (2003). Actuarial risk assessment: Commentary on Berlin et al. *Sexual Abuse: A Journal of Research and Treatment, 15*(4), 383–392.

Hawkins, D. J., Herrenkohl, T., Farrington, D. P., Brewer, D., Catalano, R. F., & Harachi, T. W. (1998). A review of predictors of youth violence. In R. Loeber & D. Farrington (Eds.), *Serious and violent juvenile offenders: Risk factors and successful interventions* (pp. 106–146). Thousand Oaks, CA: Sage.

Lipsey, M. W., & Derzon, J. H. (1998). Predictors of violent or serious delinquency in adolescence and early adulthood: A synthesis of longitudinal research. In R. Loeber & D. Farrington (Eds.), *Serious and violent juvenile offenders: Risk factors and successful interventions* (pp. 86–105). Thousand Oaks, CA: Sage.

Loeber, R., & Stouthamer-Loeber, M. (1998). Development of juvenile aggression and violence: Some common misconceptions and controversies. *American Psychologist, 53*, 242–259.

Lynam, D. R. (1996). Early identification of chronic offenders: Who is the fledgling psychopath? *Psychological Bulletin, 120*, 209–234.

Moffitt, T. E. (1993). Adolescence-limited and life-course persistent antisocial behavior: A developmental taxonomy. *Psychological Review, 100*, 674–701.

Moffitt, T. E., & Caspi, A. (2001). Childhood predictors differentiate life-course persistent and adolescence-limited antisocial pathways among males and females. *Development and Psychopathology, 13*, 355–375.

Monahan, J. (1996). Violence prediction: The last 20 years and the next 20 years. *Criminal Justice and Behavior, 23*, 107–120.

Patterson, G. R., Forgatch, M. S., Yoerger, K. L., & Stoolmiller, M. (1998). Variables that initiate and maintain an early-onset trajectory for juvenile offending. *Development and Psychopathology, 10*, 531–547.

Reppucci, N. D., Fried, C. S., & Schmidt, M. G. (2002). Youth violence: Risk and protective factors. In R. R. Corrado, R. Roesch, S. D. Hart, & J. K. Gierowski (Eds.), *Multi-problem violent youth: A foundation for comparative research on needs, intervention, and outcomes* (pp. 3–22). Amsterdam: IOS Press.

Robins, L. N. (1978). Etiological implications in studies of childhood histories relating to antisocial personality. In R. D. Hare & D. Schalling (Eds.), *Psychopathic behavior: Approaches to research* (pp. 255–271). Chichester, UK: Wiley.

U.S. Department of Health and Human Services. (2001). *Youth violence: A report of the Surgeon General.* Washington, DC: U.S. Government Printing Office.

CHAPTER 16

Washington State
Juvenile Court Assessment

Robert Barnoski
Steven Markussen

PURPOSE

In 1997, the Washington State Legislature embarked on an experiment to encourage the use of research-based programs for juvenile offenders. The state created funding for these programs contingent upon changes in certain juvenile court operating procedures. The most significant of these changes requires the use of a statewide risk assessment (Revised Code of Washington 13.40.510(4b)).

The Washington Association of Juvenile Court Administrators worked with the Washington State Institute for Public Policy (hereafter, the Institute) in 1997 and 1998 to develop and implement the Washington State Juvenile Court Assessment (WSJCA; Barnoski, 1998), now in Version 2.1 (Barnoski, 2004c). In addition to meeting the legislative requirement, the juvenile court administrators envisioned an assessment that could accomplish the following goals:

- Determine a youth's level of *risk for reoffending* as a way to allocate resources.
- Identify the specific risk and protective factors linked to criminal behavior, so that rehabilitative efforts could be tailored to address a youth's assessment profile.
- Develop a case management approach focused on reducing risk factors and increasing protective factors.
- Allow probation managers to determine whether targeted factors change as a result of the court's intervention.

BASIC DESCRIPTION

In response to these goals, Version 2.0 of the WSJCA (again, it is now in Version 2.1; Barnoski, 2004c) was created in 1999 as a comprehensive assessment consisting of 132 items. Because of resource constraints, the courts decided to implement the assessment as a multistage process involving a short prescreen assessment, an initial full assessment, one or more reassessments, and a final assessment. Each of these stages is described below.

Prescreen Assessment

The WSJCA prescreen is a shortened version of the full assessment that quickly indicates a youth's level of risk for reoffending. The prescreen contains 27 items concerning criminal history, school, family, peers, drug/alcohol use, and mental health problems. The prescreen items are not rating scales; rather, they attempt to capture factual information about the youth, such as number of felony convictions. The prescreen produces two scores demonstrated to predict felony recidivism: Criminal History scores ranging from 0 ("low-risk") to 31 ("high-risk"), and Social History scores ranging from 0 ("low-risk") to 18 ("high-risk"). These two scores, when combined, determine low, moderate, or high risk for felony recidivism.

All youth placed on probation are administered the prescreen by court staff members, usually during intake, when routine criminal and social history data are typically collected. Court staffers review each youth's criminal history in the Washington State Juvenile Information System, conduct a structured interview with the youth, and make collateral contacts with schools and social service agencies to confirm the youth-reported information (if confirmation is deemed necessary). Court staffers typically complete the prescreen within 45 minutes. During 2002, approximately 15,000 prescreens were administered in Washington State's juvenile courts.

Initial Full Assessment

The courts determined that an initial full assessment should be completed within 45 days of placement on probation, but some courts complete these assessments at earlier stages in the legal process. To reduce impacts on limited resources, the courts only complete the full assessment for youths rated as moderate- or high-risk on the prescreen. Low-risk youths, by definition, have few of the problems measured on the full assessment. Not completing a full assessment for low-risk youths presumes the absence of significant risk factors and the presence of some protective factors. The prescreen has motivated many Washington courts to assign low-risk youths to minimum supervision caseloads. This group generally includes youths who are not antisocial, but rather have made errors in conduct and have a low probability of reoffending.

A structured motivational interview is conducted with a youth and the youth's family to complete the initial full assessment. The motivational interview is the first step in the rehabilitative process; as such, it engages the youth and family to "own" the rehabilitation plan, and places the youth into an intervention appropriate for the youth's risk profile. The entire initial assessment process, including verification through collateral contacts, requires 1–3 hours.

The initial assessment includes 132 items that are organized into 13 domains (see Table 16.1). The Sex Offender domain was implemented for youths convicted of sex offenses who are on intensive parole but not on probation. Although community risk and protective factors are correlated with juvenile delinquency, a Community Risk domain was not included, because juvenile court administrators believed that use of information about a youth's neighborhood would be unfair.

The assessment items do not use a uniform rating scale. Item responses are tailored to capture behaviors or attitudes relevant to the concept being measured. For example, the "school misconduct" item has five response options: "recognition for good behavior," "no problem with school conduct," "problems reported by teachers," "problem calls to parents," and "calls to police." Item response options were based on objective facts whenever possible; however, the nature of many items dictated subjective judgments. One example is the "family willingness to help support youth" item, rated as follows (based on interviewers' assessments of a family): "consistently willing to support youth," "inconsistently willing to support youth," "little or no willingness to support youth," or "hostile, berating, and/or belittling of youth."

TABLE 16.1. WSJCA Version 2.1 Assessment Domains

Domains	Number of items
1. Criminal History	12
2. Demographics	1
3. School	15
4. Use of Free Time	5
5. Employment	8
6. Relationships	8
7. Family	20
8. Alcohol and Drugs	10
9. Mental Health	13
10. Attitudes/Behaviors	11
11. Aggression	6
12. Skills	11
13. Sex Offender: Intensive Parole	12

Each item response is recorded in a computer system that scores and presents the information in a variety of ways.

The WSJCA includes static and dynamic items referring to both risk factors and protective factors. Each domain produces four types of scores: static risk, static protective, dynamic risk, and dynamic protective factors. The dynamic factor-scoring scheme is designed to be sensitive to changes in risk and protective factors, so some item responses are scored as risks and others as protective. For example, the "belief in the value of an education" item receives 1 protective factor point for a "believes in getting an education" response, 1 risk factor point for a "does not believe in getting an education" response, and 0 risk or protective points for a "somewhat believes in getting an education" response. The *WSJCA Manual* (Barnoski, 2004c) includes the scoring scheme for each domain.

Reassessment

The third stage, reassessment, involves monitoring a youth's rehabilitation process and recording changes in the dynamic items on the initial full assessment during probation. Reassessments can be recorded when a change becomes known, after an intervention has been completed, or on a 90-day schedule. Reassessment may not involve another interview because of the probation counselor's knowledge about the youth. When a youth has improved, scores will generally result in a decreased risk score and an increased protective score. The intention is to provide feedback to both the probation counselor and the youth when progress is made.

Final Assessment

The last stage is a final assessment completed at discharge. The final assessment uses the same format as the reassessment and involves a review of all dynamic risk and protective factors to measure overall progress on probation. If a youth reoffends, the assessment cycle (prescreen, initial assessment, reassessment, and final assessment) is repeated for the subsequent period of supervision.

HISTORY OF THE METHOD'S DEVELOPMENT

The development of the WSJCA proceeded through the following phases:

- 1997: Literature review, initial item drafting, and international expert review.
- 1998: Pilot implementation, data analyses, and revisions.
- 1999: Statewide implementation of Version 2.0.
- 2003: Statewide implementation of Version 2.1, and Version 2.0 validation.

The development of the WSJCA, beginning in 1997, relied upon the juvenile delinquency and risk prediction research that had been evolving for over 30 years (e.g., Baird, Storrs, & Connelly, 1984; Farrington & Tarling, 1985; Hawkins, Catalano, & Miller, 1992; Henggeler, 1989; Hoge & Andrews, 1994, 1996; Howell, 1995; Jones, 1994; Lerner, Arling, & Baird, 1986; Loeber & Farrington, 1998). This body of research included recidivism prediction instruments, theoretical models for juvenile delinquency, identification of risk and protective factors, resiliency research, and research on effective juvenile delinquency programs. This literature was used to select items for the Criminal History scale of the prescreen and the initial full assessment. The prescreen's Social History scale was based on a modified version of Baird and colleagues' (1984) Wisconsin Risk Scale.

After the Institute created a draft instrument in 1997, over 40 Washington State juvenile court professionals conducted a series of reviews to refine terminology and provide examples. A group of international experts independently reviewed the first version of the assessment and provided written comments. These individuals included Brian Beemus (Oregon Department of Corrections); Robert DeComo, Donna Hamparian, and Patricia Hardyman (National Center on Crime and Delinquency); Jennifer Grotpeter (University of Colorado); Scott Henggeler (Medical University of South Carolina); Mark Lipsey (Vanderbilt University); Patrick Tolan (University of Illinois at Chicago); Robert Hoge (Carleton University, Ontario, Canada); Vernon Quinsey (Queen's University, Ontario, Canada); and David Farrington (University of Cambridge, England).

In 1998, the Institute created Version 1.0 of the WJSCA, following a series of focus group sessions with juvenile court professionals and a 2-day training session in the spring. The instrument was pilot-tested with 150 youths in a dozen Washington State juvenile courts. Data from these assessments were analyzed and redundant items cut to create Version 2.0. Version 2.0 was subsequently implemented statewide in 1999, and was subject to two large-scale validation studies, described in the following section.

RESEARCH EVIDENCE

Internal Consistency and Reliability

The WSJCA was designed to measure a youth's risk and protective factors comprehensively but with minimum redundancy. The items on the full assessment were not intended to be highly intercorrelated. In a recent study of the structural validity of the full assessment part of the WSJCA (Barnoski, 2004), factor analyses indicated that the domains were relatively independent, but the items from all but two domains loaded on more than one factor. That is, most domains are multidimensional. The Use of Free Time and Alcohol and Drug domains were the two single-factor domains. With regard to reliability, no studies have been conducted to measure the test–retest, interrater, or item reliability of the WJSCA.[1] In lieu of these studies, the courts have concentrated their efforts on training and integrating the assessment into their operations to ensure accuracy.

Validity

The prescreen Criminal History and Social History scales were developed empirically to predict felony recidivism (Barnoski, 1998). As such, the criterion for assessing its validity is the occurrence of reoffenses that result in convictions over an 18-month follow-up period (Barnoski, 1997). The courts agreed that for the juvenile offender population, low risk should reflect less than a 10% probability of 18-month felony recidivism, and high risk should reflect greater than a 30% probability or recidivism. Moderate risk is between 10% and 30%.

Two studies have examined the validity of the WSJCA Version 2.0 (Barnoski, 1998, 2004). Barnoski (1998) included a validation study of the Criminal History scale, using two Washington State samples comprising 21,682 youths placed on diversion, 8,265 youths on probation, and 1,365 youths sentenced to a state institution during 1995. All three groups exhibited the same associations between felony recidivism and criminal history scores. Sixty-eight percent of the diversion group had low scores, while 76% of the youths in a state institution had high scores. These results illustrated the applicability of the Criminal History score across the entire range of juvenile offenders in Washington State.

For the Social History scale validation study, Barnoski (1998) used data from a prior program evaluation with a much smaller sample than the Criminal History scale validation study (Barnoski & Matson, 1997). The sample consisted of 1,404 males and females placed on probation in Washington State for the first time during the 1997 fiscal year. Felony recidivism was linearly related to Social History scores, independently of Criminal History scores. However, because there was also an interaction between the Criminal History and Social History scores, a table of these combined scores is used to determine low-, moderate-, and high-risk status. The 6-month felony recidivism rates for the three risk levels were 6.6% for low-risk, 19.4% for moderate-risk, and 31.6% for high-risk.

In the second validation report, Barnoski (2004a) described the validity of the prescreen for youths adjudicated and placed on probation in Washington State juvenile courts during 1999. The sample included 20,339 prescreen assessments and 12,187 full assessments. The study continued to support the validity of the prescreen assessment; 29% of the sample was classified as low-risk (probability of 18-month felony recidivism less than 10%) and 42% as high-risk (probability of 18-month felony recidivism greater than 30%). The

---

[1] Currently, videotaped interviews of assessments completed by both court staff members and an assessment expert are available for a reliability study.

report presented the associations between recidivism and each item on the full assessment, as well as the domain risk and protective factor scores.

The 2004 report also assessed the validity of the prescreen for different subpopulations of juvenile offenders. Prescreen risk levels were valid for each subpopulation; recidivism rates escalated with increasing risk levels in all groups. However, there were significant group differences in recidivism rates at each level of risk. For example, males had consistently higher recidivism rates than females at each level of risk. A higher weight in the prescreen scoring for males would eliminate this difference. In addition, juveniles between 14 and 16 years old had lower recidivism rates than youths under 14 years, and higher rates than youths over 16 years. Age at adjudication could be included as a predictor variable to account for these differences. Finally, minorities had slightly higher recidivism rates at each level of risk than white youths. The juvenile courts will be reviewing the scoring of the prescreen in 2004 for the next version of the assessment.

APPLICATION

The WSJCA is designed for use with adolescents ages 12 through 18 who come into contact with juvenile justice programs and facilities. As noted earlier in this chapter, the purposes of the WSJCA are to determine a youth's level of risk, identify the risk and protective factors linked to a youth's criminal behavior, develop a case plan that focuses on reducing risk factors and increasing protective factors, and allow probation managers to determine whether targeted factors change as a result of court intervention. The prescreen can be used at a variety of points in the juvenile justice system—from the initial decision to detain a youth, to prior to adjudication, to placement on supervision following adjudication. The full assessment is most appropriately used after adjudication to guide the youth's rehabilitation, because of the more sensitive nature of the information collected. The *WSJCA Manual, Version 2.1* (Barnoski, 2004c) is available from either the Washington State Institute for Public Policy (*http://www.wsipp.wa.gov*) or the Washington Association of Juvenile Court Administrators (*http://www.wajca.org*). Since the WSJCA was developed using public funds, it is copyrighted but freely available.

Most Washington State juvenile courts now assign low-risk youths to minimum-supervision caseloads to conserve court resources. The state legislature has funded research-based programs for moderate- and high-risk youths who need more attention (Barnoski, 2004c). WSJCA domain scores provide risk profiles that match youths to programs designed to address their problems. For example, a high-risk youth with a dynamic family risk score of at least 6 out of 24 points is eligible for family-oriented interventions (see Table 16.2 for an illustration of how a risk profile can identify an intervention program). In addition to designing intervention plans, probation staffers can use the WSJCA risk profiles to guide rehabilitative efforts and support gains made by youths who have participated in a research-based program.

Accurate use of the WSJCA requires a thorough understanding of the assessment concepts, as well as an ability to elicit and interpret information. The Washington State juvenile courts addressed this issue by establishing a quality assurance process. A consultant was hired by the courts in 1998 to develop a training manual and curriculum. An experienced probation manager was assigned as the statewide expert to oversee the training effort on a full-time basis. Each court designates at least one person to become a certified assessment specialist for that court. Designated probation staff persons from across the state are trained by the consultant and statewide expert to be "certified assessment trainers." Potential trainers are required to submit a videotape of an assessment interview for critique. Only trainees who demonstrate competent interview skills and knowledge about the instrument are certified to be trainers. These certified trainers then train court staff members across the state. A quality assurance committee conducts periodic reviews of assessment systems to ensure that practices adhere to the WSJCA definitions and motivational interview principles. As of 2003, more than 700 court staffers had received assessment training. Since 1999, 10,000 to 15,000 youths in Washington State have been assessed annually.

Jurisdictions in other states have implemented the WSJCA. Utah, for example, has implemented the assessment and software statewide. Two private firms have disseminated the WSJCA widely by providing software and training services. The firm of Orbis Partners implemented a slightly modified version of the instrument, which it calls the Youth Assessment Screening Inventory (YASI), in several U.S. juvenile justice programs (e.g., the New York State Division of Probation and Correctional Alternatives in Juvenile Probation, the Administrative Office of the Illinois Courts for Juvenile Probation, the North Dakota Juvenile Court).[2] Assessments.com in Seattle, Washington, provides the software for Washington State juvenile courts and clients in California, Wyoming, Iowa, Alaska, Texas, and Idaho.

TABLE 16.2. Mapping Hypothetical Risk Profile to Appropriate Program

Problem	Program
Single parent	Mentoring
Family	Functional Family Therapy or Multisystemic Therapy
No parent	Multidimensional Treatment, Foster Care
Aggression	Aggression Replacement Training
Drug/alcohol	University of Vermont Incentive System
Mental health	Dialectical Behavior Therapy

CASE EXAMPLE

Police officers brought Josh, a 15-year-old white male, to the Snohomish County Juvenile Detention Center at 2:00 P.M. on Monday. Josh appeared on school property during school hours after being suspended for abusive language toward his teacher the previous Friday. When a school police resource officer confronted Josh to tell him he had to leave school property, Josh began hitting and fighting with the officer. Josh was admitted and confined on probable cause for third-degree assault. At 9:00 A.M. Tuesday, the presiding judge of the Superior Court, Juvenile Division found probable cause for Josh's arrest, and ordered him held for 72 hours on a $500 cash-only bail pending filing of formal charges. The following Thursday, the deputy prosecuting attorney charged Josh with felony third-degree assault. Josh appeared for his arraignment on Friday at 10:00 A.M. and was assigned a defense attorney, who entered a plea of not guilty on his behalf.

Josh was also assigned an intake juvenile probation counselor (JPC). The JPC prepared for the prescreen interview by reviewing Josh's court social file, prior police reports, school records, a parent information questionnaire, and case notes. Josh's criminal history consisted of third-degree theft (shoplifting, age 12), being a minor in possession of alcohol (age 13), and three fourth-degree assaults (ages 13, 14, and 15)—all misdemeanor offenses. Josh had three prior court-ordered detention periods totaling 30 days and one failure to appear for a court hearing warrant.

To complete the prescreen, the JPC conducted a 45-minute interview with Josh and his mother in the detention visitation area. The JPC reviewed the court's confidentiality policy and indicated that they could not talk about the pending third-degree assault. Josh described his school attendance and behavior as poor, blaming his school problems on his diagnosed attention-deficit/hyperactivity disorder (ADHD). He stated that all his friends had had contact with the court for crimes. His mother expressed disapproval of Josh's antisocial behavior. She further explained that when she would attempt to discipline Josh, he would become very angry and hostile, and rarely obeyed her rules. She stated that at the request of the school, Josh had seen an individual counselor for about 2 months 1 year ago to work on his behaviors. According to both Josh and his mother, the mental health counseling did not help. He had no formal mental health diagnosis other than ADHD. For the following week, the JPC made collateral contacts with Josh's school and the individual counselor. The JPC reviewed all the information and entered it into the computer. The software produced Josh's Summary Risk Report, identifying his level of reoffense risk as high.

---

[2]Orbis Partners is negotiating with the Ministry of Education in the province of Ontario, Canada, to use the YASI as an assessment tool in schools for students with multiple suspensions or limited or permanent expulsions.

Josh's attorney entered a plea of guilty to third-degree assault, and Josh was sentenced to 9 months of community supervision with standard conditions (attending school, maintaining a residence with a parent, attending counseling as directed, etc.). Josh was released from detention to reside with his mother. Josh's case was transferred to a JPC whose caseload consisted of moderate- to high-risk youths.

Following a review of Josh's prescreen and court social file, the JPC met with Josh and his mother during the first community supervision meeting to conduct the full initial assessment. The JPC covered the confidentiality policy and the purpose of the meeting, and employed motivational interviewing to engage Josh and his mother. Josh reported that he had been back in school since his release from detention; however, he was continuing to experience problems with teachers and other staff members. He stated that his attendance had been perfect since his return. He continued to focus blame on his ADHD for his past and current school problems. The JPC determined that Josh was experiencing success in two classes—math and art. Josh was still spending nearly all his free time with the same group of antisocial friends, however. His mother stated that she would like Josh to spend more time in some sort of organized activity. Josh stated that he had been kicked off sports teams for fighting and was currently not interested in any activities except hanging out with his friends. Josh reported using marijuana and alcohol with his friends, but said he would never spend money on either.

Josh described his home life as "boring." He said that there was nothing to do at home except watch TV with his mom, and added that his mother was always yelling at him. Josh's mother indicated that she was not employed because of medical problems. As a result, she struggled with financial obligations and the ability to give Josh material items. She said that she and Josh argued daily about chores, curfew, homework, and his friends. Josh stated that he rarely saw his father. Josh's mother said they had divorced because the father was abusive. Josh reported that he did not like being told what to do by adults. He often found himself in arguments at school with peers and the police. Josh said that once people made him mad, he found it hard to stop himself from hitting them. He was not able to identify his external or internal triggers, or the problem behaviors that got him in trouble with the law. The JPC observed that Josh had trouble communicating effectively and expressing his feelings clearly. The JPC finished the interview with Josh and his mother, and scheduled their next meeting for the following week.

A day later, the JPC made collateral contacts with Josh's school to verify Josh's self-reported progress. After reviewing all the information, the JPC completed the initial full assessment. The JPC reviewed Josh's dynamic risk and protective factors, and identified three WSJCA domains (Aggression, Attitudes/Behaviors, and Skills) as risks directly contributing to Josh's criminal behavior. The JPC added that Josh's inability to tolerate frustration could be a barrier to his making progress. The JPC matched the Aggression Replacement

Training (ART) program intervention to Josh's risk factor profile (risk scores of 3 on Aggression, 12 on Attitudes, and 15 on Skills).

At the second feedback meeting, the JPC reviewed all the information with Josh and his mother, directing the conversation toward helping Josh see the results of his aggressive behaviors. The JPC was able to help Josh understand that his aggressive behaviors caused adults, not Josh, to have more control over his life. The JPC asked Josh and his mother whether they felt Josh could benefit from learning new social skills and ways to control his anger. Both agreed that learning ways to avoid fights would help him avoid trouble with the law and teachers, and Josh agreed to attend ART intervention in 2 weeks. This became the focus of Josh's community supervision.

The JPC helped Josh use the new social skills by practicing them when problem situations arose at home and in school, and by reviewing the skills every other week throughout the intervention period. The JPC also continually encouraged Josh's mother to remind Josh to use anger reducers. At the end of the ART intervention, the JPC completed a reassessment by reviewing and changing (if warranted) items on the initial full assessment. The JPC reviewed this information with Josh and his mother to reinforce the improvements in Josh's aggressive behaviors and skills and in the associated dynamic scores. The JPC continued to encourage Josh and his mother to practice the learned social skills and anger reducers throughout the remaining months of community supervision. Both Josh and his mother saw changes in their communication. Josh's mother reported reductions in their arguments after 5 months. Josh acknowledged that when he actually used the anger reducers, he could stop himself from physically hitting people. However, he still had problems reminding himself to use the anger reducers when he became angry. Josh had not been in a physical fight for over 6 months. The focus of Josh's remaining community supervision was to continue to work on improving his ability to recognize his triggers, use anger reducers, and practice the learned social skills. At the end of Josh's community supervision, the JPC completed a final assessment and reviewed this information with Josh and his mother.

REFERENCES

Baird, S. C., Storrs, G. M., & Connelly, H. (1984). *Classification of juveniles in corrections: A model systems approach*. Washington, DC: Arthur D. Little.

Barnoski, R. (1997). *Standards for improving research effectiveness in adult and juvenile justice* (Report No. 97-12-1201). Olympia: Washington State Institute for Public Policy.

Barnoski, R. (1998). *Validation of the Washington State Juvenile Court Assessment: Interim report* (Report No. 98-11-1201). Olympia: Washington State Institute for Public Policy.

Barnoski, R. (2004a). *Assessing risk for re-offense: Validating the Washington State*

Juvenile Court Assessment (Report No. 04-03-1201). Olympia: Washington State Institute for Public Policy.

Barnoski, R. (2004b). *Outcome evaluation of Washington State's research-based programs for juvenile offenders* (Report No. 04-01-1201). Olympia: Washington State Institute for Public Policy.

Barnoski, R. (2004c). *Washington State Juvenile Court Assessment manual, Version 2.1* (Report No. 04-03-1203). Olympia: Washington State Institute for Public Policy.

Barnoski, R., & Matson, S. (1997). *Evaluating early intervention in Washington State juvenile courts: A six-month progress report* (Report No. 97-01-1202). Olympia: Washington State Institute for Public Policy.

Farrington, D., & Tarling, R. (1985). *Prediction in criminology.* Albany: State University of New York Press.

Hawkins, J. D., Catalano, R. F., & Miller, J. Y. (1992). Risk and protective factors in adolescence and early adulthood: Implications for substance abuse prevention. *Psychological Bulletin, 112,* 64–105.

Henggeler, S. W. (1989). *Delinquency in adolescence.* Newbury Park, CA: Sage.

Hoge, R. D., & Andrews, D. A. (1994). *The Youth Level of Service/Case Management Inventory and manual.* Ottawa, Ontario, Canada: Carleton University, Department of Psychology.

Hoge, R. D., & Andrews, D. A. (1996). *Assessing the youthful offender: Issues and techniques.* New York: Plenum Press.

Howell, J. C. (Ed.). (1995). *Guide for implementing the comprehensive strategy for serious, violent and chronic juvenile offenders.* Washington, DC: Office of Juvenile Justice and Delinquency Prevention.

Jones, P. R. (1996). Risk prediction in criminal justice. In A. T. Harland (Ed.), *Choosing correctional options that work: Defining the demand and evaluating the supply* (pp. 33–68). Thousand Oaks, CA: Sage.

Lerner, K., Arling, G., & Baird, S. C. (1986). Client management: Classification strategies for case supervision. *Crime and Delinquency, 32,* 254–271.

Loeber, R., & Farrington, D. P. (Eds.). (1998). *Serious and violent juvenile offenders: Risk factors and successful interventions.* Thousand Oaks, CA: Sage.

CHAPTER 17

Youth Level of Service/ Case Management Inventory

Robert D. Hoge

PURPOSE

The Youth Level of Service/Case Management Inventory (YLS/CMI; Hoge & Andrews, 2002; Hoge, Andrews, & Leschied, 2002) is a standardized inventory for use with juvenile offenders. It assesses factors associated with *risk of recidivism*, as well as *need* factors that assist in case management. The authors of the YLS/CMI designed it primarily to assist with pre- and postadjudication case planning. However, the YLS/CMI can also assist with making a wide range of decisions relating to juvenile offenders, such as preadjudication diversion and detention, waivers to adult court and the mental health system, and postadjudication dispositions.

The YLS/CMI is based on three principles of case classification (Andrews, Bonta, & Hoge, 1990; Hoge, 2001) to guide treatment interventions with offenders. The "risk principle" states that services to the offender should reflect the level of risk presented. For example, offenders at high risk of recidivism should receive intensive services, whereas lower-risk offenders should be provided with less intensive services or no services at all. Observance of this principle is important for providing appropriate services to clients while optimizing use of agency resources.

The "need principle" states that targets of service should be matched with the criminogenic needs of the client. For example, if poor parental supervision and involvement with antisocial peers seem to be the major factors contributing to a youth's delinquent behavior, then those should be the primary targets of intervention with the youth. Criminogenic needs are risk factors that are amenable to change and that, if changed, reduce the probability of continued criminal activity. Observance of this principle will also help to ensure that appropriate services are provided to clients and that agency resources are used effectively.

The "responsivity principle" states that decisions about interventions should consider other characteristics of the youth and his or her circumstances that may affect responses to the interventions. These factors may not be directly related to criminal activity, but are relevant to case planning. Examples of responsivity factors include intelligence, learning style, and motivation for treatment. Protective or strength factors may also be represented as responsivity factors, since they too are relevant to treatment planning. Examples include high levels of emotional maturity, prosocial attitudes, and the availability of a supportive adult.

Reviews and meta-analyses by Andrews, Zinger, and colleagues (1990), Lipsey (1995), and Lipsey and Wilson (1998) support the hypothesis that interventions based on these three principles are, in general, most efficacious. The YLS/CMI permits structured assessments of risk, need, and responsivity factors relevant to juvenile offenders. The selection of risk and need factors in the instrument was guided by recent research on the causes and correlates of youth crime (see Cottle, Lee, & Heilbrun, 2001; Hawkins et al., 1998; Hoge, 2001; Lipsey & Derzon, 1998). The YLS/CMI is a standardized measure that combines the principles of *actuarial* decision making (based on a scoring algorithm) and clinical decision making, and thus serves as an alternative to the purely clinical judgments that so often underlie forensic decisions (Grisso, 1998, 2003; Hoge, 1999; Hoge & Andrews, 1996b; Le Blanc, 1998).

BASIC DESCRIPTION

A probation officer or other trained professional can complete the YLS/CMI on the basis of a file review and interviews with a client and collateral sources. The measure can be completed in 20–30 minutes following the interview and file review. The following provides a brief introduction to the six sections of the YLS/CMI. More detailed descriptions are available in the *User's Manual* (Hoge & Andrews, 2002).

Part I: Assessment of Risks and Needs

Part I comprises 42 items based on the major risk and need factors identified in the literature as relevant to juvenile offending. The 42 items are divided into eight subscales: Prior and Current Offenses, Family Circumstances/Parenting, Education/Employment, Peer Associations, Substance Abuse, Leisure/Recreation, Personality/Behavior, and Attitudes/Orientation. Both static (e.g., "prior probation") and dynamic (e.g., "chronic drug use") items are included.

The scoring key in the *User's Manual* provides detailed guidelines for scoring items.

Items are listed in a checklist format, and assessors are asked to indicate whether each risk factor is present (e.g., "inadequate parental supervision"). For seven of the eight categories, the assessor is also asked to indicate whether the area is a strength. For example, although a youth may be experiencing difficulties in many areas, he or she may like school and maintain good school performance. In this case, school performance can be identified as a strength or protective factor. Space is also provided for recording comments and indicating sources of information.

Part II: Summary of Risk/Need Factors

Part II provides an opportunity to summarize the risk/need factors represented in each of the subscales. Assessors calculate subscale scores and an overall risk/need index by summing across all items. Four categories of overall risk/need level are indicated: "low" (0–8), "moderate" (9–22), "high" (23–34), and "very high" (35–42). Normative data based on a sample of 263 Canadian adjudicated offenders are reported in the *User's Manual*. The sample included male and female juveniles with both probation and custody dispositions. The average overall risk/need scores of the normative sample ranged from 2 to 35 ($M = 11.52$, $SD = 8.33$). The instrument's authors encourage users to develop norms for their own samples of juvenile offenders.

Part III: Assessment of Other Needs/Special Considerations

Part III provides an opportunity to record the presence of other factors that may be relevant to case planning. Some of the items in this section represent responsivity factors. The two categories of variables include those relevant to the family (e.g., "parental drug/alcohol abuse") and the youth (e.g., "depressed"). Items relevant to institutional adjustment are also included (e.g., "history of assault on authority figures").

Part IV: Your Assessment of the Client's General Risk/Need Level

Part IV represents the "professional override" feature of the instrument. The assessor is asked to take into account all the information available about the client and to provide an estimate of the level of risk and need represented by specifying whether it is low, moderate, high, or very high. If this estimate differs from that indicated in Part II, the assessor is asked to comment on the reasons. This section ensures that final decisions about the client rest with the responsible professional. The *User's Manual* stresses that the YLS/CMI is not to be used in a rigid fashion to dictate decisions based on a scoring algorithm.

Part V: Contact Level

Part V indicates the appropriate level of contact for a young offender. The level of contact should be linked directly to the overall risk/need level. As stated in the risk principle of case classification, intensive services should be reserved for high-risk cases, and less intensive services for lower risk cases.

Part VI: Case Management Plan

In Part VI, assessors are expected to indicate specific goals for youths and the means for achieving those goals. The major consideration in the selection of goals flows from the need principle of case classification: Targets of service should be matched with the criminogenic needs of each youth as identified in Part I. Means of achieving goals are to be expressed in explicit and concrete terms. Case planning should also take into account the strength factors identified in Part I and the responsivity considerations in Part III. For example, antisocial attitudes and beliefs may be identified as a major risk/need factor, so replacing those with more prosocial attitudes and beliefs may be a goal of treatment. Enrollment in a cognitive-behavioral attitude modification program may be specified as the means for achieving this goal. However, if the youth is of limited cognitive ability, this type of treatment may be inappropriate, so a skills training program may be recommended instead.

HISTORY OF THE METHOD'S DEVELOPMENT

The YLS/CMI is the youth version of the Level of Service Inventory—Revised (LSI–R; Andrews & Bonta, 1995). Andrews and Bonta designed the LSI–R to assess risk and need factors in adult offenders. It is widely used in adult correctional and parole systems. Considerable psychometric support is available for this instrument (Andrews & Bonta, 1995; Gendreau, Goggin, & Little, 1996).

An earlier effort to produce a youth version of the LSI–R resulted in the Youth Level of Service Inventory (YLSI; Andrews, Robinson, & Hoge, 1984), which contained 112 risk/need items based on variables identified in the research literature as showing moderate to strong associations with youthful offending. The psychometric properties of this instrument were explored in a number of studies (Andrews, Robinson, & Balla, 1986; Shields & Simourd, 1991; Simourd, Hoge, & Andrews, 1991; Simourd, Hoge, Andrews, & Leschied, 1994). In this research, 42 of the original 112 items consistently showed significant correlations with indexes of reoffending. These form the items of Part I of the YLS/CMI. These were grouped into eight subscales on the basis of previous factor analyses (Simourd et al., 1991). Many other items were incorporated into Part III. Strength items and the professional override feature (Part IV) were added, as was the case management plan (Part VI). The latter plan was included to encourage a direct link between the risk/need assessment and case planning. The usability of the instrument was evaluated through a pilot test in which the YLS/CMI was completed by a group of experienced probation officers (Hoge & Andrews, 1996b).

RESEARCH EVIDENCE

Research with the YLSI provided support for the reliability and validity of the 42 items incorporated into Part I of the YLS/CMI (Andrews et al., 1986; Shields & Simourd, 1991; Simourd et al., 1991, 1994). In particular, analyses supported the predictive validity of risk/need items for future offending. Findings concerning the psychometric properties of Part I of the YLS/CMI are briefly summarized here. All studies were based on samples of Canadian juvenile offenders between 12 and 17 years of age. Jung (1996) also included a sample of nonoffending youths See the YLS/CMI *User's Manual* (Hoge & Andrews, 2002) for additional details.

Internal Consistency and Reliability

Rowe (2002) reported a coefficient alpha value of .91 for the total risk/need score. The mean coefficient alpha value across the eight subscales was reported as .72 by Rowe and .69 by Schmidt, Hoge, and Robertson (2002). Both studies were based on samples of adjudicated offenders.

Poluchowicz, Jung, and Rawana (2000) reported an interrater agreement coefficient of .75 for the overall risk/need score, based on 33 cases scored by two independent raters. These researchers reported adequate interrater agreement for all subscales except Leisure/Recreation, ranging from .05 to .92 (median $r = .70$). Schmidt and colleagues (2002) reported interrater agreement between the independent ratings of two assessors across 29 cases. Interrater reliability for the subscales ranged from .61 to .85 (median $r = .76$).

Validity

Several concurrent validity studies have reported correlations between YLS/CMI overall risk/need scores and scores from alternative measures of externalizing disorders. One would not expect perfect agreement in these cases, because the YLS/CMI assesses a broader range of variables than the alternative measures do. However, the analyses do bear on the ability of the YLS/CMI to evaluate conduct disorder, and to this extent may be said to bear on construct validity.

Schmidt and colleagues (2002) reported significant correlations between YLS/CMI overall risk/need scores and the Total Problem and Externalizing scores of the Child Behavior Checklist (Achenbach, 1991a) and Youth Self-Report measure (Achenbach, 1991b). Rowe (2002) reported significant correlations between the YLS/CMI overall risk/need score and the total and Callous/Deceitful and Conduct Problems factor scores of an early version of the Hare Psychopathy Checklist: Youth Version (Forth, Kosson, & Hare, 2003), as well as the Conduct Disorder score of the Disruptive Behavior Disorder Rating Scales (Barkley & Murphy, 1998).

With respect to other evidence of construct validity, Hoge and Andrews (1996a) demonstrated that YLS/CMI overall risk/need scores differed significantly, depending on custody level (specifically, probation, staff-secure custody, and secure custody). Jung (1996) compared a group of adjudicated offenders to a sample of high school students who had no prior involvement with the juvenile justice system. The offender sample exhibited significantly higher YLS/CMI overall risk/need and subscale scores than the nonoffender sample did.

The predictive validity of YLS/CMI scores has been evaluated in a number of studies relating scores to indexes of reoffending. Hoge and Andrews (1996b), Rowe (2002), and Schmidt and colleagues (2002) reported significant correlations between overall risk/need YLS/CMI scores and a variety of reoffending indexes, including new charges, new convictions, and charges for serious offenses. Rowe reported that the correlations were significant for both boys and girls, whereas Schmidt and colleagues (2002) indicated a significant correlation for males but a nonsignificant correlation for a small sample of females. With one exception, all three studies reported significant correlations between YLS/CMI subscales and each reoffense index.

Two studies reported categorical analyses of predictive validity. Jung and Rawana (1999) divided their sample into two groups: those who had reoffended within 6 months of the conclusion of their disposition, and those who had not yet reoffended. The reoffending group displayed higher YLS/CMI overall risk/need scores and subscale scores than the nonreoffending group. The differences were significant for both genders and for the two ethnic groups examined (Native Canadian [Aboriginal] vs. non-Native).

Costigan (1999; Costigan & Rawana, 1999) analyzed data based on a follow-up of participants in the Jung and Rawana (1999) study. Multivariate analyses compared youths from three risk/need groups (low, moderate, or high) based on YLS/CMI overall risk/need and subscale scores. Mean reoffense scores differed significantly across the three groups. The differences among the three groups were significant for the total sample, for both males and females, and for both Native and non-Native groups.

Jung (1996; Jung & Rawana, 1999) conducted a linear discriminant analysis based on the eight YLS/CMI subscale scores to predict reoffending. The analysis yielded a 75.38% correct classification value. Schmidt and colleagues (2002) reported an accuracy rate of 57% in the prediction of general reoffending and 56% in the prediction of serious reoffending. All of these decision accuracy rates were statistically significant. Rowe (2002) assessed the predictive power of YLS/CMI total scores through survival analysis. Youths classified as high-risk recidivated at a significantly faster rate (likelihood ratio = 60.50, p < .001) than low-risk youths did over time.

Rowe (2002) evaluated the dynamic predictive validity of YLS/CMI scores by analyzing the association between changes in YLS/CMI scores (assessed at intake and again at termination) and reoffending levels. In general, cases showing increases in YLS/CMI scores exhibited higher reoffending rates than cases with reductions or no changes in YLS/CMI risk levels. Hoge and Andrews (1996a) reported correlations of YLS/CMI overall risk/need and subscale scores with adjustment ratings made by probation officers subsequent to intake. YLS/CMI scores correlated significantly with ratings of compliance with probation conditions and overall adjustment.

APPLICATION

The YLS/CMI assists probation officers, child care workers, psychologists, and others working in juvenile justice settings with assessing the risk and need factors of youths and with developing case plans. The major strengths of the instrument are as follows:

- Provides a standardized and empirically validated basis for assessing risk and need factors.
- Helps to ensure consistency in the assessment of clients, thereby reducing the operation of bias in data collection.
- Helps ensure consistency in decisions about clients.
- Facilitates communication among workers.
- Incorporates a professional override.
- Provides protection where judgments are questioned.
- Assists in allocation of resources within agencies.
- Helps in collecting and recording data on client characteristics and services for agency and external funding accountability purposes.

The YLS/CMI can be administered and scored by front-line staff members of juvenile justice and correctional agencies, although some initial training is required. A background in child development and experience with youths who have conduct disorder are also useful, though not required. The *User's Manual*, available from Multi-Health Systems, provides detailed guidance regarding administration and scoring procedures. The YLS/CMI is normally completed on the basis of an interview with a youth, but information collected in the interview should be supplemented with file information and data from collateral sources such as parents, teachers, and police. A Case Management Review Form is also available for reassessing the client.

There are some cautions to be observed in using the YLS/CMI. First, only professionals trained in administration and scoring procedures should use the instrument. Second, the risk/need scores should not dictate decisions about offenders; final decisions rest with the responsible professionals. This is the purpose of the professional override feature. Third, care should be taken to ensure that use of the measure does not result in the use of inappropriate dispositions ("net widening"). Higher levels of risk/need do not indicate that punitive dispositions are appropriate. Fourth, where needs are identified, the agency should recognize an obligation to provide services that will meet those needs. Finally, agencies adopting the YLS/CMI should consider the impact of the measure on the larger judicial or correctional system in which agencies are operating. Guidelines for introducing and supporting use of the inventory within agencies are included in Table 17.1.

CASE EXAMPLE

Lucy, a 14-year-old female, was convicted of malicious assault. The YLS/CMI was completed at the request of the family court judge to assist in the disposition decision. The inventory was completed by Lucy's probation officer on the basis of interviews with Lucy and her guardian (grandmother) individually

TABLE 17.1. Implementation Guidelines for the YLS/CMI

- A commitment to the use of standardized assessments with clients should be included in the agency's mission statement.
- All relevant administrative and judicial personnel should be provided with an orientation to the YLS/CMI. The latter should include judges, lawyers, and other court officials. The orientation should familiarize these professionals with the purpose of the instrument and its role in the processing of offenders.
- Policy regarding the use of the YLS/CMI in agency procedures should be established in collaboration with personnel who will use the measure. The instrument should be incorporated into the system in a rational manner that takes account of existing procedures, with the goal of reducing redundant activities. The instrument should be introduced gradually.
- The instrument should be integrated into a computerized automated system that facilitates the work of the individual probation officer, ensures effective communication among agency personnel, and facilitates data collection and analysis.
- Comprehensive training in administering the instrument should be provided to all relevant personnel. This should be supported by resource personnel in the agency for answering queries and by periodic retraining sessions. The resource personnel should also be responsible for monitoring the quality of assessments.
- The benefits of utilizing the instrument should be evaluated periodically.

and together, with Lucy's school principal, and with one of Lucy's teachers. The following is a summary of scores for the six sections of the YLS/CMI.

Risk/Need Scores (Parts I and II)

Lucy's overall risk/need score was 20, placing her at the high end of the moderate category. Her subscale risk/need levels were low for Prior and Current Offenses, Family Circumstances/Parenting, and Substance Abuse; moderate for Personality/Behavior and Attitudes/Orientation; and high for Education, Peer Associations, and Leisure/Recreation. Strengths were indicated in Family Circumstances/Parenting and Personality/Behavior.

Briefly, Lucy was a first-time offender with no history of criminal activity. Her conviction related to an assault on another girl, with whom she was in conflict over her boyfriend. Lucy's behavior had been generally prosocial until about a year ago, when it began to deteriorate significantly. She obtained a low score on Prior and Current Offenses.

Lucy had no contact with her biological father and only intermittent contact with her mother, who had serious drug and alcohol problems. Lucy lived with her maternal grandmother, who was a prosocial individual, fully committed to Lucy. The grandmother made efforts to provide Lucy with direction, but Lucy's behavior was becoming increasingly difficult to control. A low score was indicated for the Family Circumstances/Parenting subscale. Family strengths were the grandmother's determination to help Lucy through her problems and Lucy's affection for her grandmother.

Lucy's performance and behavior in school had been satisfactory until about a year ago, when they significantly deteriorated. She received a high risk/need score in the Education category because of poor academic performance, conflicts with teachers and other students, and truancy. Lucy was also given a high risk/need score on Peer Associations. Part of the deterioration in her behavior related to a new boyfriend acquired about a year ago. He was older than Lucy, and both he and his associates represented poor social influences. Lucy no longer had contact with her prosocial friends. Although her boyfriend and his associates drank and used drugs on a casual basis, Lucy did not exhibit any problem in this respect. A high risk/need score was recorded as well for the Leisure/Recreation subscale, because Lucy was not engaged in any type of positive activity or sport. She spent most of her time hanging out with her new friends.

Lucy received a moderate risk/need score for the Personality/Behavior subscale, based on her displays of verbal and physical aggression and lack of guilt for the harm caused to the victim. A strength in this category was that adults responded positively to her, despite all her problems. There was a general feeling that her hostility and defiance were relatively shallow, and people seemed motivated to help her. She also obtained a moderate score on the Attitudes/Orientation subscale, because of her defiance of authority and apparent lack of motivation to change.

Other Needs/Special Considerations (Part III)

Two items were checked under Family Circumstances/Parenting: "drug/alcohol abuse" because of the mother's history of substance abuse, and "financial/accommodation" because the grandmother's income was low and they have had to move several times.

The Probation Officer's Assessment (Part IV)

The probation officer agreed with the overall risk/need level of moderate.

Contact Level (Part V)

The probation officer recommended a term of probation under medium supervision (once-weekly contact), accompanied by the interventions outlined below.

Case Management Plan (Part VI)

The selection of goals and of means for achieving those goals was based on the risk/need factors identified in Part I and the responsivity considerations indicated in Part III. Although peer relations constituted a major risk/need factor in Lucy's case, the decision was to focus on other goals initially. The first goal involved an effort to address Lucy's emotional problems relating to her mother. She agreed with some reluctance to begin sessions with a counselor from a family service center. The grandmother agreed to participate in some of these sessions. The second goal focused on improving Lucy's school performance and behavior. Lucy agreed to meet with the school social worker two mornings per week to address some of her problems. The final goal focused on addressing the leisure/recreation issue. Lucy indicated that she would like to join a badminton group held at the YMCA two evenings per week. Lucy's activities would be monitored weekly, and her progress would be reviewed in 3 months.

REFERENCES

Achenbach, T. M. (1991a). *Manual for the Child Behavior Checklist and 1991 Profile.* Burlington: University of Vermont, Department of Psychiatry.

Achenbach, T. M. (1991b). *Manual for the Youth Self-Report and 1991 Profile.* Burlington: University of Vermont, Department of Psychiatry.

Andrews, D. A., & Bonta, J. (1995). *Level of Service Inventory—Revised.* North Tonawanda, NY: Multi-Health Systems.

Andrews, D. A., Bonta, J., & Hoge, R. D. (1990). Classification for effective rehabilitation: Rediscovering psychology. *Criminal Justice and Behavior, 17,* 19–52.

Andrews, D. A., Robinson, D., & Balla, M. (1986). Risk principle of case classification and the prevention of residential placements: An outcome evaluation of the Share the Parenting Program. *Journal of Consulting and Clinical Psychology, 54*, 203–207.

Andrews, D. A., Robinson, D., & Hoge, R. D. (1984). *Manual for the Youth Level of Service Inventory.* Ottawa, ON, Canda: Department of Psychology, Carleton University.

Andrews, D. A., Zinger, I., Hoge, R. D., Bonta, J., Gendreau, P., & Cullen, F. T. (1990). Does correctional treatment work?: A psychologically informed meta-analysis. *Criminology, 28*, 369–404.

Barkley, R. A., & Murphy, K. R. (1998). *Attention-deficit hyperactivity disorder: A clinical workbook* (2nd ed.). New York: Guilford Press.

Costigan, S. (1999). *Critical evaluation of the long-term validity of the risk/need assessment and its young offender typology.* Unpublished master's thesis, Lakehead University, Thunder Bay, ON, Canada.

Costigan, S., & Rawana, E. (1999, June). *Critical evaluation of the long-term validity of the risk/need assessment.* Paper presented at the annual conference of the Canadian Psychological Association, Montreal.

Cottle, C. C., Lee, R. J., & Heilbrun, K. (2001). The prediction of criminal recidivism in juveniles: A meta-analysis. *Criminal Justice and Behavior, 28*, 367–394.

Forth, A. E., Kosson, D. S., & Hare, R. D. (2003). *The Hare Psychopathy Checklist: Youth Version.* Toronto: Multi-Health Systems.

Gendreau, P., Goggin, C., & Little, T. (1996). A meta-analysis of predictors of adult offender recidivism. *Criminology, 34*, 401–433.

Grisso, T. (1998). *Forensic evaluation of juveniles.* Sarasota, FL: Professional Resource Press.

Grisso, T. (2003). Forensic evaluation in delinquency cases. In I. B. Weiner (Series Ed.) & A. M. Goldstein (Vol. Ed.), *Handbook of psychology: Vol. 11. Forensic psychology* (pp. 315–334). New York: Wiley.

Hawkins, J. D., Herrenkohl, T., Farrington, D. P., Brewer, D., Catalano, R. F., & Harachi, T. W. (1998). A review of predictors of youth violence. In R. Loeber & D. P. Farrington (Eds.), *Serious and violent juvenile offenders: Risk factors and successful interventions* (pp. 106–146). Thousand Oaks, CA: Sage.

Hoge, R. D. (1999). An expanded role for psychological assessments in juvenile justice systems. *Criminal Justice and Behavior, 26*, 251–266.

Hoge, R. D. (2001). *The juvenile offender: Theory, research, and applications.* Boston: Kluwer Academic.

Hoge, R. D., & Andrews, D. A. (1996a, August). *Assessing risk and need factors in the youthful offender.* Paper presented at the annual conference of the American Psychological Association, Toronto.

Hoge, R. D., & Andrews, D. A. (1996b). *Assessing the youthful offender: Issues and techniques.* New York: Plenum Press.

Hoge, R. D., & Andrews, D. A. (2002). *Youth Level of Service/Case Management Inventory: User's manual.* North Tonawanda, NY: Multi-Health Systems.

Hoge, R. D., Andrews, D. A., & Leschied, A. W. (2002). *Youth Level of Service/Case Management Inventory.* North Tonawanda, NY: Multi-Health Systems.

Jung, S. (1996). *Critical evaluation of the validity of the risk/need assessment with Aboriginal young offenders in northwestern Ontario.* Unpublished master's thesis, Lakehead University, Thunder Bay, ON, Canada.

Jung, S., & Rawana, E. P. (1999). Risk–need assessment of juvenile offenders. *Criminal Justice and Behavior, 26*, 69–89.

Le Blanc, B. (1998). Screening of serious and violent juvenile offenders: Identification, classification, and prediction. In R. Loeber & D.P. Farrington (Eds.), *Serious and violent juvenile offenders: Risk factors and successful interventions* (pp. 167–193). Thousand Oaks, CA: Sage.

Lipsey, M. W. (1995). What do we learn from 400 research studies on the effectiveness of treatment with juvenile delinquents? In J. McGuire (Ed.), *What works: Reducing reoffending* (pp. 63–78). Chichester, UK: Wiley.

Lipsey, M. W., & Derzon, J. H. (1998). Predictors of violent or serious delinquency in adolescence and early adulthood: A synthesis of longitudinal research. In R. Loeber & D. P. Farrington (Eds.), *Serious and violent juvenile offenders: Risk factors and successful interventions* (pp. 86–105). Thousand Oaks, CA: Sage.

Lipsey, M. W., & Wilson, D. B. (1998). Effective intervention for serious juvenile offenders: A synthesis of research. In R. Loeber & D. P. Farrington (Eds.), *Serious and violent juvenile offenders: Risk factors and successful interventions* (pp. 313–345). Thousand Oaks, CA: Sage.

Poluchowicz, S., Jung, S., & Rawana, E. P. (2000, June). *The interrater reliability of the Ministry Risk/Need Assessment Form for juvenile offenders*. Paper presented at the annual conference of the Canadian Psychological Association, Montreal.

Rowe, R. (2002). *Predictors of criminal offending: Evaluating measures of risk/needs, psychopathy, and disruptive behavior disorders*. Unpublished doctoral dissertation, Carleton University, Ottawa, ON, Canada.

Schmidt, F., Hoge, R. D., & Robertson, L. (2002, May). *Assessing risk and need in youthful offenders*. Paper presented at the annual conference of the Canadian Psychological Association, Vancouver, BC, Canada.

Shields, I.W., & Simourd, D. J. (1991). Predicting predatory behavior in a population of young offenders. *Criminal Justice and Behavior, 18*, 180–194.

Simourd, L., Hoge, R. D., & Andrews, D. A. (1991, June). *The Youth Level of Service Inventory: An examination of the development of a risk/needs instrument*. Paper presented at the annual conference of the Canadian Psychological Association, Calgary, AB, Canada.

Simourd, D. J., Hoge, R. D., Andrews, D. A., & Leschied, A. W. (1994). An empirically-based typology of young offenders. *Canadian Journal of Criminology, 447–461*.

CHAPTER 18

Early Assessment Risk Lists for Boys and Girls

Leena K. Augimeri
Christopher J. Koegl
Kathryn S. Levene
Christopher D. Webster

PURPOSE

The Early Assessment Risk List for Boys (EARL-20B), Version 2 (Augimeri, Koegl, Webster, & Levene, 2001), and the Early Assessment Risk List for Girls (EARL-21G), Version 1, Consultation Edition (Levene et al., 2001), are risk assessment devices for children under 12 years of age who are exhibiting disruptive behavior problems that may be indicative of future antisocial, aggressive, or violent conduct. The intended purpose of these instruments is threefold: (1) to provide a platform for increasing clinicians' and researchers' general understanding of early childhood risk factors for violence and antisocial behavior; (2) to help construct violence or antisocial behavior risk assessment schemas for particular children, according to an acceptable structured format; and (3) to assist in the creation of effective clinical risk management plans for high-risk children and their families.

The assessments cover a wide range of variables related to the child, the family, neighborhood, responsiveness to treatment, and other social factors (e.g., poverty, negative peer influence) that the scientific literature has shown to be positively related to antisociality. Although there is no shortage of dependable information on this subject (see, e.g., Burke, Loeber, Mutchka, & Lahey, 2002; Loeber & Farrington, 2001; Loeber & Stouthamer-Loeber, 1998; Wasserman et al., 2003), little has been done in the way of harnessing this knowledge and making it available to clinicians in a practical and usable format. To this end, a properly conceived and scientifically based assessment device would be of considerable value to clinical and educational practice. Like others concerned with the life course of aggressive and antisocial young children (Loeber & Farrington, 2001), we have found that the sooner at-risk children get the help they need, the better their life chances.

Over the years, the necessity of developing risk assessment tools became increasingly evident to clinicians and researchers at Earlscourt Child and Family Centre (currently known as the Child Development Institute)—an accredited, family-focused treatment center in Toronto for children under the age of 12 exhibiting serious behavior problems. Referred children and their families participate in a thorough screening process conducted by trained child and family workers to determine suitability for admission. Since many of these children are known at the time of initial evaluation to be committing seriously antisocial and aggressive acts, and experience has taught us that more than a few of these children go on to have serious troubles with the law in young adulthood, it became imperative to focus attention on developing an interdisciplinary assessment scheme that might possess some predictive power. Our aim was to place a concise and testable scheme in the hands of clinicians. We thought that a systematic risk assessment scheme might be of great benefit in this regard, since mental health workers could "red-flag" seemingly high-risk children at an early age and direct interventions accordingly. Second, a tool of this sort could help ensure that the intensity of services matches each child's level of need and risk (Hrynkiw-Augimeri, 1998). Potential "savings" associated with such early interventions might be realized, not only at the level of the individual child, but also at the societal level (Hoge & Andrews, 1996). A key recommendation of the U.S. Office of Juvenile Justice and Delinquency Prevention Study Group on Serious and Violent Offenders was the development and validation of screening instruments to identify children at risk of committing serious and violent offenses (Loeber & Farrington, 1998).

The EARL-20B and EARL-21G were developed with this purpose in mind and were among "the first of the structured assessment instruments being developed and studied for assessing violence risk in youth" (Borum, Bartel, & Forth, 2002, p. 5). Prior to the development of Version 1 of the EARL-20B (Augimeri, Webster, Koegl, & Levene, 1998), there were no known devices available to assess violence or future antisocial behavior in young children, although relevant measures were available for adolescents (e.g., the Youth Level of Service/Case Management Inventory [YLS/CMI]—Hoge & Andrews, 1996) and adults (i.e., the Hare Psychopathy Checklist—Revised [PCL-R]—Hare, 1991; the Violence Risk Appraisal Guide [VRAG]—Quinsey, Harris, Rice, & Cormier, 1998; and the 20-item Historical/Clinical/Risk Management scheme [HCR-20]—Webster, Douglas, Eaves, & Hart, 1997). This may have been due to the fact that in many jurisdictions, including Canada, children under the age of 12 cannot be held criminally liable and, for the most part, typically do not get involved in incidents that require the attention of the police. In fact, of those incidents investigated by police services in Canada, only a fraction (fewer than 1.5%) are purportedly committed by children under the age of 12, and most of these incidents fall at the less serious end of the continuum (Statistics Canada, 2003a). Other reasons for the lack of focus on this population include the concern over the detrimental effects of labeling children "high-risk," as well as the influence of maturation and the developmental trajectory of antisocial behaviors (Augimeri et al., 2001; Hrynkiw-Augimeri, 1998).

BASIC DESCRIPTION

The EARL-20B and the EARL-21G were modeled after the HCR-20 (Webster et al., 1997), a widely used device for assessing adults' violence risk in forensic, civil, and correctional settings. Like the HCR-20, the EARL-20B contains 20 items that are used to assess risk and guide clinical risk management across a number of specific domains. The EARL-20B and EARL-21G are divided into three main categories of items (see Table 18.1). The Family Items category (6 items in the EARL-20B and 7 in the EARL-20G) is used to assess the extent to which the child has or has not been effectively nurtured, supported,

TABLE 18.1. Comparison of the EARL-20B and EARL-21G

EARL-20B, Version 2	EARL-21G, Version 1, Consultation Edition
Family Items	
F1. Household Circumstances	F1. Household Circumstances
F2. Caregiver Continuity	F2. Caregiver Continuity
F3. Supports	F3. Supports
F4. Stressors	F4. Stressors
F5. Parenting Style	F5. Parenting Style
F6. Antisocial Values and Conduct	F6. Caregiver–Daughter Interaction
	F7. Antisocial Values and Conduct
Child Items	
C1. Developmental Problems	C1. Developmental Problems
C2. Onset of Behavioral Difficulties	C2. Onset of Behavioral Difficulties
C3. Abuse/Neglect/Trauma	C3. Abuse/Neglect/Trauma
C4. Hyperactivity/Impulsivity/Attention Deficits (HIA)	C4. HIA
C5. Likeability	C5. Likeability
C6. Peer Socialization	C6. Peer Socialization
C7. Academic Performance	C7. Academic Performance
C8. Neighborhood	C8. Neighborhood
C9. Authority Contact	C9. Sexual Development
C10. Antisocial Attitudes	C10. Antisocial Attitudes
C11. Antisocial Behavior	C11. Antisocial Behavior
C12. Coping Ability	C12. Coping Ability
Responsivity Items	
R1. Family Responsivity	R1. Family Responsivity
R2. Child Responsivity	R2. Child Responsivity

supervised, and encouraged. Assessors must also gauge the level of support and amount of stress the family is encountering, and the extent to which its members may or may not endorse or participate in antisocial activities. The Child Items category (12 items) focuses on individual risk factors associated with the child and the extent to which the child performs social roles and acts responsibly. The third category, Responsivity Items (2 items), focuses on the ability and willingness of both the child and family to engage in treatment and benefit from planned interventions.

As indicated in Table 18.1, there is considerable overlap between the devices for boys and girls. The EARL-20B and the EARL-21G follow the same format and are both grounded in the scientific literature. The within-item content differs between the two manuals because, although considerably more evidence exists for boys, literature reviews revealed that some risk factors are manifested differently for boys and girls. There are also gender differences in the way antisociality is expressed (Pepler, Madsen, Webster, & Levene, 2005). For this reason, we included one additional family item in the EARL-21G (F6, "Caregiver–Daughter Interaction") and replaced one EARL-20B child item (C9 in the EARL-21G, "Sexual Development," replaced C9 in the EARL-20B, "Authority Contact").

In both manuals, each item description is limited to two pages and contains all the pertinent information for a single factor. The condensed literature review is located on the left-hand page, and coding directions are outlined on the right-hand page. Both manuals are printed with spiral bindings to allow assessors to keep each item description easily available to them as they conduct evaluations. Each item is rated on a 3-point scale. A rating of 0 indicates that the "characteristic or circumstance is not evident." A rating of 2 indicates that the "characteristic or circumstance is present," and a rating of 1 indicates there is "some, but not complete, evidence" for the factor. Scores may be totaled to yield a maximum of 40 for the EARL-20B and 42 for the EARL-21G. The devices can be completed by a single clinician (with or without the parent) or by a clinical team. The assessor must evaluate each of the items carefully, based on the information obtained through a structured interview process or case conference and a file review. Evaluators must obtain and assess information from multiple agents (e.g., teachers, parents, child caregivers, doctors) and multiple sources (e.g., clinical records, school reports, standardized tests) prior to completing an EARL assessment. This process ensures that the evaluator has the most up-to-date and accurate information before rendering a clinical risk judgment. Depending on the rater's or team's knowledge of the child and familiarity with the EARL, these assessments take approximately 15 minutes to complete.

A one-page Summary Sheet is located in the back of each manual to shape assessments that are to the point, without sacrificing accuracy. The Summary Sheets are to be used in conjunction with their corresponding manuals. At the completion of either EARL, after item scores are totaled, clinicians render a global index of risk ("Overall Clinical Judgment"). This three-choice box allows assessors to use information covered in the EARL-20B or EARL-

21G assessment process to assign a global summary rating of low, moderate, or high risk. This feature of the assessment was intended to provide additional clinical freedom to assessors, and it assumes that the EARL instruments (like any structured tool) cannot perfectly attend to *all* relevant factors for *all* individuals. Ostensibly, the higher the total score, the more likely a child is to be at risk for engaging in future antisocial or aggressive behavior, because violence risk factors are additive (Hall, 2001). However, it is probably more important to focus on the individual violence or antisocial behavior risk summary rating, which involves some clinical judgment, than on a total score. In the vast majority of cases, the clinical rating will correlate with the EARL total score, even though it may be informed by factors not covered explicitly in the EARL schemes. As stated by Webster and Hucker (2003), a "simple additive model will likely not suffice" (p. 104). Professionals using the EARL-20B and EARL-21G are expected to provide an explanation in the "Notes" section of the Summary Sheet when an Overall Clinical Judgment diverges considerably from the EARL total score.

No single risk factor can predict future antisocial behavior, because risk factors are probably both cumulative and interactive (Monahan et al., 2001). Yet it is possible for a single risk factor to play a disproportionate role in contributing to a particular child's overall level of risk. For example, a child may have a relatively low total EARL score, yet may display one category of behaviors (e.g., antisocial friends) that places him or her at greater risk for an antisocial trajectory. Therefore, "Critical Risk" checkboxes are provided beside each item on the Summary Sheet to denote factors of particularly high concern. Although it is typically the case that items checked as critical also receive a rating of 2, items rated 1 or 0 can be marked as critical if the assessor believes that the factor requires focused clinical attention or ongoing monitoring.

HISTORY OF THE METHOD'S DEVELOPMENT

With the decriminalization of children under 12 years of age by the Young Offenders Act in Canada in 1984, Earlscourt introduced the Under 12 Outreach Project (ORP), a model intervention for boys under 12 years of age who have come into police contact for engaging in antisocial activities.[1] The ORP is Canada's only sustained, multifaceted intervention designed for boys under age 12 who have committed offenses (Augimeri, Farrington, Koegl, & Day, 2004; Hrynkiw-Augimeri, Pepler, & Goldberg, 1993; Webster, Augimeri, & Koegl, 2002). During the early stages of the program's development, it became evident that the assessment process lacked a systematic method of

---

[1] Prior to 1996, the ORP served both boys and girls. In 1996, Earlscourt developed the Girls Connection, a gender-specific intervention for girls under the age of 12 with conduct problems—the first reported gender-specific intervention for young girls with disruptive behavior problems (Walsh, Pepler, & Levene, 2002).

assessing the risk level of children. As a result, we created an informal risk assessment list called "Risk Factors Associated with Possible Conduct Disorders and Non-Responders" (Augimeri & Levene, 1994, 1997) to assist clinicians in differentiating between high and low risk children. Although this 53-item list was helpful for clinicians in "red-flagging" potentially high-risk children during the treatment-planning phase, it had not been tested for reliability or validity, and the items were not defined or explicitly connected to the empirical literature (Hrynkiw-Augimeri, 1998).

In 1997, Christopher Webster joined Earlscourt as a senior research consultant. Given his expertise and knowledge in the area of violence risk assessment (e.g., his role in the development of the HCR-20; Webster et al., 1997), as well as funding from the National Crime Prevention Centre of Canada, we spent a year condensing the list to a manageable number of items and subsequently issued a Consultation Edition (Version 1) of the EARL-20B (Augimeri et al., 1998). This required a thorough review of the child developmental literature, as well as extensive assistance from the ORP clinical staff. Staff members participated in extensive discussions about identifying risk factors for aggressive, antisocial, and violent behavior, and in exercises to test the device for interrater reliability and clinical utility. Our challenges were to isolate 20 variables pertinent to the assessment of antisocial behavior in boys under 12 years of age, and to produce a scientifically sound and practical device, aimed at fostering a scientist-practitioner model by integrating research and clinical practice (see Webster et al., 1997). Consistent with Hart (2001), our goal was to develop a sound risk assessment procedure that produced consistent results, was prescriptive in terms of interventions that might be introduced to manage individual violence risk, and was transparent in the sense that key terms and decisions about assigning risk were clearly defined and examinable.

Using the HCR-20 as a template, we grouped the 53 items into 20 factors. Initially we attempted to group the items into "Historical," "Clinical," and "Risk Management" categories, using a "past, present, future" method of organizing the items. However, in contrast to adults, many risk factors for children are dynamic and oriented to the present. Since the major treatment components in the ORP are parent and child groups (Earlscourt Child and Family Centre, 2001a, 2001b), and many of the factors that place children at risk are child and parent factors, we thought these categories would be more appropriate. The third category of items (Responsivity Items) was introduced into the scheme to reflect the reality that very high-risk children and their families can be hard to engage clinically and often drop out of treatment prematurely (Kazdin & Wassell, 1998). Knowing a family's past treatment successes and failures is important for clinicians to consider—not only for gauging risk, but also for taking steps to build rapport with the child and his or her parents.

The evolution of the EARL-20B involved a five-step consultation and evaluation process. Initially we hosted an in-house research day, to which practitioners, researchers, teachers, parents and the media were invited to discuss the new device. Each participant received a complimentary copy, and all were asked to review it and provide opinions as to whether the device was clinically worthwhile, user-friendly, scientifically sound, and ethical. Following these discussions, Earlscourt hosted an in-house consultation day with leading experts in the field (i.e., David Farrington, Rolf Loeber, and Debra Pepler) to review and offer criticisms about the tool. Subsequently, we distributed the EARL-20B to other researchers, clinicians, and government officials, who provided additional remarks about content, layout, and ways to improve the readability and usability of the device.

With this valuable information in hand, we were confident about testing the reliability and validity of the EARL-20B through a retrospective file study of 447 children who had come through the ORP from 1985 to 1999 and were eligible for youth or adult court contact (i.e., were ages 12 and older). The dual goals of the study were to find out what level of interrater reliability could be achieved via the item descriptions in the manual, and to relate EARL-20B scores to subsequent youth and adult court conviction data (a cursory summary of these findings is available in Appendix C of the manual for the EARL-20B, Version 2). The last step of the evaluation process involved further consultations with practitioners, researchers, and policy makers to determine the utility of refining the manual for the EARL-20B, Version 1 (Consultation Edition).

The EARL-20B, Version 2 (Augimeri et al., 2001) was published in early 2001. Many of the changes from Version 1 to Version 2 were subtle, within-item content changes. Based on feedback from clinicians and consultants, we edited the 20 coding sections to make them as clear as possible. Other changes focused on broadening the content of items to draw a closer tie to published research, eliminating item overlap, changing the scope of items to increase relevance to other settings (including a greater emphasis on ecological risk factors), and renaming items to make them more consistent with a client-centered treatment approach.

Following the same initial development process of the EARL-20B, we then produced a companion, gender-specific device for girls: the EARL-21G, Version 1 (Consultation Edition) (Levene et al., 2001). Although we remain in the beginning stages of evaluating the device for girls, preliminary opinions from Earlscourt Girls Connection clinicians (see footnote 1) suggest that the EARL-21G brings together scientific knowledge and clinical practice, is practical, and enhances clinical risk management decisions during the assessment process (see Levene, Walsh, Augimeri, & Pepler, 2004).

RESEARCH EVIDENCE

Several studies have focused specifically on the EARL-20B and EARL-21G. Below, is a summary of the studies that have been conducted to date. An up-to-date list of research projects can be found at *http://www.childdevelop. ca.*

Internal Consistency and Reliability

The first evaluation of the EARL-20B (Hrynkiw-Augimeri, 1998) was a small prospective study using a draft (i.e., prepublication) version of the EARL-20B on a sample of 21 boys from the ORP. Five clinical staff members participated in the study, which demonstrated that most items achieved acceptable interclinician agreement on the total EARL-20B score.

Our first formal test of the reliability of the EARL-20B (Augimeri et al., 2001) was a retrospective file study of 447 children (379 boys and 68 girls) who had been involved in the ORP from 1985 to 1999. Interrater reliability was tested with three different raters, each of whom coded 229 randomly selected files (120 were common, 109 were unique), using Version 1 of the EARL-20B. Raters were unaware of which files were considered common files for interrater reliability purposes. The study revealed a highly acceptable level of agreement among the three raters on the total EARL-20B score for the common files, with an intraclass correlation coefficient of .80 (Augimeri, 2004).

In Sweden, researchers tested the interrater reliability of Version 2 of the EARL-20B across seven child and adolescent psychiatric units (Enebrink, Långström, Neij, Grann, & Gumpert, 2001) with children referred to child and psychiatric facilities for behavioral or emotional problems. Kappa statistics indicated good agreement for most of the individual EARL-20B items (M = 0.62, range 0.30–0.87). Intraclass correlation coefficients for total, Child Items, and Family Items subscale scores indicated excellent agreement (.90–.92). As a continuation of this study, Enebrink, Långström, Hultén, and Gumpert (in press) extended the scope to nine child psychiatric clinics in central Sweden. Again, good interrater reliability was achieved for most of the individual EARL-20B items (with an average of .62), and excellent interrater agreement was obtained for the EARL-20B total score (.92).

The EARL-21G has also undergone retrospective and prospective studies to assess interrater reliability. Encouragingly, one of the EARL-21G retrospective studies found a moderate to high level of agreement (.64 to .84) among three raters (Levene et al., 2001). In addition, prospective studies on use of the device have also found statistically significant agreement among raters (Levene et al., 2004).

Validity

The first investigation of the validity of the EARL-20B for "predicting" official criminal conviction involvement was the retrospective study of the 447 children involved in the ORP from 1985 to 1999 (Augimeri et al., 2001). We accessed correctional records of all former clients for an average follow-up period of 7.8 years after each child's 12th birthday (i.e., the age at which one can be charged with a criminal offense in Canada). There was a statistically significant relationship between high EARL-20B scores and subsequent adolescent and adult criminal contact for both boys and girls (Webster et al., 2002). When only the 379 boys in the sample were considered, 164, or 43%, were found guilty of at least one offense at follow-up. These offenses ranged from minor mischief (e.g., causing a disturbance) to attempted murder. When a median split on total EARL-20B scores was used to group children into low- and high-risk categories, a chi-square analysis revealed that 38% of the low-risk group had been found guilty of an offense, compared to 49% of the high-risk group ($p < .02$). In addition, high-risk boys had an average of 1.6 more appearances in court for sentencing ($p < .02$), and were found guilty of three more charges on average ($p < .03$), than low-risk boys (Augimeri, 2004).

Enebrink and colleagues (in press) found moderate to high convergent validity between the EARL-20B and parent ratings of antisocial and aggressive behavior. The authors of this study concluded that "Decision-tools such as the EARL-20B might help in identifying children and families at risk for problem behavior or psychopathology and help professionals focus limited resources on evidence-based risks and needs."

APPLICATION

As stated in each manual, the EARL devices are to be used only by clinicians, researchers, and professionals experienced in working with high-risk children. These include professionals working in children's mental health centers, hospitals, juvenile assessment centers, child protection agencies, schools and student support services, and correctional settings in jurisdictions where children under the age of 12 are subject to criminal liability. Training in the application of the tools is not mandatory, as the manuals provide direction and explanation, but it is strongly recommended that users receive at least initial training to ensure that the tools are being used in the intended manner. Because we have only partially validated each device, we continue to urge users of the EARL-20B and EARL-21G to be cautious with respect to their application.

It is worth repeating that although it is important to pay attention to the total score in determining overall risk for future antisocial behavior, assessors are advised to focus as much or more on the individual risk patterns and clusters of risk items. Particular risk patterns may require different clinical strategies to alleviate risk. It is likely that two individuals with the same total score will have different scores on the various EARL items and exhibit different kinds of offending (i.e., overt, covert, or authority conflict) (Stouthamer-Loeber & Loeber, 2002). For this reason, while awaiting research on predictive validity of these tools, we advise users to employ the EARL manuals as a means of arriving at a thorough understanding of the static and dynamic factors that contribute to each child's risk pattern, and to use this knowledge to implement culturally sensitive clinical risk management plans that reduce or eliminate violence risk. Furthermore, the EARL devices should not be used in a mechanical way to determine the availability or intensity of treatment (e.g., the total score should not be used as the sole determinant).

Because the EARL devices grew out of the experience of treating children at the former Earlscourt, which serves the multicultural city of Toronto, one may reasonably expect that they can be successfully applied to a wide range of client groups. Over half of the client population at the former Earlscourt is born outside of Canada, and roughly 40% are from visible minority groups (Statistics Canada, 2003a). Users must be sensitive to cultural factors that may influence how information is gathered and considered during an EARL assessment. The fact that over 1,600 EARL manuals have been distributed and successfully used on varied populations in both urban and rural jurisdictions in Europe, Canada, and the United States, and that they are in different stages of translation into various languages (e.g., Swedish, Norwegian, Dutch, and Finnish), lend some support to their universal applicability. As we continue to work with colleagues in other jurisdictions, we anticipate that these experiences, in addition to carefully collected research data, will expand our understanding of how we can maximize the clinical and predictive utility of the EARL devices.

The EARL-20B (Augimeri et al., 2001) and EARL-21G (Levene et al., 2001) are available from the Child Development Institute, Toronto (*http:// www.childdevelop.ca*). Users of the devices are asked to register with the Institute, using a form located at the back of each manual. The purpose of the registry is to inform users of the EARL-20B and EARL-21G of any changes or developments to the manuals, to solicit information regarding experiences with the devices, to disseminate research findings about use of the tools, and to provide an opportunity to engage in clinical and collaborative research.

CASE EXAMPLE

Javar's teacher suggested to his mother, Maxine, that she seek treatment for her son at a local family treatment center to address his problems with managing his anger. When Maxine called to inquire about services, she was asked to participate in the Brief Child and Family Phone Interview (BCFPI; Cunningham, Pettingill, & Boyle, 2002) with an intake worker as a routine part of intake. The BCFPI report indicated that Javar met the basic program admission criteria, and that the family's only previous involvement had been with a child welfare agency. A face-to-face screening interview was scheduled with Maxine, so that she could complete standardized assessment measures, sign third-party disclosure forms, and complete a basic family history. A face-to-face meeting was also held between Javar and a child and youth worker, to determine Javar's perception of the problem and cross-validate information from his mother. Data from these meetings, assessments, standardized measures, collateral reports, and discussions with other key informants (e.g., Javar's teacher) form the basis of the following case synopsis.

Javar is an energetic, creative, and likeable 7-year-old boy who is enrolled in the second grade. Although he seems to be functioning adequately in many areas and displays some positive social skills, he is often stubborn, oppositional, and violent at home and school. Current problems include difficulty concentrating and sleeping, as well as destructiveness and at times displaying a tendency toward antisocial thinking. His mother, Maxine, finds it hard to set effective limits with Javar, and is distressed that he never listens to her. At school he is reported to be impulsive, unable to control his anger, and easily frustrated. For example, he was recently suspended for assaulting a classmate with a chair, sending the child to the hospital. The police were called in to investigate the incident. Javar wrote a letter of apology to the child and expressed remorse and sadness about what he had done. Academically, he is functioning at grade level but has trouble reading, which his teacher attributes to his difficulty with concentrating and staying on task.

No developmental problems were identified during Javar's early years. Maxine fondly describes him as having always been a "busy and active" child. However, since his father's incarceration for domestic violence (which Javar witnessed on several occasions) 2 years ago, she has observed an escalation in her son's aggressive behaviors. Maxine has been quoted as saying, "I have lost control of my child," and sometimes has resorted to spanking him. She feels guilty about this, because it reminds her of the physical and emotional abuse she experienced from Javar's father. There are also concerns that she occasionally leaves Javar and his younger siblings unattended for extended periods of time, is inconsistent with respect to discipline, does not enforce "house rules," and has become lax in her parenting—allowing her children to do what they want. Child welfare authorities have been engaged with this family on two occasions, conducting investigations related to domestic violence and alleged neglect. The family resides in a rented, poorly maintained home in a neighborhood that is characterized as a densely populated, high-crime area. Dependent on government financial support, the family remains on a long waiting list for improved housing through a governmental subsidy program.

Maxine indicates feeling "alone and stressed," but is optimistic that things will get better. While saying that she would like to get help for herself and her three children, she is also aware that she has not followed through in the past with such recommendations. Also, she identifies obstacles to her attending sessions at the treatment center, such as the financial and emotional burdens of travelling on public transportation to and from sessions with her children.

This family enjoys doing activities together, such as playing games, going for walks, reading, and having family meals. Maxine has few supports other than her husband's parents, who are very good to her children but critical of her. They blame Maxine for their son's being incarcerated. Maxine has one close friend—a woman she met at her part-time cleaning job. They talk on the phone frequently, but do not see each other outside of work.

Javar does not take part in structured community activities in the neighborhood. Although he has difficulty getting along with other kids, he has one close friend at school who is a positive influence. He would like to play basketball and make more friends. He acknowledges that he needs to learn how to deal with his anger; in fact, he has identified this as his treatment goal, because he does not like "feeling mad" all the time.

The completed EARL-20B Summary Sheet demonstrates how assessors should summarize key information directly on the form for each of the 20 items (see the "handwritten" responses in Figure 18.1). This provides a convenient, one-page transparent summary of the case at hand and helps to ensure that items are rated accurately. As can also be seen in Figure 18.1, in the "Notes" section of the EARL-20B Summary Sheet, a prescription of suggested clinical risk management strategies follows from Javar's overall EARL-20B assessment.

As noted on the EARL-20B Summary Sheet, the overall clinical risk judgment based on Javar's EARL assessment indicates, based on findings to date, that he is at moderate risk of engaging in future antisocial activities (he has received a total score of 25/40). Although he has many positive attributes (i.e., he is likeable, does not display an antisocial attitude, and is responsive to treatment), he also has some very worrisome risk factors (i.e., lack of supports, inconsistent parenting style, early onset of behavioral difficulties, abuse/neglect/trauma, high-risk neighborhood, authority contact, and antisocial behavior). His responsivity to treatment (R2), as indicated by his ability to set a realistic treatment goal and his desire to learn how to control his anger, is a positive marker. Based on his EARL-20B Summary Sheet, the intervention should focus on building on his identified strengths (see the "Notes" section of the Summary Sheet); addressing the problem areas (i.e., building family supports, teaching Maxine effective child management strategies, advocating for better housing in a safer neighborhood, and teaching Javar strategies to deal more effectively with his anger, such as Stop Now And Plan [SNAP™][2]); and conducting more in-depth assessment. In particular, a thorough psychological assessment is indicated to determine whether his problems are indicative of hyperactivity/impulsivity/attention deficits (C4), anxiety (as a result of witnessing family violence, neglect issues, and punitive discipline), or a combination of both risk areas.

The assessor also considers those items that are checked in the "Critical Risk" column. This is used to flag items that are especially worrisome with regard to the child's overall risk for engaging in antisocial behavior. Flagging of these items is vital for treatment planning, as it provides a clinician with direction regarding what clinical risk management strategies should be highlighted in the treatment plan and addressed as soon as possible. In Javar's case, for example, Family Responsivity (R1) has been designated as a Critical Risk item, even though it has received a rating of 1 rather than 2. Assisting Maxine with instrumental issues (i.e., transportation to and from group sessions, child care assistance) is a concrete and meaningful way to address this salient area of risk and to facilitate treatment compliance.

---

[2] SNAP is a self-control and problem-solving technique originally developed at Earlscourt (Augimeri, 2000; Earlscourt Child and Family Centre, 2001a).

The EARL-20B Version 2 Summary Sheet
(To be used in association with the EARL-20B, Version 2 manual)

Child's Name or ID#: _____Javar JONES_____ Date: _2004-03-02_
(First name SURNAME)   (YYYY-MM-DD)

Assessor: ___L. K. A.___ Child's DOB: __1997-02-15__ Age: _7_
                                        (YYYY-MM-DD)

Family Items		Rating (0–1–2)	Critical Risk
F1	**Household Circumstances**—decrepit, government assistance, subsidized housing	2	
F2	**Caregiver Continuity**—mother stable caregiver; father left home 2 years ago	1	
F3	**Supports**—one close friend, in-laws, no structured community activities	2	√
F4	**Stressors**—parenting distress, isolated, in-laws (critical of Maxine)	1	
F5	**Parenting Style**—inconsistent, "out of control," spanking, lack of supervision	2	√
F6	**Antisocial Values and Conduct**—father in jail (domestic violence—Maxine)	1	

Child Items		Rating (0–1–2)	Critical Risk
C1	**Developmental Problems**—no identified concerns	0	
C2	**Onset of Behavioral Difficulties**—5 years of age	2	
C3	**Abuse/Neglect/Trauma**—witnessing extreme family violence, neglect, spanking	2	√
C4	**Hyperactivity/Impulsivity/Attention Deficits (HIA)**—impulsive, concentration problems	1	
C5	**Likeability**—creative, likeable, pleasant demeanor (however can be stubborn)	0	
C6	**Peer Socialization**—one close positive friend, history of problems with peers	1	
C7	**Academic Performance**—regular Grade 2 class, behind in reading	1	
C8	**Neighborhood**—high crime, densely populated	2	
C9	**Authority Contact**—police, principal, teachers	2	
C10	**Antisocial Attitudes**—remorseful, able to write apology letter, evidence—some antisocial thinking	1	
C11	**Antisocial Behaviour**—assault with a weapon causing bodily harm, suspensions	2	
C12	**Coping Ability**—functioning adequately, sleep problems, easily frustrated	1	√

Responsivity Items		Rating (0–1–2)	Critical Risk
R1	**Family Responsivity**—wants help, guarded (past—did not follow through)	1	√
R2	**Child Responsivity**—would like to deal with his anger	0	

Overall Clinical Judgment	LOW	MOD	HIGH		TOTAL SCORE	25
		√				

Notes: Javar has some very positive attributes. He is a likeable boy who is interested in learning how to control his anger. He attends school and is in a regular class. The goal would be to continue buildingin on these strengths. Based on the risk summary above, the following clinical risk management strategies are recommended. (1) connect Maxine to a parent management training program, to help her learn effective parenting strategies; (2) build a support system for this family; (3) promote family responsivity by helping Maxine with instrumental challenges (i.e., transportation, child care); (4) enroll Javar in an anger management program; (5) connect him to a structured community activity (i.e., basketball), to build on his social skills and encourage him to make some new friends; (6) further assess items C4 and C12—HIA versus anxiety. It is suspected that the sleep, impulsivity and concentration problems may be tied in with C3 (Abuse/Neglect/Trauma).

FIGURE 18.1. Completed EARL-20B Summary Sheet for Javar. The Summary Sheet itself is copyright 2004 by Child Development Institute. Reprinted by permission of the Child Development Institute, Toronto.

REFERENCES

Augimeri, L. K. (2000). *SNAP*. Toronto: Earlscourt Child and Family Centre.

Augimeri, L. K. (2004). *Aggressive and antisocial young children: Risk, assessment and management: Utilizing the Early Assessment Risk List for Boys (EARL-20B)*. Unpublished doctoral dissertation, University of Toronto.

Augimeri, L. K., Farrington, D. P., Koegl, C. J., & Day, D. M. (2004). *A community based program for children with conduct problems: Immediate and long-term effects*. Manuscript submitted for publication.

Augimeri, L. K., Koegl, C. J., Webster, C. D., & Levene, K. S. (2001). *Early Assessment Risk List for Boys: EARL-20B, Version 2*. Toronto: Earlscourt Child and Family Centre.

Augimeri, L. K., & Levene, K. S. (1994, 1997). *Risk factors associated with possible conduct disorders and non-responders*. Toronto: Earlscourt Child and Family Centre.

Augimeri, L. K., Webster, C. D., Koegl, C. J., & Levene, K. S. (1998). *Early Assessment Risk List for Boys: EARL-20B, Version 1, Consultation Edition*. Toronto: Earlscourt Child and Family Centre.

Borum, R., Bartel, P., & Forth, A. (2002). *Manual for the Structured Assessment of Violence Risk in Youth (SAVRY): Version 1, Consultation Edition*. Tampa: Louis de la Parto Florida Mental Health Institute, University of South Florida.

Burke, J. D., Loeber, R., Mutchka, J. S., & Lahey, B. B. (2002). A question for DSM-V: Which better predicts persistent conduct disorder—delinquent acts or conduct symptoms? *Criminal Behaviour and Mental Health, 12*, 37–52.

Cunningham, C. E., Pettingill, P., & Boyle, M. (2002). *The Brief Child and Family Phone Interview: BCFPI-3*. Hamilton, ON, Canada: Canadian Centre for the Study of Children at Risk, Hamilton Health Sciences.

Earlscourt Child and Family Centre. (2001a). *SNAP children's group manual*. Toronto: Author.

Earlscourt Child and Family Centre. (2001b). *SNAP parent group manual*. Toronto: Author.

Enebrink, P., Långström, N., Hultén, A., & Gumpert, C. H. (in press). Swedish validation of the Early Assessment Risk List for Boys (EARL-20B), a decision-aid for use with children presenting with conduct-disordered behaviour. *Nordic Journal of Psychiatry*.

Enebrink, P., Långström, N., Neij, J., Grann, M., & Gumpert, C.H. (2001). *Brief report: Interrater reliability of the Early Assessment Risk List: EARL-20B: A new guide for clinical evaluation of conduct-disordered boys*. Huddinge, Sweden: Karolinska Institutet.

Hall, H. V. (2001). Violence prediction and risk analysis: Empirical advances and guides. *Journal of Threat Assessment, 1*, 1–39.

Hare, R. D. (1991). *Manual for the Hare Psychopathy Checklist—Revised*. Toronto: Multi-Health Systems.

Hart, S. D. (2001). Assessing and managing violence risk. In K. S. Douglas, C. D. Webster, S. D. Hart, D. Eaves, & J. R. P. Ogloff (Eds.), *HCR-20 violence risk management companion guide* (pp. 13–25). Burnaby, BC, Canada: Mental Health, Law, and Policy Institute, Simon Fraser University.

Hoge, R. D., & Andrews, D. A. (1996). *Assessing the youthful offender: Issues and techniques.* New York: Plenum Press.

Hrynkiw-Augimeri, L. K. (1998). *Assessing risk for violence in boys: A preliminary risk assessment study using the Early Assessment Risk List for Boys: EARL-20B.* Unpublished master's thesis, Ontario Institute for Studies in Education, University of Toronto.

Hrynkiw-Augimeri, L. K., Pepler, D., & Goldberg, K. (1993). An outreach project for children having police contact. *Canada's Mental Health, 41,* 7–12.

Kazdin, A. E., & Wassell, G. (1998). Treatment completion and therapeutic change among children referred for conduct disorder. *Journal of Clinical Child Psychology, 28,* 160–172.

Levene, K. S., Augimeri, L. K., Pepler, D., Walsh, M., Webster, C. D., & Koegl, C. J. (2001). *Early Assessment Risk List for Girls: EARL-21G, Version 1, Consultation Edition.* Toronto: Earlscourt Child and Family Centre.

Levene, K. S., Walsh, M. M., Augimeri, L. K., & Pepler, D. (2004). Linking identification and treatment of early risk factors for female delinquency. In M. Moretti, C. Odgers, & M. Jackson (Eds.), *Perspectives in law and psychology: Vol. 19. Girls and aggression: Contributing factors and intervention principles* (pp. 131–146). New York: Kluwer Academic/Plenum.

Loeber, R., & Farrington, D. P. (Eds.). (1998). *Serious and violent juvenile offenders: Risk factors and successful interventions.* Thousand Oaks, CA: Sage.

Loeber, R., & Farrington, D. P. (Eds.). (2001). *Child delinquents: Development, interventions and service needs.* Thousand Oaks, CA: Sage.

Loeber, R., & Stouthamer-Loeber, M. (1998). Development of juvenile aggression and violence: Some common misconceptions and controversies. *American Psychologist, 53*(2), 242–259.

Monahan, J., Steadman, H. J., Silver, E., Appelbaum, P. S., Robbins, P. C., Mulvey, E. P. et al. (2001). *Rethinking risk assessment: The MacArthur study of mental disorder and violence.* New York: Oxford University Press.

Pepler, D. J., Madsen, K., Webster, C. D., & Levene, K. S. (Eds.). (2005). *The development and treatment of girlhood aggression.* Mahwah, NJ: Earlbaum.

Quinsey, V. L., Harris, G. T., Rice, M. E., & Cormier, C. A. (1998). *Violent offenders: Appraising and managing risk.* Washington, DC: American Psychological Association.

Statistics Canada. (2003a). *2001 community profiles.* Retrieved from *http://www12. statcan.ca/english/profil01/Search/PlaceSearch1.cfm?SEARCH=BEGINS&LANG=E &Province=35&PlaceName=Toronto*

Statistics Canada. (2003b). *2002 uniform crime report.* Retrieved from *http://stcwww. statcan.ca/english/sdds/3302.htm#Datafile*

Stouthamer-Loeber, M., & Loeber, R. (2002). Lost opportunities for intervention: Undetected markers for the development of serious juvenile delinquency. *Criminal Behaviour and Mental Health, 12,* 69–82.

Walsh, M. M., Pepler, D. J., & Levene, K. S. (2002). A model intervention for girls with disruptive behaviour problems: The Earlscourt Girls Connection. *Canadian Journal of Counselling, 36*(4), 297–311.

Wasserman, G. A., Keenan, K., Tremblay, R. E., Coie, J., Herrenkohl, T. I., Loeber, R., et al. (2003, April). *Risk and protective factors of child delinquency* (Child Delinquency Bulletin Series). Washington, DC: U.S. Department of Justice.

Webster, C. D., Augimeri, L. K., & Koegl, C. J. (2002). The Under 12 Outreach Project for antisocial boys: A research based clinical program. In R. R. Corrado, R. Roesch, S. D. Hart, & J. K. Gierowski (Eds.), *Multi-problem violent youth: A foundation for comparative research needs, interventions, and outcomes* (pp. 207–218). Amsterdam: IOS Press.

Webster, C. D., Douglas, K. S., Eaves, D., & Hart, S. D. (1997). *HCR-20: Assessing risk for violence, Version 2*. Burnaby, BC, Canada: Mental Health, Law, and Policy Institute, Simon Fraser University.

Webster, C. D., & Hucker, S. J. (2003). *Release decision making*. Hamilton, ON, Canada: St. Joseph's Healthcare, Hamilton Centre for Mountain Health Services.

CHAPTER 19

Structured Assessment of Violence Risk in Youth

Randy Borum
Patrick A. Bartel
Adelle E. Forth

PURPOSE

The Structured Assessment of Violence Risk in Youth (SAVRY; Bartel, Borum, & Forth, 2000; Borum, Bartel, & Forth, 2002, 2003), as its title indicates, is a guide to help focus and structure assessments of violence risk in adolescents. Adolescence is a peak risk period for initiating or participating in acts of serious violence (U.S. Department of Health and Human Services, 2001); yet in the late 1990s, the absence of guidelines for assessing violence risk in adolescents became strikingly apparent. Risk assessments with juvenile offenders became more common when many states lowered the age at which juveniles could be transferred to the jurisdiction of adult court, and implemented future risk to the community as one factor commonly considered in these decisions (Grisso, 1996, 1998; Grisso & Schwartz, 2000). Today, appraisals of future risk are often required for adolescents in juvenile justice, psychiatric emergency service, civil psychiatric hospital, and outpatient clinic settings (Borum, 1996, 2000). Indeed, professionals in juvenile justice and behavioral health are responsible for supervising and managing in the community nearly 500,000 youths each year who are at increased risk for delinquency or violent offenses (Borum, 2003; Puzzanchera, Stahl, Finnegan, Tierney, & Snyder, 2002).

In an early effort to move the field forward, some researchers and clinicians attempted to apply adult risk assessment tools to adolescents. On their face, some of them appeared broadly applicable to the task. Unfortunately, this approach neglected developmental differences in the nature of risk, relevance of risk factors, and operation of risk factors (Borum & Verhaagen, 2003; Hoge, 2001, 2002; Hoge & Andrews, 1996), which are critical determinants of youths' behavior (Griffin & Torbet, 2002; McCord, Widom, & Crowell, 2001; Rosado, 2000). Violence risk in adolescents differs from that in adults, because the base rates and risk factors for violence are different, behavioral norms are different, individual factors are less stable, and psychosocial immaturity is more central (Borum, 2000, 2002, in press; Borum & Verhaagen, 2003). Even among youths, predictors of violent behavior can vary across developmental stages (Howell, 1997). Consequently, while applied risk assessment measures and technology have advanced considerably for adult populations since the 1980s, progress with juvenile populations has been much slower.

Over the years, the behavioral sciences, including criminology, psychology, and sociology, have amassed a substantial amount of research identifying factors associated with increased risk of violent and delinquent offending in juveniles (Borum, 2000; Borum & Verhaagen, in press; Howell, 1997; Lipsey & Derzon, 1998). Unfortunately, practitioners in juvenile justice and behavioral health are often not educated in this research base; nor are they given guidance about how best to *apply* the research to their youth assessments. In developing the SAVRY, our goal was to draw on the strengths of existing risk assessment technology and empirical findings with youths to create an instrument that would help to structure and improve violence risk assessment practice—as well as risk management—with adolescents receiving "treatment" from a variety of service systems. In the SAVRY, a developing juvenile's risk for reoffending is viewed as the result of dynamic and reciprocal interplay between factors that increase, and factors that decrease, the likelihood of violent offending over time (Borum & Verhaagen, in press). Violence as a criterion, for purposes of using the SAVRY, is defined as "an act of physical battery sufficiently severe to cause injury that would require medical attention, a threat with a weapon in hand, or any act of forcible sexual assault."

With our objective in mind, we concluded that the instrument would need to be the following (Borum et al., 2003, p. 15):

1. *Systematic*. It would need to cover the primary domains of known risk and protective factors, with clear operational definitions provided for each.
2. *Empirically grounded*. Items needed to be based on the best available research and guidelines for juvenile risk assessment practice.
3. *Developmentally informed*. Risk and protective factors would need to be selected on the basis of how they operate with adolescents, as opposed to children or adults.
4. *Treatment-oriented*. The risk assessment should have direct implications for treatment, which would include considering dynamic factors that could be useful targets for intervention in risk reduction.

5. *Flexible.* The instrument would need to allow consideration of idiographic or case-specific factors, as well as those derived from research.
6. *Practical.* Using the guide should not require much additional time beyond that needed to collect information in a competent assessment. It should be inexpensive and easy to learn, and should not require diagnostic judgments.

BASIC DESCRIPTION

The SAVRY is based on the "structured professional judgment" (SPJ) risk assessment framework, and is designed for use with adolescents between the approximate ages of 12 and 18 who have been detained or referred for an assessment of violence risk. Evaluators conduct systematic assessments of predetermined risk factors that are empirically associated with violence, consider the applicability of each risk factor to a particular examinee, and classify each factor's severity. The ultimate determination of an examinee's overall level of violence risk is based on the examiner's professional judgment as informed by a systematic appraisal of relevant factors. In this way, the SPJ model draws on the strengths of both the clinical and actuarial (formula-driven) approaches to decision making, and attempts to minimize their respective drawbacks (Borum & Douglas, 2003).

The SAVRY protocol is composed of 6 items defining Protective Factors and 24 items defining Risk Factors (see Table 19.1 for a list of SAVRY items). Risk items are divided into three categories: Historical, Individual, and Social/Contextual. The coding form also includes a section for listing "Additional Risk Factors" and "Additional Protective Factors," because the SAVRY is not exhaustive in identifying all potential risk and protective factors for any given individual. In the course of conducting a risk assessment or assessing patterns in past violent episodes, additional factors or situational variables may emerge that are important in understanding potential for future violence. In such situations, the additional factors should be documented and weighed in final decisions of risk.

The SAVRY is coded on the basis of reliable, available information. In most nonemergency circumstances, it is helpful to include information from an interview with the examinee and a review of records (e.g., police or probation reports, mental health and social service records). The time required to gather this information will vary according to the complexity of the case. Once the information is gathered, however, it typically takes only 10–15 minutes to code all the SAVRY items.

For each Risk Factors item, the manual contains specific guidelines for rating the severity according to a three-level coding structure ("high," "moderate," or "low"). For example, on the "History of Violence" item, a youth is coded as low if he or she has committed no prior acts of violence, moderate if the youth is known to have committed one or two violent acts, and high if there have been

TABLE 19.1. Items from the Structured Assessment of Violence Risk in Youth (SAVRY)

Historical Risk Factors

- History of Violence
- History of Nonviolent Offending
- Early Initiation of Violence
- Past Supervision/Intervention Failures
- History of Self-Harm or Suicide Attempts
- Exposure to Violence in the Home
- Childhood History of Maltreatment
- Parental/Caregiver Criminality
- Early Caregiver Disruption
- Poor School Achievement

Social/Contextual Risk Factors

- Peer Delinquency
- Peer Rejection
- Stress and Poor Coping
- Poor Parental Management
- Lack of Personal/Social Support
- Community Disorganization

Individual Risk Factors

- Negative Attitudes
- Risk Taking/Impulsivity
- Substance Use Difficulties
- Anger Management Problems
- Low Empathy/Remorse
- Attention-Deficit/Hyperactivity Difficulties
- Poor Compliance
- Low Interest/Commitment to School

Protective Factors

- Prosocial Involvement
- Strong Social Support
- Strong Attachments and Bonds
- Positive Attitude toward Intervention and Authority
- Strong Commitment to School
- Resilient Personality Traits

three or more. Protective Factors are coded as "present" or "absent." Although the severity of items is graded, items are not scored in the traditional sense, so no numerical values are assigned. The primary objective of the SAVRY is not to "quantify" risk, but to provide operational definitions for key (empirically and professionally supported) risk factors for evaluators to *apply* across different assessments. Accordingly, when examiners are faced with uncertainty, how they decide to code any given risk item is less critical than their assessment of that factor's association with violence. After carefully weighing the risk and protective factors relevant to a particular examinee, an evaluator must ultimately form an opinion or make a judgment about the nature and degree of the juvenile's risk for violence. Though the SAVRY is sufficiently flexible to accommodate varying styles of risk communication, the coding form prompts evaluators to make a final "summary risk rating" of low, moderate, or high. This summary risk rating is a professional judgment based on the results of the entire SAVRY assessment of risk and protective factors.

HISTORY OF THE METHOD'S DEVELOPMENT

To address the gap in applied risk assessment technology with juveniles, two separate efforts were undertaken simultaneously in the late 1990s; both of these were based on the SPJ framework, which was then emerging as a "best-practice model" for violence risk assessments (Webster, Hucker, & Bloom, 2002; Webster, Mueller-Isberner, & Fransson, 2002). Randy Borum at the University of South Florida developed a prototype for an SPJ adolescent risk assessment tool, initially referred to as the Youth Risk Checklist. Patrick Bartel and Adelle Forth in Canada had begun a similar effort with a tool they had been calling the Adolescent Violence Risk Assessment. Having ties to both efforts, Christopher Webster—affectionately known as the "godfather" of the SPJ model—suggested that we contemplate coordination. After a joint review of the status of the projects, the nascent tools were sufficiently similar that we decided our efforts would be directed more productively by collaborating on a single instrument, which came to be known as the SAVRY.

In 2000, items from the two assessment prototypes were pooled and evaluated for inclusion in the final version (Bartel et al., 2000). The primary criterion for item selection was the robustness of the empirical relationship between each factor and violence, identified through prior reviews, meta-analyses, and original studies with adolescent populations (e.g., Hann & Borek, 2001; Hawkins et al., 1998, 2000; Howell, 1997; Lipsey & Derzon, 1998). The research base on protective factors for violence in adolescents was much less extensive (U.S. Department of Health and Human Services, 2001), so we selected those with the greatest promise. Though all included items demonstrated some empirical link to violence, a few (such as "Poor Compliance" remained despite a lack of robust research because of their clinical relevance. Next, we constructed operational coding definitions for each test item, drawing from definitions used in prior studies where possible, and developed criteria to anchor the levels of severity.

The items were revised, tightened, and integrated into a manual—the Consultation Edition of the SAVRY manual (Borum et al., 2002), released in February 2002—as a result of two efforts. First, in 2001, the pilot version of the items and coding criteria were circulated to several risk assessment professionals for comments, and applied in a couple of preliminary studies where researchers provided feedback about item clarity and language. Simultaneously, the SAVRY items underwent translation into Dutch by Henny Lodewijks, who provided valuable feedback about item definitions. Second, we conducted a validation study using a retrospective analysis of 104 incarcerated male delinquents (Bartel, Forth, & Borum, 2003), described in more detail below (see "Research Evidence"). Since the manual's dissemination, the only substantive change involved one risk item, "Psychopathic Traits," for which coding was linked directly to scores on the Hare Psychopathy Checklist: Youth Version (PCL:YV; Forth, Kosson, & Hare, 2003). There were several reasons for this. First, the PCL:YV is a psychometric instrument designed to assess the construct of psychopathy. For applied risk assessment, however, we were mainly interested in assessing the relevant cluster of traits as a "risk marker" for violence, rather than the diagnostic construct per se in juveniles. Second, the user qualifications for the SAVRY (a risk assessment tool) are less stringent than those for the PCL:YV (a clinical test). Third, the connotations of the term "psychopathy" are uniformly negative, and the label itself is so powerful that any information about a youth as an individual may be lost once this language is applied. Furthermore, given that several SAVRY items overlapped substantially with PCL:YV items, we sought to construct an item that captured only the otherwise unaccounted variance in the cluster of personality/behavioral traits. The "Low Empathy/ Remorse" item was the product of those efforts.

Although scores are not used with the SAVRY, we examined whether this item modification would affect a hypothetical "SAVRY risk total score" by comparing original SAVRY total scores to modified SAVRY total scores that replaced "Psychopathic Traits" (coded from PCL:YV total scores) with "Low Empathy/Remorse" (coded from PCL:YV affective items) in a sample of male adolescents. The SAVRY risk total scores using modified coding criteria correlated with the original total scores at .99 for both the total sample and the offender-only sample, suggesting no meaningful change in the aggregate construct of risk. The new "Low Empathy/Remorse" item was included in a second printing of the SAVRY manual, designated as Version 1.1 (Borum et al., 2003). No other substantive changes were made to the instrument or manual.

RESEARCH EVIDENCE

Research pertaining to the reliability and validity of the SAVRY is somewhat limited for two reasons. First, the SAVRY manual has not been available for very long. Second, since SPJ instruments are not numerically driven, interpretation of findings and speculation regarding implications for practice are more complex than for traditional psychometric tests. Examiner summary risk ratings are the foci, rather than total scores or classifications based on cutoff scores. Nonetheless, SPJ instrument "scores" can be generated to conduct traditional analyses as points of reference for item performance. Some of the research described has used the SAVRY risk total variable, calculated by transposing item ratings of low, moderate, and high to values of 0, 1, and 2, respectively, and summing the values.

Reliability and Internal Consistency

While the SAVRY and its component domains are not intended to be unidimensional "scales," for heuristic purposes we analyzed the internal consistency of SAVRY risk total scores in our initial validation samples. Internal consistency was .82 for young offenders and .84 for a sample of community youths (Bartel et al., 2003). However, the primary issue for SPJ instruments is interrater reliability. In one study using trained student raters, the single-rater intraclass correlation coefficient was .81 for the SAVRY total scores and .77 for the summary risk ratings (Catchpole & Gretton, 2003). Comparably, McEachran (2001) found relatively high reliability for SAVRY total scores (.83) and moderate coefficients (.72) for summary risk ratings.

Validity

The concurrent validity of the SAVRY has been examined in relation to the Youth Level of Service/Case Management Inventory (YLS/CMI; Hoge & Andrews, 2002) and the PCL:YV (Forth et al., 2003). In our initial validation study, the SAVRY risk total scores correlated significantly with both instruments among offenders (YLS/CMI = .89, PCL:YV = .78), and the Protective Factors domain negatively correlated with both measures. Catchpole and Gretton (2003) found that the SAVRY summary risk ratings correlated .64 with YLS/CMI summary classifications and .68 with PCL:YV total scores.

With regard to criterion validity, numerous studies have found significant correlations between SAVRY scores and various measures of violence in juvenile justice and high-risk community-dwelling populations (Bartel et al., 2003; Catchpole & Gretton, 2003; Fitch, 2002; Lodewijks, 2002; McEachran, 2001). In our validation sample, SAVRY risk total scores were all significantly related to behavioral measures of institutional aggressive behavior (.40) and aggressive conduct disorder symptoms (.52). The Protective Factors domain, again, was negatively related. Significant correlations (.32 and .25) between SAVRY risk total scores and measures of violence have been reported in other studies of male offenders (Catchpole & Gretton, 2003; Gretton & Abramowitz, 2002) and high-risk Native American youths (.56 for sample, .72 for females; Fitch, 2002). Summary risk ratings have been shown to correlate with violence by McEachran (2001; $r = .67$) and Gretton and Abramowitz (2002; $r = .35$). Retrospective studies using hierarchical regression analyses have shown that the SAVRY improves the YLS/CMI's and PCL:YV's postdictive power for both institutional aggression and aggressive conduct disorder symptoms. The SAVRY accounted for a large proportion of the explained variance in each type of violence (Bartel et al., 2003).

Other retrospective studies have used receiver operating characteristics (ROC) to assess the SAVRY's accuracy according to its relative improvement over chance. Areas under the curve (AUCs) for the total score's retrospective prediction of violent recidivism (the probability that a randomly selected juvenile scoring high on the SAVRY will be more likely to recidivate than a randomly selected juvenile with a low SAVRY score) average .74 to .80 across studies. Interestingly, examiner summary risk ratings have performed as well as, if not better than, the linear combination of scores. For example, McEachran (2001) found an AUC of .70 for SAVRY total scores, but an AUC of .89 for summary risk ratings. This finding has been evident in research with other SPJ tools (e.g., Dempster & Hart, 2002), and it provides the first empirical evidence that clinical judgments—properly structured and based on sound assessments—can achieve levels of accuracy that rival those of other known predictors while maintaining latitude for case-specific analysis.[1]

Finally, two prospective studies have been conducted to examine the link between summary risk ratings and actual recidivism. Catchpole and Gretton (2003) found that juveniles classified as low risk had a 6% violent recidivism rate, those classified as moderate risk had a rate of 14%, and those classified as high risk had a violent recidivism rate of 40% over a 1-year period. Similarly, Gretton and Abramowitz (2002) found that low-risk young offenders had a 5.7% violent recidivism rate, moderate-risk youths had a rate of 13.1%, and high-risk youths had a rate of 40.4%. Among those who did recidivate, 69.7% were rated as high risk, 24.2% as moderate risk, and only 6.1% as low risk. The high-risk group also recidivated more quickly than other youths.

Concerning generalizability, although the results of these studies support the use of the SAVRY for assessing violence risk in adolescents, more research is clearly needed to clarify its applicability across genders and different ethnic groups. Of particular importance is the dearth of data on African American and Hispanic youths, who are largely over-represented in many juvenile justice systems throughout the U.S. Two SAVRY studies focusing on Hispanic and female youths are currently underway at the California Youth Authority.

---

[1] One cautionary note is necessary for interpreting some of these findings. The author of this study used a scoring strategy in which the SAVRY total score was calculated by adding the converted codes for the 24 Risk Factors, then subtracting from that the sum of the converted codes for the Protective Factors. This deviates somewhat from the intended protocol, where the SAVRY total score simply represents the sum of the Risk Factors items. The Protective Factors are considered separately and are not subtracted. The effect that this scoring variation may have had on the study results is unknown.

APPLICATION

The question of whether and when to assess an adolescent for risk of violence is often determined by policy or legal mandate. When such assessments are required or when professionals are concerned about potential violence, the SAVRY is available for use by professionals from a variety of disciplines who conduct assessments and/or make intervention and supervision plans concerning violence risk in youths. More information can be found at *http:// www.fmhi.usf.edu/mhlp/savry/statement.htm*. Copies of the SAVRY can be ordered from Specialized Training Services, P.O. Box 28181, San Diego, CA 92198; (858) 675-0860; or *http://www.specializedtraining.com*. At a minimum, those who use the SAVRY should have expertise (i.e., training and experience) in conducting individual assessments and in child/adolescent development and youth violence. In general, psychologists, psychiatrists, trained juvenile probation officers, and social workers with requisite expertise will be qualified to use the SAVRY. There is no required training course to use the SAVRY. Professionals who meet the general user qualifications can often learn how to use the instrument by studying the manual and learning collaboratively with colleagues by comparing ratings and rationales to identify "weak spots" or rating biases.

It is difficult to estimate the extent to which the SAVRY is used in actual practice. Over 1,500 SAVRY manuals were sold/distributed internationally between February 2002 and February 2004. The SAVRY is used regularly at Youth Forensic Psychiatric Services in Burnaby, British Columbia and at detention facilities in the state of Connecticut, which adopted the SAVRY as its official tool for assessing violence risk in juveniles admitted into detention facilities. The SAVRY and its manual have been translated into Dutch (by Henny Lodewijks), Swedish (by Niklas Langstrom), and Finnish (by Riittakerttu Kaltiala-Heino), and are being used to some extent in The Netherlands, Sweden, and Finland. It is being applied in practice and in research studies in the United Kingdom (most prominently in Manchester, England) and at the Psychological Service Unit at the Ministry of Community Development, Youth and Sports in Singapore. The decision about whether or when to use the SAVRY (or any SPJ instrument, for that matter) in a correctional, clinical, or forensic evaluation involves a somewhat different calculus and standard from those employed in decisions to use traditional tests. The SAVRY, fundamentally, is an organizing scheme to guide a violence risk judgment. It is not a tool that "produces" a decision with a cutoff or specific formula. Viewed in this way, the applied use of the tool is appropriate to the extent that the risk and protective factors are appropriate predictors of relevant outcomes in the population. As noted above, the SAVRY items were drawn from a substantial body of empirical research, based on their known associations with violent behavior in adolescents ages 13 and older. The majority of these studies were conducted with male offenders ages 14–17 who were incarcerated or under correctional supervision.

In general, our view is that is appropriate for qualified users to incorporate the SAVRY in adolescent risk assessments for general violence risk (i.e., potential for engaging in some violent act toward anyone during a specified time period), including assessments intended to prevent violent behavior through supervision or intervention (e.g., probation/community supervision). Assessments of "general violence risk" differ from assessments of "targeted violence," defined as circumstances where a youth comes to the official attention of a school, clinical, or juvenile justice professional because of a concern about the potential for acting violently toward an identified or identifiable person (Borum, Fein, Vossekuil, & Berglund, 1999; Borum & Reddy, 2001; Fein & Vossekuil, 1998; Fein, Vossekuil, & Holden, 1995; Reddy et al., 2001). Here, the objective is typically to appraise the likelihood of a violent act against an identified person, not general violence. These cases require reliance on case-specific facts rather than general nomothetic risk factors, making the SAVRY less relevant.

CASE EXAMPLE

Jason was a 16-year-old European American male who was referred to a psychologist for a violence risk assessment after being expelled from school as a result of a violent altercation. The index incident involved a physical fight with another student in the school hallway. After one teacher attempted unsuccessfully to stop the fight, four additional staff members were required to restrain Jason, who was reported to be extremely belligerent and resistant. Jason was arrested and convicted on a criminal charge of assault, and sentenced to a period of probation. The purpose of this assessment was to assist in community treatment planning. The consulting psychologist interviewed Jason and reviewed his school, probation, and mental health records. In the past year, juvenile justice and school disciplinary records showed that Jason had a prior assault conviction in connection with a community incident, and collateral sources reported that he had physically threatened other students on two occasions. Jason reported being suspended for fighting several times in elementary school, and stated that he had been in four serious fights over the past 3 years. He stated that he enjoyed the "rush" of fighting.

Jason reported being somewhat of a loner, with no close friends. He was not involved in sports or organized groups/activities and admitted to frequent marijuana abuse. Jason had little parental supervision, and parental management was consistently permissive and overindulgent. Jason had at times been verbally abusive and threatening toward his mother. His academic performance was generally poor. Throughout much of his school career, there had been concerns about Jason's nonattendance and failure to complete class assignments. He failed his last school year. Jason had also had had several contacts with mental health professionals over the course of his life. In March of the current year, Jason was involuntarily placed in the inpatient psychiatric ward of the city general hospital for a 5-day period after threatening to burn himself or kill someone, reportedly in response to being prevented from seeing his girlfriend. During the period of probation for the index offense, however, he attended all probation appointments and was generally compliant with probation orders.

The SAVRY was used to assist in estimating the nature and degree of risk for future violence that Jason might pose. Based on a systematic appraisal and consideration of the SAVRY's Historical, Social/Contextual, and Individual Risk Factors domains balanced against the Protective Factors domain, Jason was rated as being "high risk" for serious violence (i.e., punching, hitting kicking) at the time of the assessment. The basis for this judgment included the presence of a history of serious violence, early initiation of violence, and academic difficulties. Social/Contextual factors evident in this case included low commitment to school, poor parental management, and lack of social support. Individual factors included negative attitudes, anger management problems, low empathy/remorse, poor compliance, and substance use difficulties. In addition, there were moderate tendencies in the Historical domain toward peer rejection, history of self-harm, and stress/poor coping, along with a marked absence of protective factors. In essence, serious difficulties were noted in each of the major Risk Factor domains and were not mitigated by any items in the Protective Factors domain.

Jason's "high risk" was specifically linked to the likelihood of perpetrating violence against peers, and to a lesser extent against his mother. He reported no current grievances (plans or intentions to harm other persons), suggesting that his risk might be more long-term than imminent. It was also important to note, however, that his current risk level was contingent upon the continued presence of the identified risk factors. Should these factors (particularly his anger management problems) be mitigated through circumstance or intervention, Jason's risk could decrease substantially. Recommendations for risk reduction focused on interventions to improve family/parental management and self-management of negative affect and behavior.

REFERENCES

Bartel, P., Borum, R., & Forth, A. (2000). *Structured Assessment for Violence Risk in Youth (SAVRY): Consultation Edition*. Tampa: Louis de la Parte Florida Mental Health Institute, University of South Florida.

Bartel, P., Forth, A., & Borum, R. (2003). *Development and concurrent validation of the Structured Assessment for Violence Risk in Youth (SAVRY)*. Manuscript submitted for publication.

Borum, R. (1996). Improving the clinical practice of violence risk assessment: Technology, guidelines and training. *American Psychologist, 51*, 945–956.

Borum, R. (2000). Assessing violence risk among youth. *Journal of Clinical Psychology, 56*, 1263–1288.

Borum, R. (2002, March). *Why is assessing violence risk in juveniles different than in adults?* Paper presented at the biennial conference of the American Psychology–Law Society, Austin, TX.

Borum, R. (2003). Managing at risk juvenile offenders in the community: Putting evidence based principles into practice. *Journal of Contemporary Criminal Justice, 19*, 114–137.

Borum, R. (in press). Assessing risk for violence among juvenile offenders. In S. Sparta & G. Koocher (Eds.), *The forensic assessment of children and adolescents: Issues and applications.* New York: Oxford University Press.

Borum, R., Bartel, P., & Forth, A. (2002). *Manual for the Structured Assessment for Violence Risk in Youth (SAVRY): Version 1, Consultation Edition.* Tampa: Louis de la Parte Florida Mental Health Institute, University of South Florida.

Borum, R., Bartel, P., & Forth, A. (2003). *Manual for the Structured Assessment for Violence Risk in Youth (SAVRY): Version 1.1.* Tampa: Louis de la Parte Florida Mental Health Institute, University of South Florida.

Borum, R., & Douglas, K. (2003, March). New directions in violence risk assessment. *Psychiatric Times, 20*(3), 102–103.

Borum, R., Fein, R., Vossekuil, B., & Berglund, J. (1999). Threat assessment: Defining an approach for evaluating risk of targeted violence. *Behavioral Sciences and the Law, 17*, 323–337.

Borum, R., & Reddy, M. (2001). Assessing violence risk in *Tarasoff* situations: A fact-based model of inquiry. *Behavioral Sciences and the Law, 19*, 375–385.

Borum, R., & Verhaagen, D. (2003). *A practical guide to assessing and managing violence risk in juveniles.* Manuscript in preparation.

Catchpole, R., & Gretton, H. (2003). The predictive validity of risk assessment with violent young offenders: A 1-year examination of criminal outcome. *Criminal Justice and Behavior, 30*, 688–708.

Dempster, R. J., & Hart, S. D. (2002). The relative utility of fixed and variable risk factors in discriminating sexual recidivists and nonrecidivists. *Sexual Abuse: A Journal of Research and Treatment, 14*, 121–138.

Fein, R. A., & Vossekuil, B. (1998). *Protective intelligence and threat assessment investigations: A guide for state and local law enforcement officials* (Publication No. NCJ 170612). Washington, DC: U.S. Department of Justice.

Fein, R. A., Vossekuil, B., & Holden, G. A. (1995, September). Threat assessment: An approach to prevent targeted violence. *National Institute of Justice: Research in Action*, pp. 1–7.

Fitch, D. (2002). *Analysis of common risk factors for violent behavior in Native American adolescents referred for residential treatment.* Unpublished doctoral dissertation, Texas Southern University.

Forth, A. E., Kosson, D. S., & Hare, R. D. (2003). *Hare Psychopathy Checklist—Revised: Youth Version.* Toronto: Multi-Health Systems.

Gretton, H., & Abramowitz, C. (2002, March). *SAVRY: Contribution of items and scales to clinical risk judgments and criminal outcomes.* Paper presented at the biennial conference of the American Psychology–Law Society, Austin, TX.

Griffin, P., & Torbet, P. (2002). *Desktop guide to good juvenile probation practice.* Washington, DC: Office of Juvenile Justice and Delinquency Prevention.

Grisso, T. (1996). Society's retributive response to juvenile violence: A developmental perspective. *Law and Human Behavior, 20*, 229–247.

Grisso, T. (1998). *Forensic evaluation of juveniles.* Sarasota, FL: Professional Resource Press.

Grisso, T., & Schwartz, R. (Eds.). (2000). *Youth on trial: A developmental perspective on juvenile justice.* Chicago: University of Chicago Press.

Hann, D. A., & Borek, N. (2001). *Taking stock of risk factors for child/youth externalizing behavior problems.* Bethesda, MD: National Institute of Mental Health.

Hawkins, J., Herrenkohl, T., Farrington, D., Brewer, D., Catalano, R., & Harachi, T. (1998). A review of predictors of youth violence. In R. Loeber & D. Farrington (Eds.), *Serious and violent juvenile offenders: Risk factors and successful interventions* (pp. 106–146). Thousand Oaks, CA: Sage.

Hawkins, J., Herrenkohl, T., Farrington, D., Brewer, D., Catalano, R., Harachi, T., & Cothern, L. (2000, April). *Predictors of youth violence* (Bulletin). Washington, DC: Office of Juvenile Justice and Delinquency Prevention.

Hoge, R. D. (2001). *The juvenile offender: Theory, research, and applications.* Boston: Kluwer Academic.

Hoge, R. D. (2002). Standardized instruments for assessing risk and need in youthful offenders. *Criminal Justice and Behavior, 29,* 380–396.

Hoge, R. D., & Andrews, D. A. (1996). *Assessing the youthful offender: Issues and techniques.* New York: Plenum Press.

Hoge, R. D., & Andrews, D. A. (2002). *Youth Level of Service/Case Management Inventory.* North Tonawanda, NY: Multi-Health Systems.

Howell, J. (1997). *Juvenile justice and youth violence.* Thousand Oaks, CA: Sage.

Lipsey, M., & Derzon, J. (1998). Predictors of violent or serious delinquency in adolescence and early adulthood: A synthesis of longitudinal research. In R. Loeber & D. P. Farrington (Eds.), *Serious and violent juvenile offenders: Risk factors and successful interventions* (pp. 86–105). Thousand Oaks, CA: Sage.

Lodewijks, H. (2002, July). *The reliability and predictive validity of the SAVRY (Structured Assessment of Violent Risk in Youth) in a Dutch population of male adolescent delinquents.* Paper presented at the International Congress of Law and Mental Health, Amsterdam.

McCord, J., Widom, C. S., & Crowell, N. A. (Eds.). (2001). *Juvenile crime, juvenile justice.* Washington, DC: National Academy Press.

McEachran, A. (2001). *The predictive vailidity of the PCL-YV and the SAVRY in a population of adolescent offenders.* Unpublished master's thesis, Simon Fraser University, Burnaby, BC, Canada.

Puzzanchera, C., Stahl, A., Finnegan, T., Tierney, N., & Snyder, H. (2002). *Juvenile court statistics 1999.* Washington, DC: Office of Juvenile Justice and Delinquency Prevention.

Reddy, M., Borum, R., Vossekuil, B., Fein, R., Berglund, J., & Modzeleski, W. (2001). Evaluating risk for targeted violence in schools: Comparing risk assessment, threat assessment, and other approaches. *Psychology in the Schools, 38*(2), 157–172.

Rosado, L. (Ed.). (2000). *Kids are different: How knowledge of adolescent development theory can aid decision-making in court.* Washington, DC: American Bar Association Juvenile Justice Center.

U.S. Department of Health and Human Services. (2001). *Youth violence: A report of the Surgeon General.* Washington, DC: U.S. Government Printing Office.

Webster, C., Hucker, S., & Bloom, H. (2002). Transcending the actuarial versus clinical polemic in assessing risk for violence. *Criminal Justice and Behavior, 29*(5), 659–665.

Webster, C., Mueller-Isberner, R., & Fransson, G. (2002). Violence risk assessment: Using structured clinical guides professionally. *International Journal of Forensic Mental Health, 1*(2), 185–193.

CHAPTER 20

Hare Psychopathy Checklist: Youth Version

Adelle E. Forth

PURPOSE

Research with adults indicates a strong relationship between psychopathy on the one hand and serious repetitive crime, violent behavior, and a poor treatment response on the other (Hare, Clark, Grann, & Thornton, 2000; Hemphill, Hare, & Wong, 1998; Rice, Harris, & Cormier, 1992; Richards, Casey, & Lucente, 2003; Seto & Barbaree, 1999). Psychopathy does not emerge suddenly in adulthood; researchers and clinicians believe that psychopathic traits are manifested early in life (Forth & Mailloux, 2000; Johnstone & Cooke, 2004; Lynam, 2002; Saltaris, 2002). Consequently, researchers have designed various measures to identify psychopathic traits early. These measures use youth self-reports (e.g., Youth Psychopathic Traits Inventory [YPI]—Andershed, Gustafson, Kerr, & Stattin, 2002; Psychopathy Content Screening Scale [PCS]—Murrie & Cornell, 2000) or parent and teacher reports (Child Psychopathy Scale [CPS]—Lynam, 1997; Antisocial Process Screening Device [APSD]—Frick & Hare, 2001). This chapter focuses on the Hare Psychopathy Checklist: Youth Version (PCL:YV; Forth, Kosson, & Hare, 2003). The PCL:YV is an instrument designed to assess psychopathic traits and behaviors in adolescents via a structured clinical rating approach. It was adapted from the Hare Psychopathy Checklist—Revised (PCL-R; Hare, 2003), considered to be the most reliable and valid measure of psychopathy in adults (Fulero, 1995).

BASIC DESCRIPTION

The PCL:YV is a rating scale designed to measure psychopathic traits and behaviors in male and female adolescents ages 12–18 years. The PCL:YV emphasizes the need for multidomain and multisource information in order to assess psychopathic traits adequately. It consists of 20 items that measure the interpersonal, affective, and behavioral dimensions considered to be fundamental to the construct of psychopathy (see Table 20.1 for a list of items). The PCL:YV manual provides detailed item descriptions and examples of sources of information to use when rating items. Each item is scored a 2 (the item "definitely applies"), 1 (the item "applies to some extent"), or 0 (the item "definitely does not apply"). The items are summed to obtain a total score ranging from 0 to 40. Up to five items can be omitted when insufficient information is available to score an item. If items are omitted, tables are available to prorate total and factor scores.

Several sources of information are needed to score the PCL:YV—namely, a semistructured interview with the youth, and a review of available file and collateral information. The interview takes between 90 and 120 minutes. It covers information about past history and current functioning, including school history and adjustment, work history and goals, family background and current functioning, interpersonal relationships, substance use, attitudes

---

TABLE 20.1. Items in the Hare Psychopathy Checklist: Youth Version (PCL:YV)

1. Impression management
2. Grandiose sense of self-worth
3. Stimulation seeking
4. Pathological lying
5. Manipulation for personal gain
6. Lack of remorse
7. Shallow affect
8. Callous/lack of empathy
9. Parasitic orientation
10. Poor anger control
11. Impersonal sexual behavior
12. Early behavior problems
13. Lacks goals
14. Impulsivity
15. Irresponsibility
16. Failure to accept responsibility
17. Unstable interpersonal relationships
18. Serious criminal behavior
19. Serious violations of conditional release
20. Criminal versatility

and emotions, and childhood and adolescent antisocial behaviors. The type and amount of file information will vary across settings; however, adequate information from a variety of social contexts (e.g., institutional files, mental health evaluations, police reports, social worker reports, school records, court records, and interviews with parents or other caregivers) is required for clinical purposes. Depending on the amount of information and familiarity with a case, file reviews will vary from 30 minutes to several hours, and the entire assessment will require approximately 3 hours.

Some researchers (Campbell, Porter, & Santor, 2004; Gretton, Hare, & Catchpole, 2004; Gretton, McBride, Hare, O'Shaughnessy, & Kumka, 2001; Marczyk, Heilbrun, Lander, & DeMatteo, 2003; O'Neill, Lidz, & Heilbrun, 2003a) have used extensive file information exclusively to generate PCL:YV scores, meaning that no interviews with youths were conducted. Although not optimal, file-only PCL:YV scores are acceptable when an archival study is being conducted and/or when it is impossible to do an interview. File-only assessments limit the information necessary for scoring items dealing with affective and interpersonal styles. A clinician who bases a PCL:YV assessment solely on chart/collateral information must acknowledge the limitations of such a procedure (e.g., difficulties in scoring some of the items) and indicate in his or her report that the youth was not directly examined.

Raters record item scores on the PCL:YV QuikScore Form. Total scores are generally the scores of primary interest, but factor scores can provide more fine-grained descriptions (see the "Research Evidence" section). The PCL:YV total score provides a dimensional measure of the number and severity of psychopathic features. No categorical cutoff score exists for the diagnosis of psychopathy. The manual provides T-scores and percentiles for total and factor scores for institutionalized male offenders, male probationers, and small samples of female offenders and community males. Raters should obtain T-scores and percentile ranks based on the most appropriate comparison sample.

HISTORY OF THE METHOD'S DEVELOPMENT

A key decision made by the test's authors was to use the item content of the PCL-R to guide development of the PCL:YV. In the first study to examine psychopathic traits in youths (Forth, Hart, & Hare, 1990), several modifications were made to the PCL-R. For instance, items 9 ("Parasitic lifestyle") and 17 ("Many short-term marital relationships") were deleted because of adolescents' limited work histories and few marital relationships. Items 18 ("Juvenile delinquency") and 20 ("Criminal versatility") were modified because adolescent offenders had fewer opportunities than adult offenders to come into contact with the judicial system. This original version of the scale, often referred to as the "modified PCL-R" or "18-item PCL-R," has been used in several other studies (Brandt, Kennedy, Patrick, & Curtin, 1997; Murrie & Cornell, 2000; Myers, Burket, & Harris, 1995).

Subsequently, the authors made more extensive modifications to the PCL-R. First, to ensure that the assessment of psychopathy was sensitive to the ways in which normative behaviors change with age, raters were advised to evaluate individuals' behavior in the context of normative behavior of same-age peers. Second, to tailor the assessment of psychopathy to the specific life experiences of adolescents, item descriptions were modified to place more emphasis on peers, family, and school in the lives of adolescents. Third, items 9 (now labeled "Parasitic orientation") and 17 (now labeled "Unstable interpersonal relationships") were modified to permit assessments in youths. Fourth, the focus was placed on relatively enduring features of a youth, displayed across settings and situations since late childhood. This modified version of the PCL-R was named the PCL:YV.

The PCL:YV was made available to researchers, and data from these researchers are summarized in the technical manual for the PCL:YV. Experience with the PCL:YV, as well as feedback from other researchers, led to some minor modifications to the PCL:YV item descriptions. These modifications are described in the manual, which was published in 2003 (Forth et al., 2003).

RESEARCH EVIDENCE

The research reviewed was based on the PCL:YV normative sample and some more recent publications. The test manual contains data from 2,438 youths in three countries (Canada, the United States, and the United Kingdom) across 19 different samples. Samples include young offenders from custodial institutions, probation, psychiatric inpatient facilities, and the community. In most cases, data represent convenience samples made up of volunteers. Studies based on file reviews, however, used representative samples including all cases with sufficient information.

Internal Consistency and Reliability

The interrater reliability of PCL:YV total scores is generally high, with a single-rater intraclass correlation (ICC_1) of .90 to .96 (Forth et al., 2003). Recent research has reported that the ICC_1 ranges from .82 ($n = 10$; Spain, Douglas, Poythress, & Epstein, 2004) to .89 ($n = 30$; Salekin, Neumann, Leistico, DiCicco, & Duros, 2004). This high level of agreement may be due to the level of training provided to the raters in the research studies that formed the basis for the manual. Whether this high level of interrater reliability will be maintained once the PCL:YV is used for clinical purposes will need to be investigated.

Confirmatory factor analyses across all the normative samples suggested that a model with four correlated factors provided a good explanation for the pattern of covariation among PCL:YV item scores (Forth et al., 2003). Four items loaded on Factor 1, an interpersonal dimension (e.g., "Impression management," "Pathological lying"), and four items on Factor 2, an affective dimension (e.g., "Lack of remorse," "Callous/lack of empathy"). Five items loaded on Factor 3, a behavioral dimension (e.g., "Impulsivity," "Lacks goals"), and five items on Factor 4, an antisocial dimension (e.g., "Poor anger control," "Serious criminal behavior").

The internal consistency of PCL:YV total scores is acceptable, with alpha coefficients ranging from .85 to .94 (Forth et al., 2003; O'Neill et al., 2003a), although other researchers have reported somewhat lower alphas of .73 (Skeem & Cauffman, 2003) and .79 (Lee, Vincent, Hart, & Corrado, 2003). Across settings, the mean interitem correlations in the normative data were all above .20. The internal consistency of the four factors ranged from .74 to .81. These values are consistent with the view that the PCL:YV is a homogeneous scale.

Skeem and Cauffman (2003) evaluated the test–retest reliability of the PCL:YV over a 1-month period in a sample of 114 male adolescent offenders. Adequate levels of test–retest reliability were obtained (intraclass correlation of .66 for PCL:YV total score). Studies are currently underway to examine the test–retest reliability of the PCL:YV over longer periods.

Validity

Face Validity

Face validity is a basic component of any theoretical construct. Studies have investigated how child clinicians (Salekin, Rogers, & Machin, 2001) and juvenile justice personnel (Cruise, Colwell, Lyons, & Baker, 2003) conceptualize psychopathy in male and female adolescents. Both studies asked respondents to rate prototypical features of a male and a female adolescent described as having psychopathy. Respondents considered a wide range of indicators, including interpersonal (e.g., "Lies easily and skillfully"), affective (e.g., "Emotions seem shallow"), behavioral (e.g., "Dangerous or risky activities"), and antisocial (e.g., "Juvenile delinquency") traits—the majority of which are captured in the PCL:YV.

Generalizability

PCL:YV total scores vary across samples and settings, with incarcerated youths scoring the highest ($M = 24.4$), followed by youths on probation ($M = 20.1$), and lower-scoring youths in the community ($M = 3.2$). Average scores of incarcerated youths are slightly higher than average scores of incarcerated adult offenders. There is a small negative correlation between age at assessment and PCL:YV total scores among youths pooled across samples ($r = -.11$). This reflects the tendency of younger adolescents (ages 14 or below) to obtain higher PCL:YV total scores than older adolescents (ages 15 or higher).

The degree of association between PCL:YV total scores and ethnicity has been small across studies, ranging from correlations of .03 in probation samples to .17 in institutionalized samples. In the normative sample, African American youths scored slightly higher than youths from other ethnic backgrounds. Females scored slightly lower (about 1 point), on average, than males in incarcerated and probation samples. Recent research has reported no gender differences in the prevalence of youths scoring high on the PCL:YV (Campbell et al., 2004; Salekin et al., 2004). Despite findings from the normative data, the results presented here suggest that PCL:YV total scores are not unduly influenced by youths' age, ethnicity, or sex.

Rogers, Vitacco, Jackson, and colleagues (2002) examined whether the PCL:YV was susceptible to response styles. The researchers conducted two PCL:YV assessments with youth participants. All youths were first assessed under a standard condition, and then were randomly assigned to simulate "social desirability" (a prosocial attitude toward authority and parental figures, with expressed regret for past behaviors) or to simulate "social nonconformity" (a tough criminal attitude, with expressed defiance toward authority) for the second assessment. PCL:YV scores were lower than the standard assessment in the social desirability condition and higher in the social nonconformity condition.[1]

Concurrent Validity

Research pertaining to the concurrent (convergent and discriminant) validity of the PCL:YV provides evidence that PCL:YV scores are related in appropriate ways to a variety of clinical, psychosocial, and criminological variables. In addition, scores are unrelated or only weakly related to variables that theoretically should not be associated with psychopathy.

Convergent validity studies have included self-report questionnaires designed to assess psychopathic traits in youths. The PCL:YV is moderately correlated (r = .30, Murrie & Cornell, 2002; r = .40, Lee et al., 2003) with the self-report version of the *APSD* (Caputo, Frick, & Brodsky, 1999) and the *PCS* (r = .49, Murrie & Cornell, 2002) from the Millon Adolescent Clinical Inventory (Millon, 1993). However, it is only weakly associated with the *YPI* (Skeem & Cauffman, 2003).

Kosson, Cyterski, Steuerwald, Neumann, and Walker-Matthews (2002) examined the construct validity of the PCL:YV in a sample of 115 male adolescents on probation. They found weak correlations with oppositional defiant disorder symptoms, attention-deficit/hyperactivity disorder symptoms, and anxiety scores. PCL:YV total scores were correlated with adolescents' ratings of familial emotional distance. In a sample of 226 male and female adolescent offenders, Campbell and colleagues (2004) found that prorated PCL:YV total scores were positively correlated with externalizing symptoms (r = .23), such as delinquency and aggression, and unrelated to internalizing

---

[1] The authors acknowledged that the interviewers knew that participants had been told to simulate during the second session, and this may have influenced their scoring of the PCL:YV.

symptoms ($r = -.\ 03$), such as anxiety, depression, and suicidal ideation. Mailloux, Forth, and Kroner (1997) examined the association between psychopathy and substance use in 40 male adolescent offenders. PCL:YV total scores were positively correlated with scores on the Michigan Alcohol Screening Test (Selzer, 1971) and on the Drug Abuse Screening Test (Skinner, 1982). PCL:YV total scores also correlated with age of initial alcohol use, age of initial drug use, and with the number of drugs tried. Gretton and colleagues (2004) found that high PCL:YV scorers had more conduct disorder (CD) symptoms and violent offense histories than low scorers.

O'Neill, Lidz, and Heilbrun (2003b) measured the association among childhood abuse and neglect, parental substance use, and PCL:YV scores in a sample of 64 males with substance abuse. Childhood abuse/neglect and parental drug or alcohol use were rated on 5-point scales (ranging from "none" to "extreme or severe") on the basis of interview and file information. The PCL:YV was not correlated with parental substance use or with youths' number of previous substance offenses, but was moderately correlated with child abuse/neglect ratings. Similarly, Campbell and colleagues (2004) found that higher prorated PCL:YV total scores were related to experiencing physical abuse and histories of nonparental living arrangements.

Criterion-Related and Predictive Validity

Although the PCL:YV was not designed as a measure for predicting institutional or criminal behavior, a growing body of research suggests that it is a strong predictor, particularly with respect to violent behavior (Forth & Mailloux, 2000). Kosson and colleagues (2002) found that psychopathic traits were related to past nonviolent and violent offenses, the number of different types of offenses, and use of a weapon. Murrie, Cornell, Kaplan, McConville, and Levy-Elkon (2004) examined the association between PCL:YV scores and violent behavior in a sample of 133 incarcerated adolescents. PCL:YV scores were moderately associated with violent offense history, nonadjudicated violence, severity of violence, and instrumental motives for violence. In a prospective 4- to 6-week follow-up period, PCL:YV scores were significantly associated with institutional charges for physical aggression.

Several retrospective follow-up studies have examined the *postdictive* validity of the PCL:YV, using scores based on extensive file information available up until discharge. Gretton and colleagues (2001) investigated the postdictive validity of the PCL:YV in a sample of 220 adolescent sex offenders referred to a sexual offender treatment program. High scorers (30 or higher on file-rated PCL:YV total scores) were more likely to have attempted or committed an escape from custody, and to have breached conditions of release, than medium-scoring (18 to 29) and low-scoring (18 or less) juveniles. Recidivism data were obtained approximately 5 years after discharge from the treatment program. Total scores were significantly correlated with general and violent recidivism, but not with sexual recidivism. Gretton and colleagues created four groups based on a median split of PCL:YV scores and evidence of deviant sexual arousal. The group with high PCL:YV scores and high deviant sexual arousal was most likely to reoffend generally and violently.

Gretton and colleagues (2004) examined the postdictive validity of PCL:YV file ratings in a sample of 157 adolescent offenders. Criminal offending was coded for a maximum 10-year retrospective period. The PCL:YV made a significant contribution to the postdiction of violent recidivism and time to first offense after CD symptoms and criminal history variables were controlled for. Another retrospective study extended this association to females. Catchpole and Gretton (2003) found that file-only PCL:YV scores were moderately related to general and violent recidivism in a sample of 74 male and female violent young offenders. In contrast to the preceding studies, Marczyk and colleagues (2003) found no association between PCL:YV total scores and rearrests in a retrospective study of 95 juvenile defendants.[2]

A few *prospective* studies have recently reported the predictive validity of the PCL:YV. Corrado, Vincent, Hart, and Cohen (2004) examined the past antisocial correlates and average 1-year predictive validity of the PCL:YV in a sample of 182 male adolescent offenders. Retrospectively, PCL:YV scores were associated with the age of first conviction, age of first drug use, and age of onset of conduct problems at school. Prospectively, PCL:YV total scores significantly predicted any recidivism (including violations), nonviolent recidivism, and violent recidivism. In addition, youths scoring higher on the PCL:YV committed a new offense about twice as quickly as lower-scoring youths. The behavioral features of the PCL:YV were more strongly related to reoffending than the interpersonal and affective features. Vincent, Vitacco, Grisso, and Corrado (2003) found a cluster of incarcerated male adolescents with combined interpersonal, affective, and behavioral features of psychopathy; relative to offenders with only behavioral, only affective, or no psychopathic features, those with the combined features were most likely to reoffend violently and had the highest imminence of reoffending over an average 1-year follow-up.

O'Neill and colleagues (2003a) investigated treatment participation and outcome by following a sample of 64 juveniles released from a substance abuse treatment facility for 1 year. PCL:YV scores were negatively correlated with days in the program, quality of participation, number of consecutive clean urine screens, and researchers' ratings (from discharge summaries) of clinical improvement; they were positively correlated with the number of subsequent arrest dates. In contrast, Spain and colleagues (2004) reported that PCL:YV scores were not strongly related to treatment progress in a sample of 85 male adolescent offenders.

---

[2] PCL:YV scores were based on file information, and the average score was unusually low ($M = 9.12$). The reason for such a low score in a sample of juvenile defendants being evaluated for certification to the adult criminal justice system is unclear. Only youths who have a history of committing a serious offense or who are charged with a serious offense are potentially subject to the adult criminal justice system.

APPLICATION

The PCL:YV technical manual, interview guide, and QuikScore Forms are available for commercial purchase from Multi-Health Services, Inc. (*http:// www.mhs.com*). The manual recommends that a clinical user of the PCL:YV possess an advanced graduate degree and the appropriate professional credentials in the social, medical, or behavioral sciences; be familiar with the empirical literature pertaining to psychopathy and adolescent development; and receive adequate training and experience. Training on the PCL:YV should cover three major topics: (1) a review of the psychopathy concept, as well as uses, potential misuses, and psychometric properties of the PCL:YV; (2) the assessment procedures; and (3) a scoring of PCL:YV items. Raters should complete 5 to 10 practice cases and compare scores with an experienced rater prior to clinical use. Institutions and agencies can provide their own in-house training or can attend a PCL:YV training workshop (see *http:// www.hare.org*).

The PCL:YV provides researchers and clinical users with a tool to assess psychopathic traits and behaviors in youths. Within the juvenile justice context, this information may be useful in identifying youths who represent more serious management problems within institutions, who need intensive interventions, and who require more resources for risk management in the community. Reservations have been raised concerning the appropriateness of applying the construct of psychopathy to youths and the consequences of doing so (Edens, Guy, & Fernandez, 2003; Edens, Skeem, Cruise, & Cauffman, 2001; Seagrave & Grisso, 2002). These concerns have focused on (1) the issue of labeling a youth as a "psychopath"; (2) the possibility that characteristics of psychopathy are common features of typically developing youths; (3) the stability of psychopathic traits from late childhood to early adulthood; and (4) the implications of the PCL:YV for classification, sentencing, and treatment.

The PCL:YV manual addresses the issue of labeling, stating that "users not use the PCL:YV to diagnose adolescents as psychopaths for clinical or forensic purposes" (Forth et al., 2003, p. 16). Although some adolescents may exhibit some features of psychopathy in certain contexts or for a limited time, in order for a youth to obtain a high score on the PCL:YV, evidence for the trait or behavior must exist across social contexts over substantial time periods. High ratings of psychopathy are rare in community youths (80% of community males score below 5; Forth et al., 2003). Longitudinal research examining constellations of personality traits, including psychopathic-like traits, have provided some evidence for stability from childhood to adolescence to early adulthood (Block, 1993; Caspi et al., 2003; Crawford, Cohen, & Brook, 2001; McCrae et al., 2002). Nonetheless, research is needed to examine the relationship between PCL:YV ratings of adolescents and subsequent PCL-R ratings in adulthood. A danger exists that limitations in the availability of treatment resources may tempt some administrators to use high PCL:YV scores to exclude young offenders from treatment, given that adults described as having psychopathy do not seem amenable to treatment. It is important that the PCL:YV not be used to exclude adolescents with psychopathic traits from intervention. We do not yet know enough about the malleability of psychopathic traits in adolescents who are provided treatment programs.

CASE EXAMPLE

Kevin was a 16-year-old African American male adolescent offender who was convicted of sexual assault and burglary. An assessment of psychopathic traits was requested to aid in recommendations regarding risk for future criminal behavior and appropriate level of intervention. A forensic psychologist completed the PCL:YV in a detention facility on the basis of file information; an interview with Kevin's mother and probation officer; and a 2-hour interview with Kevin, during which he was talkative, suspicious, and at times angry. He was somewhat controlling, often interrupting and questioning the evaluator about her qualifications.

Kevin reported that his father had left his mother prior to his birth, and that his mother had raised him. When Kevin was 6 years old, his mother married his stepfather, who ultimately died in a car accident when Kevin was 12 years old. Kevin reported experiencing a serious loss at this stepfather's death and claimed that it triggered his disruptive childhood behavior. He stated, "Everything was fine until my stepdad died. I wanted to be in control, and was pissed off at authority 'cause I lost the dominant force in my life."

According to file information, Kevin began acting out at an early age. His first contact with the local police was at age 8 for running away from home. By the age of 13, he was made a ward of the juvenile court for being beyond the control of his mother and running away from home. According to his mother's report, Kevin would lie to her "about everything."

Academically, Kevin was doing quite poorly. School records indicated that he complained he was bored by classes and skipped school frequently. He was suspended several times for fighting in elementary school (beginning in Grade 3), but he was never expelled. He was placed in a structured full-time behavioral program at age 12. He often threatened the teacher and other students. He failed Grade 6, but blamed his teacher for picking on him unfairly. He reported wanting to drop out of school, since he could learn everything he needed to know on the street.

Kevin had minimal employment history in the community. When he was 14, he worked part of the summer for his uncle's plumbing business, but was often late for work and occasionally didn't show up at all. When his uncle confronted him about this, he always had an excuse. When Kevin was asked about his future goals, he believed he could easily get a job in computers. He acknowledged that he might need to get his high school diploma, but then stated that it was unlikely he would get one, because he "had other plans." When asked what these plans involved, he smirked and said, "That is not something you need to know." In one report, Kevin denied a history of substance abuse except the social use of alcohol; he said he had only tried marijuana once, when he was 14 years old, but did not like it. During the current assessment, however, he stated that he had started sniffing glue when he was 11 and had tried pot, hash, amphetamines, and cocaine, but that the only drug he used and liked was pot. He said he had first tried alcohol at age 10 and that he was drinking regularly prior to his current offenses. He denied ever being addicted to any drug.

With respect to his sexual history, Kevin reported having first experienced sexual intercourse when he was 11 years old. Later in the interview, Kevin claimed to have started dating at 13 years old and reported five past girlfriends. He described most of these relationships as lasting a couple of weeks. His longest relationship with a girlfriend had been 4 months; he ended that relationship when she accused him of sleeping with other girls. He acknowledged that he had been having sex with other girls, but that she knew he had a reputation for being a "slut."

Kevin's previous convictions included driving without a license, burglary (two counts), and assault causing bodily harm. The first burglary had occurred when he was 13 and was caught in a neighbor's house stealing a camera and a wallet. The second had occurred when Kevin burglarized a home and, when surprised by finding the victim at home, forced her into her bedroom at knifepoint and stole her purse. The assault causing bodily harm was against Kevin's Big Brother, who was assigned as part of his probation. After four outings with no apparent conflict, the Big Brother took Kevin to lunch and then to his office. There, the victim "lectured" Kevin on the importance of staying in school and out of trouble. When the Big Brother drove Kevin home, Kevin told the victim that he wanted to give him something. Kevin went into his house and got a hockey stick. He hit the victim three times across the head with the stick. Kevin reported that the assault would not have happened if the victim had "kept his mouth shut." To date, Kevin had spent a total of 14 months in juvenile facilities as a result of his juvenile offending.

Kevin had committed 10 rule violations over the course of his last two juvenile terms, including disobeying orders, possession of alcohol, and destroying state property. He was known to stare at female custody officers in an intimidating fashion, and he told one to "kiss my ass, you fat bitch." He was demanding and confrontational with staff members and other offenders. Kevin had also violated conditions of his probation following both earlier burglary convictions. During the first probation, he missed three appointments and regularly violated his curfew. He was on probation when he committed the assault on his Big Brother.

Kevin admitted to his most recent offenses, the sexual assault and burglary, at his trial. The victim was a 21-year-old female who returned to her home at 10:30 P.M. She entered her residence and went into her bedroom. Kevin came out from behind the door, grabbed her, and held a knife to her neck. She started to scream, and he threatened to kill her if she screamed again. He stuffed a pair of socks in her mouth, raped her, and told her he would come back if she called the police. He then stole her purse and cell phone, and cut the in-house telephone line. A neighbor called the police and reported he heard someone screaming. Police arrived, and Kevin was apprehended in the neighborhood. Kevin stated that he didn't feel distressed or scared after the offense, and felt that he had "not really harmed" the victim. Kevin denied committing any other sexual crimes, described this offense as impulsive, and claimed he did not burglarize the house with the intention of raping. He initially agreed to submit to a penile plethysmograph as part of this assessment, but when he arrived at the testing room he refused. He also refused to admit any deviant sexual problems or any sexual motivation for the rape.

Kevin's PCL:YV total score was very high, indicating that he exhibited many psychopathic traits. Among institutionalized male offenders, he scored at the 84th percentile, meaning that 84% of other male offenders would receive a score similar to or lower than his score. Among male probationers, he would score at the 94th percentile, indicating that he had more psychopathic features than most offenders in such a setting. Kevin also had elevated factor scores, relative to other institutionalized male offenders. He had many of the interpersonal characteristics in Factor 1 (86th percentile), and many of the affective characteristics in Factor 2 (84th percentile). His score on the behavioral factor (Factor 3) was at the 70th percentile, and his score on the antisocial factor (Factor 4) was at the 66th percentile. Overall, Kevin's score on the PCL:YV was within the range associated with institutional adjustment problems, treatment noncompliance, and increased risk of future violence. The evaluator recommended that Kevin attend both a program for violent offenders and a high-intensity cognitive-behavioral program for sexual offenders.

REFERENCES

Andershed, H. A., Gustafson, S. B., Kerr, M., & Stattin, H. (2002). The usefulness of self-reported psychopathy-like traits in the study of antisocial behaviour among non-referred adolescents. *European Journal of Personality, 16,* 383–402.

Block, J. (1993). Studying personality the long way. In D. Funder, R. Parke, C. Tomlinson-Keasy, & K. Widaman (Eds.), *Studying lives through time: Personality and development* (pp. 9–41). Washington, DC: American Psychological Association.

Brandt, J. R., Kennedy, W. A., Patrick, C. J., & Curtin, J. J. (1997). Assessment of psychopathy in a population of incarcerated adolescent offenders. *Psychological Assessment, 9,* 429–435.

Campbell, M. A., Porter, S., & Santor, D. (2004). Psychopathic traits in adolescent offenders: An evaluation of criminal history, clinical, and psychosocial correlates. *Behavioral Sciences and the Law, 22,* 23–47.

Caputo, A. A., Frick, P. J., & Brodsky, S. L. (1999). Family violence and juvenile sex offending: Potential mediating roles of psychopathic traits and negative attitudes toward women. *Criminal Justice and Behavior, 26,* 338–356.

Caspi, A., Harrington, H., Milne, B., Amell, J. W., Theodore, R. F., & Moffitt, T. E. (2003). Children's behavioral styles at age 3 are linked to their adult personality traits at age 26. *Journal of Personality, 71,* 495–513.

Catchpole, R. E. H., & Gretton, H. M. (2003). The predictive validity of risk assessment with violent young offenders: A 1-year examination of criminal outcome. *Criminal Justice and Behavior, 30,* 688–708.

Corrado, R. R., Vincent, G. M., Hart, S. D., & Cohen, I. M. (2004). Predictive validity of the Psychopathy Checklist: Youth Version for general and violent recidivism. *Behavioral Sciences and the Law, 22,* 5–22.

Crawford, T. N., Cohen, P., & Brook, J. S. (2001). Dramatic–erratic personality disorder symptoms: I. Continuity from early adolescence into adulthood. *Journal of Personality Disorders, 15,* 319–335.

Cruise, K. R., Colwell, L. H., Lyons, P. M., & Baker, M. D. (2003). Prototypical analysis of adolescent psychopathy: Investigating the juvenile justice perspective. *Behavioral Sciences and the Law, 21,* 829–846.

Edens, J. F., Guy, L. S., & Fernandez, K. (2003). Psychopathic traits predict attitudes toward a juvenile capital murderer. *Behavioral Sciences and the Law, 21,* 807–828.

Edens, J. F., Skeem, J. L., Cruise, K. R., & Cauffman, E. (2001). Assessment of "juvenile psychopathy" and its association with violence: A critical review. *Behavioral Sciences and the Law, 19,* 53–80.

Forth, A. E., Hart, S. D., & Hare, R. D. (1990). Assessment of psychopathy in male young offenders. *Psychological Assessment: A Journal of Consulting and Clinical Psychology, 2,* 342–344.

Forth, A. E., Kosson, D. S., & Hare, R. D. (2003). *The Hare Psychopathy Checklist: Youth Version.* Toronto: Multi-Health Systems.

Forth, A. E., & Mailloux, D. L. (2000). Psychopathy in youth: What do we know? In C. B. Gacono (Ed.), *The clinical and forensic assessment of psychopathy: A practitioner's guide* (pp. 25–54). Mahwah, NJ: Erlbaum.

Frick, P. J., & Hare, R. D. (2001). *The Antisocial Process Screening Device.* Toronto: Multi-Health Systems.

Fulero, S. M. (1995). Review of the Hare Psychopathy Checklist—Revised. In J. C. Conoley & J. C. Impara (Eds.), *Twelfth mental measurements yearbook* (pp. 453–454). Lincoln, NE: Buros Institute.

Gretton, H. M., Hare, R. D., & Catchpole, R. E. H. (2004). Psychopathy and offending from adolescence to adulthood: A ten year follow-up. *Journal of Consulting and Clinical Psychology, 72,* 636–645.

Gretton, H., McBride, M., Hare, R. D., O'Shaughnessy, R., & Kumka, G. (2001). Psychopathy and recidivism in adolescent sex offenders. *Criminal Justice and Behavior, 28,* 427–449.

Hare, R. D. (2003). *The Hare Psychopathy Checklist—Revised* (2nd ed.). Toronto: Multi-Health Systems.

Hare, R. D., Clark, D., Grann, M., & Thornton, D. (2000). Psychopathy and the predictive validity of the PCL-R: An international perspective. *Behavioral Sciences and the Law, 18,* 623–645.

Hemphill, J. F., Hare, R. D., & Wong, S. (1998). Psychopathy and recidivism: A review. *Legal and Criminological Psychology, 3,* 139–170.

Johnstone, L., & Cooke, D. J. (2004). Psychopathic-like traits in childhood: Conceptual and measurement concerns. *Behavioral Sciences and the Law, 22*, 103–125.

Kosson, D. S., Cyterski, T. D., Steuerwald, B. L., Neumann, C. S., & Walker-Matthews, S. (2002). Reliability and validity of the Psychopathy Checklist: Youth Version (PCL:YV) in nonincarcerated adolescent males. *Psychological Assessment, 14*, 97–109.

Lee, Z., Vincent, G. M., Hart, S. D., & Corrado, R. R. (2003). The validity of the Antisocial Process Screening Device as a self-report measures of psychopathy in adolescent offenders. *Behavioral Sciences and the Law, 21*, 771–786.

Lynam, D. R. (1997). Pursuing the psychopath: Capturing the fledgling psychopath in a nomological net. *Journal of Abnormal Psychology, 106*, 425–438.

Lynam, D. R. (2002). Fledgling psychopathy: A view from personality theory. *Law and Human Behavior, 26*, 255–269.

Mailloux, D. L., Forth, A. E., & Kroner, D. G. (1997). Psychopathy and substance use in adolescent male offenders. *Psychological Reports, 81*, 529–530.

Marczyk, G. R., Heilbrun, K., Lander, T., & DeMatteo, D. (2003). Predicting juvenile recidivism with the PCL:YV, MAYSI, and YLS/CMI. *International Journal of Forensic Mental Health, 2*, 7–18.

McCrae, R. R., Costa, P. T., Terracciano, A., Parker, W. D., Mills, C. J., De Fruyt, F., & Mervielde, I. (2002). Personality trait development from age 12 to age 18: Longitudinal, cross-sectional and cross-cultural analyses. *Journal of Personality and Social Psychology, 83*, 1456–1468.

Millon, T. (1993). *The Millon Adolescent Clinical Inventory (MACI)*. Minneapolis, MN: National Computer Systems Assessments.

Murrie, D. C., & Cornell, D. G. (2000). The Millon Adolescent Clinical Inventory and psychopathy. *Journal of Personality Assessment, 75*, 110–125.

Murrie, D. C., & Cornell, D. G. (2002). Psychopathy screening of incarcerated juveniles: A comparison of measures. *Psychological Assessment, 14*, 390–396.

Murrie, D. C., Cornell, D. G., Kaplan, S., McConville, D., & Levy-Elkon, A. (2004). Psychopathy scores and violence among juvenile offenders: A multi-measure study. *Behavioral Sciences and the Law, 22*, 49–67.

Myers, W. C., Burket, R. C., & Harris, H. E. (1995). Adolescent psychopathy in relation to delinquent behaviors, conduct disorder, and personality disorders. *Journal of Forensic Sciences, 40*, 436–440.

O'Neill, M. L., Lidz, V., & Heilbrun, K. (2003a). Adolescents with psychopathic characteristics in a substance abusing cohort: Treatment process and outcomes. *Law and Human Behavior, 27*, 299–313.

O'Neill, M. L., Lidz, V., & Heilbrun, K. (2003b). Predictors and correlates of psychopathic characteristics in substance abusing adolescents. *International Journal of Forensic Mental Health, 2*, 35–46.

Rice, M. E., Harris, G. T., & Cormier, C. A. (1992). An evaluation of a maximum security therapeutic community for psychopaths and other mentally disordered offenders. *Law and Human Behavior, 16*, 399–412.

Richards, H. J., Casey, J. O., & Lucente, S. W. (2003). Psychopathy and treatment response in incarcerated female substance abusers. *Criminal Justice and Behavior, 30*, 251–276.

Rogers, R., Vitacco, M. J., Jackson, R. L., Martin, M., Collins, M., & Sewell, K. W. (2002). Faking psychopathy?: An examination of response styles with antisocial youth. *Journal of Personality Assessment, 78*, 31–46.

Salekin, R. T., Neumann, C. S., Leistico, A. R., DiCicco, T., & Duros, R. L. (2004). Construct validity of the psychopathy in a young offender sample: Taking a closer look at psychopathy's potential importance over disruptive behavior disorders. *Journal of Abnormal Psychology, 113,* 416–427.

Salekin, R. T., Rogers, R., & Machin, D. (2001). Psychopathy in youth: Pursuing diagnostic clarity. *Journal of Youth and Adolescence, 30,* 173–194.

Saltaris, C. (2002). Psychopathy in juvenile offenders: Can temperament and attachment be considered as robust developmental precursors? *Clinical Psychology Review, 22,* 729–752.

Seagrave, D., & Grisso, T. (2002). Adolescent development and the measurement of juvenile psychopathy. *Law and Human Behavior, 26,* 219–239.

Selzer, M. L. (1971). The Michigan Alcoholism Screening Test: The quest for a new diagnostic instrument. *American Journal of Psychiatry, 127,* 1653–1658.

Seto, M. C., & Barbaree, H. E. (1999). Psychopathy, treatment behavior, and sex offenders recidivism. *Journal of Interpersonal Violence, 14,* 1235–1248.

Skeem, J. L., & Cauffman, E. (2003). View of the downward extension: Comparing the Youth Version of the Psychopathy Checklist with the Youth Psychopathic Traits Inventory. *Behavioral Sciences and the Law, 21,* 737–770.

Skinner, H. (1982). The Drug Abuse Screening Test. *Addictive Behavior, 7,* 363–371.

Spain, S. E., Douglas, K. S., Poythress, N. G., & Epstein, M. (2004). The relationship between psychopathic features, violence, and treatment outcome: The comparison of three youth measures of psychopathic features. *Behavioral Sciences and the Law, 22,* 85–102.

Vincent, G. M., Vitacco, M. J., Grisso, T., & Corrado, R. R. (2003). Subtypes of adolescent offenders: Affective traits and antisocial behavior patterns. *Behavioral Sciences and the Law, 21,* 695–712.

PART VI

Forensic Assessment Tools

The tools reviewed in Part V have been described as used often in treatment and placement planning for delinquent youths. Sometimes, however, they are used to assist courts in addressing specific legal questions. For example, if high risk of future violence is required as a matter of law for transfer (waiver) of a youth to criminal court, risk-of-violence instruments may be used to address this "forensic" question ("forensic" means that it addresses a specific legal criterion).

In Part VI, we review some instruments that were developed specifically as forensic assessment instruments to address legal questions in the adjudication process. In contrast to the instruments reviewed in Part V, these are far less often used to develop treatment plans. Instead, they are designed to address other questions in the justice system's adjudication process. We say "the justice system" as opposed to "the juvenile justice system," because one of the following chapters describes an instrument that was not originally designed for juveniles but has received some study with adolescents, and a second was designed for both juveniles and adults. Their uses and relevant research are limited, relative to those of most other tools included in this book. Therefore, these two chapters contain some commentary on cautions and limitations.

Each tool in this part should be applied only in unique circumstances where juvenile courts order these evaluations. Thus, like the instruments for assessing risk of violence/recidivism covered in Part V, each of the following instruments requires some form of comprehensive data collection—either collateral information and examinee interviews or specialized testing—by a qualified clinician or specialized mental health professional. Unlike others in this book, these instruments will not be applied or adopted routinely, because their applications are less dependent on entry points of the juvenile justice system. Finally, each chapter begins with a review of the statute or case law that directly relates to the legal question under consideration.

Salekin and colleagues describe the Risk–Sophistication–Treatment Inventory (RSTI) in Chapter 21. The RSTI was created to assist juvenile courts with juvenile courts with decisions related to the transfer or waiver of juveniles for adjudication in adult courts. As we have discussed in Chapter 3, the issues of amenability to rehabilitation within the juvenile justice system and danger to the community are at the heart of these decisions. The RSTI guides comprehensive assessments and clinical ratings in these areas for youths ages 9–18.

In Chapter 22, Goldstein, Condie, and Kalbeitzer review the Instruments for Assessing Understanding and Appreciation of *Miranda* Rights and their revision, the *Miranda* Rights Comprehension Instruments–II (MRCI-II), designed to evaluate issues related to due process. These instruments evaluate the potential interference of mental illnesses and developmental difficulties on misunderstandings of *Miranda* rights that may lead to uninformed or nonconsensual waivers of rights (and sometimes confessions) during police questioning.

Finally, Woolard and Harvell describe issues related to assessments of juveniles' competence to stand trial (see Chapter 3) in Chapter 23. This chapter is a significant departure from others in this handbook. There are no screening or assessment instruments available for assessing adjudicative competence in juvenile populations. Therefore, Woolard and Harvell describe the MacArthur Competence Assessment Tool—Criminal Adjudication (MacCAT-CA), an adult assessment tool, and review research illustrating the potential for its use with adolescents. Due to the limited state of instruments in this area, Chapter 23 reviews the complexities and developmental complications inherent in juvenile adjudicative competence evaluations, and it concludes with clinical recommendations rather than a case example.

CHAPTER 21

Risk–Sophistication–
Treatment Inventory

Randall T. Salekin
Karen L. Salekin
Carl B. Clements
Anne-Marie R. Leistico

PURPOSE

The Office of Juvenile Justice and Delinquency Prevention (2002) suggests that at least 2,369,400 juveniles are arrested per year. But not all of these youths will be long-term offenders. Delinquency in some cases is an extreme form of typical adolescent development that is transient in nature, but in other cases it is a steppingstone to more serious and chronic offending. For instance, Loeber (1991) and Moffitt (2003) have provided evidence that antisocial behavior occurs in a step-like fashion, with early onset and frequency being two factors that account for escalating levels of delinquency.

Because young offenders are a diverse group (e.g., Loeber, 1991; Moffitt, 1993; Teplin, Abram, McClelland, Dulcan, & Mericle, 2002), mental health professionals and legal decision makers are frequently faced with difficulties in distinguishing youths whose delinquent/antisocial behaviors pose a potential danger to society from youths who are malleable to treatment interventions. In addition, questions occasionally arise in the juvenile justice system as to whether youths are best managed in rehabilitation-focused programming or crime-control-focused systems. As a result, decision makers within the legal system often grapple over the level of treatment that certain juvenile offenders require—and, in more severe cases, questions about whether the youths can be dealt with in the juvenile system or must be referred to the adult criminal justice system (Grisso, 1998; Grisso, Tomkins, & Casey, 1986; Leistico &

Salekin, 2003; Melton, Petrila, Poythress, & Slobogin, 1997). Although these questions are always asked in cases involving possible transfer to criminal court, they also underlie many "dispositional" cases (i.e., cases in which the court must decide on placement within the juvenile justice system).

At the heart of many forensic evaluations of these types are questions about risk for dangerousness, sophistication–maturity, and treatment amenability. These constructs were first delineated in the U.S. Supreme Court case of *Kent v. United States* (1966), and they are frequently cited in the juvenile transfer literature (e.g., Grisso, 1998; Salekin, 2001). However, the concepts appear applicable to a broader range of dispositional cases, in which they might facilitate clinical and legal decisions.

Kruh and Brodsky (1997) reviewed the empirical status of various assessment tools and psychological constructs used to evaluate the factors of risk for dangerousness, sophistication, and treatment amenability. These authors provided useful guidelines for assessment, but also called for the development of empirically supported, standardized assessment tools, because they concluded that the clinical and legal applications of these constructs were underdeveloped. Although these guidelines (see also those of Ewing, 1990) have been of clear value, it is difficult to address questions of dangerousness, sophistication–maturity, and treatment amenability in the absence of assessment technology designed specifically for the measurement of these constructs.

The Risk–Sophistication–Treatment Inventory (RST-I; Salekin, 2004) was designed to meet the specific needs of mental health professionals who provide dispositional and transfer assessments for the juvenile courts. The RST-I addresses the three important psychological constructs mentioned above,—namely, (1) a juvenile's level of *dangerousness*, (2) the youth's level of *maturity or sophistication*, and (3) the degree to which the youth is *amenable to treatment*. It provides a focused assessment by producing ratings that offer a basis for nuanced descriptions of the complex prongs delineated in the *Kent* decision that inform court placement and treatment decisions. The RST-I can be used prior to disposition decisions or to assist with legal decisions about treatment and design of individualized treatment plans.

BASIC DESCRIPTION

The RST-I is a semistructured interview (60–90 minutes) and rating scale designed to help clinicians assess juvenile offenders (ages 9–18 years) in three important areas. First, "risk for dangerousness" refers to the likelihood of committing future acts of violence or recidivism. Second, "sophistication–maturity" refers to emotional and cognitive maturity. Finally, "treatment amenability" refers to the likelihood of being responsive to treatment.

The RST-I measures these areas with three scales composed of 15 items each. Items are rated on 3-point scales (0 = "absence of the characteristic/ability," 1 = "subclinical/moderate," 2 = "presence of the characteristic/ability"), which reflect the extent to which the individual demonstrates the specific characteristic or ability. Each scale contains three subscales, referred to as "clusters." The Risk for Dangerousness scale comprises the Violent and Aggressive Tendencies (R-VAT), Planned and Extensive Criminality (R PEX), and Psychopathic Features (R-PPF) clusters. The clusters of the Sophistication–Maturity scale are Autonomy (S-AUT), Cognitive Capacities (S-COG), and Emotional Maturity (S-EMO). The Sophistication–Maturity scale is neither prosocial nor antisocial. It measures maturity broadly, while also allowing clinicians to rate the extent to which the related emotional/cognitive skills are used for criminological purposes, and the degree to which the criminological lifestyle has become ingrained. Finally, the Treatment Amenability clusters are Psychopathology—Degree and Type (T-PAT), Responsibility and Motivation to Change (T-RES), and Consideration and Tolerance of Others (T-CAT). Table 21.1 lists the items for each RST-I scale and cluster.

The RST-I materials include the *Professional Manual*, the semistructured Interview Booklet, and the Rating Form. The Interview Booklet contains queries designed to obtain background, clinical, and historical information, as well as a sample of the juvenile's behavioral and psychological functioning. Items on the rating form reflect information central to the three scales. Scoring of items involves reviewing and synthesizing information from an interview and collateral sources (e.g., school, police, detention, and previous treatment records, and consultations with parents or guardians). Proper administration and coding of the RST-I require considerable professional knowledge, skill, and experience with juvenile offenders. Scores are derived for each subscale and scale by a simple sum of the items.

Raw scores on each cluster are compared to a norm sample of juvenile offenders to establish the descriptive categories of "low," "medium," or "high." Data for the RST-I standardized sample represent young offenders (ages 9–18 years) from a variety of juvenile justice facilities and settings, including both detained and nondetained youths, and juveniles transferred to adult court. Normative data are provided by gender in the appendices of the *Professional Manual* to convert raw scale scores to percentile ranges or *T*-scores. Approximately two-thirds of individuals in juvenile justice settings will obtain *T*-scores between 41 and 59 on any of the RST-I scales. This *T*-score should be considered typical or "middle range." *T*-scores above 70 or below 30 occur in approximately 1% to 3% of the normative juvenile justice sample. Table 21.2 illustrates the meaning of scores on each scale's clusters by providing clinical descriptions of hypothetical youths scoring within the high offender range. The *Professional Manual* provides detailed information regarding the reliability and validity of the instrument, and also includes six case studies that provide examples of appropriate interpretation of the results.

TABLE 21.1. Items for the RST-I Scales and Clusters

Risk for Dangerousness

Violent and Aggressive Tendencies (R-VAT)
Engage in unprovoked violent behavior
Violence toward individuals
Violence toward animals
Easily angered and physically aggressive
Generally oppositional and cruel

Planned and Extensive Criminality (R-PEX)
Severe antisocial behavior
Premeditated crimes
Leadership role in crimes
Frequency of past criminal acts
Age of onset of antisocial behavior
Delinquent peer group

Psychopathic Features (R-PPF)
Lacks remorse
Lacks empathy
Egocentricity
Manipulative

Sophistication–Maturity

Autonomy (S-AUT)
Autonomy
Internal locus of control
Development of self-concept
Self-reflection

Cognitive Capacities (S-COG)
Aware of wrongfulness of crimes
Understanding of behavioral norms
Able to identify alternative actions
Foresight (has future time perspective)
Cost–benefit analysis in decision making
Ability to anticipate consequences

Emotional Maturity (S-EMO)
Able to delay gratification
Moral development
Self-regulation of emotion
Conflict resolution
Interpersonal skills

(continued)

TABLE 21.1. *(continued)*

Treatment Amenability

    Psychopathology—Degree and Type (T-PAT)
      Degree of psychopathology
      Treatability of psychopathology
      Aware of difficulties and problems
      Insight into cause of problems
      Limited police/court/probation involvement

    Responsibility and Motivation to Change (T-RES)
      Motivated to engage in treatment
      Takes responsibility for actions
      Open to change
      Expects change
      Positive involvement by parents

    Consideration and Tolerance of Others (T-CAT)
      Anxiety about the circumstance
      Feels guilt/remorse
      Considers and generally cares about others
      Has protective factors
      Has positive attachments

HISTORY OF THE METHOD'S DEVELOPMENT

Salekin (2004) developed the RST-I according to the scale construction procedures outlined by Anastasi (1998), Clark and Watson (1995), and others (Floyd & Widaman, 1995; Foster & Cone, 1995; Haynes, Richard, & Kubany, 1995). This involved three primary steps. First, items were generated to operationalize risk for dangerousness, sophistication–maturity, and treatment amenability. This process entailed an extensive search for items in both case law and the psychological literature (e.g., Griffin, 2000; Griffin, Torbet, & Szymanski, 1998; Grisso et al., 1986; Heilbrun, Leheny, Thomas, & Huneycutt, 1997; Sanborn, 1994). Descriptions of juveniles and their families were drawn from three main sources: (1) relevant statutes pertaining to transfer criteria, (2) appellate cases (both successful and unsuccessful), and (3) research (both psychological studies and law reviews) related to the primary constructs and to transfer decisions. Two psychologists and six doctoral students evaluated the resulting pool of items for redundancy and lack of relevance.

    The second step involved two separate prototypical analyses. Salekin and his colleagues solicited expert ratings from 75 forensic diplomates, 240 child and adolescent clinicians, and 430 juvenile court judges. Clinical child and adolescent psychologists were asked to rate the items they considered to be

TABLE 21.2. Interpretation of the RST-I Scales

Cluster	Description of individuals in the high offender range

Risk for Dangerousness (R) clusters

Violent and Aggressive Tendencies (R-VAT)	These individuals have an extensive history of violence and have shown that they are easily angered and prone to use physical aggression. They tend to be frequently aggressive, and their violence can appear unprovoked. They also may brag about their involvement in violent acts and may have a history of cruelty to animals.
Planned and Extensive Criminality (R-PEX)	These individuals have extensive criminal histories and demonstrate a leadership role in their crimes. These individuals typically start offending at a young age, and their criminal behavior is frequent and severe. Their crimes tend to be premeditated, and they also may have a delinquent peer group.
Psychopathic Features (R-PPF)	These individuals are egocentric, manipulative, and deceptive. They also tend to lack remorse for their actions and typically do not feel guilt for their reckless and antisocial acts. If they express remorse, it is often short-lived. They tend to have little regard for the opinions of others or for society in general. Such individuals also tend to place little importance on the roles of their parents/guardians, on the law, or on being a law-abiding citizen.

Sophistication–Maturity (S) clusters

Autonomy (S-AUT)	These individuals have started to develop a good sense of who they are, and have a good command of their willpower. They view themselves as in control of their own lives, are conscious of their ability to take independent action, and exercise their ability with confidence. They increasingly tend to do things their own way, and take comfort in knowing that they can make their own decisions. They are also able to maintain their convictions, even in the face of criticism. These individuals feel comfortable in their sense of self-control and have developed a self-concept. They also may demonstrate a sense of purpose and a vision of what they want in life.
Cognitive Capacities (S-COG)	These individuals have the capacity to make decisions with sound judgment. That is, they have relatively good foresight; they tend to weigh, to a reasonable degree, the costs and benefits of given behaviors before acting; and they can distinguish right from wrong. Although judgment is never perfect for any of us, these individuals tend to have the abilities necessary to arrive at reasonably good judgments most of the time.
Emotional Maturity (S-EMO)	These individuals are aware of their emotions and have some reasonable understanding of the emotions of others. Moreover, they are capable of managing and regulating emotions in order to attain important goals. They are reasonably clear about their values and are morally mature.

(continued)

TABLE 21.2. *(continued)*

Cluster	Description of individuals in the high offender range
Treatment Amenability (T) clusters	
Psychopathology— Degree and Type (T-PAT)	These individuals have a low degree of psychopathology, and their type of psychopathology is not particularly difficult to treat. They may have symptoms of a disorder but do not fully meet the criteria for a formal diagnosis, or they may meet the criteria for a diagnosis but the symptoms overall are not marked. For example, the individual may have conduct disorder, but the symptoms are not severe or they do not fully meet the criteria for a diagnosis. Similarly, the individual may show psychopathic features, but the features are not marked and the criminal lifestyle does not appear to be ingrained.
Responsibility and Motivation to Change (T-RES)	These individuals acknowledge major difficulties in their functioning and perceive an acute need for help in dealing with these problems. They also have a positive attitude toward the possibility of personal change. In addition, these individuals accept the importance of personal responsibility. These individuals generally have significant motivation to enter into psychotherapy, and they believe that psychotherapy is likely to have a positive effect.
Consideration and Tolerance of Others (T-CAT)	These individuals are considerate and tolerant of others. They feel guilt and remorse regarding negative events they caused in the past. They experience anxiety about their current circumstance and/or about past events. They have demonstrated prosocial maturity in the past through considerate and thoughtful behaviors/actions for others.

central to dangerousness, sophistication–maturity, and treatment amenability. Forensic diplomates were asked to provide ratings of juveniles they had evaluated who had subsequently been transferred to adult criminal courts. Next, in order to expand the perspective on these constructs, judges from the National Council of Juvenile and Family Court Judges were asked to rate core characteristics for the three loosely defined concepts, as well as the underlying dimensions of these constructs. Prototypical items for each of the constructs aligned across the raters, indicating that there was general agreement regarding the central components of risk for dangerousness, sophistication–maturity, and treatment amenability (Salekin, Rogers, & Ustad, 2001; Salekin, Yff, Neumann, Leistico, & Zalot, 2002).

The final step involved both exploratory factor analysis (EFA) and confirmatory factor analysis (CFA) of the prototypical ratings. CFA results formed the basis for the development of the RST-I scales. Assignment of items to specific scales relied heavily on consideration of prototypical ratings and factor structures. Items with low prototypical ratings were not included on scales, even though they might have loaded on a factor. For example, the instrument did not include reckless and hyperactive characteristics, although they loaded onto one of the original factors that constituted dangerousness, because such characteristics received low prototypical ratings. Highly prototypical items should be most indicative of dangerous activity. In addition, CFA results revealed that inclusion of these items did not result in good model fit. Once expert ratings were obtained and analyses were completed, the interview and rating scale were developed and refined. Data collection with the RST-I began shortly thereafter, resulting in the studies described below, and eventually in the normative sample and calculation of percentile ranks and T-scores by gender.

RESEARCH EVIDENCE

This section reports findings from the normative sample, including studies that sampled youths from a variety of juvenile justice settings. Salekin conducted two studies using interview and file-based RST-I scores—one with 131 preadjudicated juveniles receiving court evaluations in an assessment unit (Salekin, 1998), and another using 222 juveniles in a pretrial detention facility (Salekin, 2002). Leistico (2002; Leistico & Salekin, 2003) conducted a retrospective file review of 130 juvenile offenders (some with adult charges) referred from correctional boys' schools to Mendota Juvenile Treatment Center, Madison, Wisconsin, because of behavioral problems. Finally, Zalot (2002a, 2002b) completed file-based RST-I ratings on a sample of 145 juvenile offenders at the Taylor Hardin Secure Medical Facility in Tuscaloosa, Alabama, for transfer to adult court evaluations.

Internal Consistency and Reliability

As reported in the manual (Salekin, 2004), alpha coefficients for the three RST-I factors produced from the combined normative sample ($N = 640$) ranged from .78 to .83. There were no substantive differences in internal consistency on the basis of race (i.e., black, white, nonwhite Hispanic, and Asian), gender, or age. Item–total correlations ranged from .20 to .68 for the various scales.

With regard to interrater reliability, intraclass correlations (ICCs) for the RST-I scales ranged from .74 to .94, indicating good agreement (Salekin, 2004) across types of raters and scoring methods. Specifically, two studies of serious delinquents tested agreement between graduate student raters on file-based ratings. Zalot (2002a, 2002b) found interrater ICCs of .84, .73, and .83, and Leistico (2002) found ICCs of .94, .74, and .91, on the Risk of Dangerousness, Sophistication–Maturity, and Treatment Amenability scales, respectively. Comparing interview-based RST-I ratings between clinicians and trained graduate student raters (Salekin, 1998, 2002) resulted in slightly higher reliability, ranging from .81 to .94; this indicates that interviews may increase the reliability of ratings.

Validity

The normative sample was used to examine differences in the distribution of scores by gender and race. Analyses with the sufficient proportion of girls in the normative sample demonstrated significant gender differences. To account for this difference, the manual reports separate norms for girls and boys, allowing examiners to calculate percentile ranks and T-scores for girls separately. In general, scores did not differ according to examinees' race, but more studies are needed in this area.

Several studies have reported evidence for the RST-I's concurrent validity, using other measures of psychological constructs to which the RST-I constructs should be related (Leistico & Salekin, 2003; Salekin, 2000; Zalot, 2002a, 2002b). The RST-I Risk for Dangerousness scale appears to correlate positively with conduct disorder (CD), violent CD, psychopathic traits (as measured by the Hare Psychopathy Checklist: Youth Version; Forth, Kosson, & Hare, 2003), and both reactive and total aggression. The Treatment Amenability scale was associated with older ages at onset of CD and negatively associated with CD symptoms.

The RST-I also appears to correlate in meaningful ways with personality inventories. Specifically, when the five-factor model of personality was examined via the Interpersonal Adjectives Scale—Revised—Big 5 Version (IASR-B5; Trapnell & Wiggins, 1990), Dangerousness significantly correlated positively with Dominance, but negatively with Nurturance and Conscientiousness. In addition, when IASR-B5 scales based on the interpersonal circumplex personality model were used, Dangerousness correlated most highly with the Cold-Hearted, Assured–Dominant, and Arrogant–Calculating octants.

Two studies (Salekin, 2000; Zalot, 2002) indicated that the Sophistication–Maturity scale was positively and significantly related to both traditionally defined intelligence, as measured by the Kaufman Brief Intelligence Test (Kaufman & Kaufman, 1990), and contemporary theories of intelligence, as measured by the Bar-On Emotional Quotient Inventory: Youth Version (Bar-On & Parker, 2000) and the Sternberg Triarchic Abilities Test (Sternberg, 1993). The Treatment Amenability scale correlated positively with the Nurturance and Neuroticism personality factors, and negatively with the Cold-Hearted octant of the IASR-B5.

Researchers have also tested the criterion-related validity of the RST-I scales. With respect to treatment amenability, it is important to note that there are relatively few empirical data to suggest which factors may be related to either excellent or poor treatment outcomes. Nevertheless, theory can suggest factors that should be related to treatment prognosis and that may help to test (and perhaps bolster) the validity of the Treatment Amenability scale. Leistico and Salekin (2003) examined the criterion validity of the Treatment Amenability scale by testing the association between file-based RST-I ratings and later treatment compliance and other criteria among male juveniles at the Mendota Juvenile Treatment Center. They found that the scale was associated

with positive interactions with staff and maintenance of appropriate boundaries, both of which are important to the therapeutic relationship. Alternatively, the Risk for Dangerousness scale was negatively associated with maintenance of appropriate boundaries, and the Sophistication–Maturity scale was
associated with excellent classroom behaviors.

Finally, two studies of youths facing transfer to adult court tested criterion validity by measuring outcomes retrospectively (Leistico & Salekin,
2003; Zalot, 2002a, 2002b). As predicted, relative to nontransferred youths,
transferred youths received significantly higher average Risk for Dangerousness and Sophistication–Maturity scores, and significantly lower average
Treatment Amenability scores. In Zalot's retrospective study, a computer-
based tracking system was used to record transfer decisions following RST-I
ratings, and findings indicated that the RST-I "postdicted" decisions. With
respect to criminal activity, other data sets demonstrated that the Risk for
Dangerousness scale was related to previous criminal involvement and was
predictive of future criminal involvement 3 years after RST-I assessments (see
Salekin, 2004).

APPLICATION

The RST-I manual (Salekin, 2004) is available from Psychological Assessment
Resources. The RST-I is copyrighted and can be purchased as a kit, which
includes the manual, 25 semistructured Interview Booklets, and 25 Rating
forms. Mental health professionals with experience in juvenile justice settings
can administer the RST-I. Ideally, a mental health professional examiner
should be trained in structured interviewing, and should have some knowledge of juvenile offenders, adolescent development, and forensic psychology
as it is applied to children and adolescents.

The RST-I can be administered in court evaluation units, in detention
centers, and by consulting clinicians in outpatient settings. As mentioned previously, the RST-I can be used in evaluations related to recommendations for
disposition decisions, hearings concerning transfer to adult court and reverse
transfer, treatment recommendations, and development of individualized
treatment plans. The RST-I should not be the sole measure utilized in evaluations related to legal decisions; rather, forensic assessments should incorporate
a battery of measures (including standard intelligence tests, measures of child
and adolescent psychopathology, and other tools). The RST-I's scoring design
allows for systematic follow-up regarding recidivism, treatment compliance,
and other outcome indicators.

Although the RST-I has a normative sample, it intentionally does not provide, or suggest, cutoff scores that would dictate or exclude a particular disposition for a given youth. It is necessary for mental health professionals to use
scores in conjunction with their clinical acumen to arrive at decisions regarding youths' levels of dangerousness, maturity, and treatment amenability.

Examiners are encouraged to consider contextual factors, for example, not only when scoring the RST-I items, but also when interpreting scale scores within the broader clinical context. For instance, as a result of their predominant environment, youths may lead a lifestyle that relies on dangerous behaviors for survival. The RST-I interview allows clinicians to obtain this information, which should be brought to light in the context of evaluations and testimony.

In alpha and beta testing of the RST-I, benefits often mentioned include its ability to provide examiners and legal professionals with a systematic approach to gathering information on meaningful and pertinent constructs for dispositional and transfer-related decision making. The constructs assessed via the RST-I are not readily assessed in other psychological measures. This is especially true for the sophistication–maturity and treatment amenability constructs. Surveys of clinicians also indicate that they generally appreciate the RST-I's comprehensive approach, easily administered structured interview, and user-friendly scoring format.

The RST-I has some limitations and potential misuses. First, there is limited information about its use with child offenders below the age of 11 and with youths of Asian descent. Second, although the RST-I was designed within a specific psycholegal context, its resulting scores should not trigger specific decisions per se. Only clinicians with the proper qualifications, as outlined in the manual, should administer the RST-I. Proper administration requires a semistructured interview and gathering of data from collateral sources to ensure accurate ratings. Clinicians should not take shortcuts. All evidence, both confirming and disconfirming, should be examined before arriving at decisions about any particular rating. Finally, the RST-I is not a thorough assessment of mental health problems; as such, it should not be utilized as the sole measure for differential psychiatric diagnoses.

CASE EXAMPLE

Timothy Kaine, a juvenile probation officer, referred 16-year-old Tommy Jackson for a psychological evaluation to assist the court in the formulation of treatment needs and assess the presence of psychological disorders. Tommy's current evaluation was initiated as the result of his most recent involvement with the judicial system, concerns regarding his risk for future offending (particularly violent offending), and questions about his need for treatment. Information for this assessment was obtained via interview and psychological testing of Tommy, consultation with collateral sources, and review of file information provided to the examiner by the court.

Tommy was currently charged with use/possession of drug paraphernalia. This arrest resulted from an incident in which John Rainer, Tommy's stepfather, contacted the police in relation to Tommy's verbally abusive behavior toward him and consistent pattern of disrespect and disobedience in the home.

According to the incident/offense report, Mr. Rainer stated that he could no longer control the behavior of his stepson, and that he was filing the report with the goal of curbing Tommy's disrespectful and threatening behavior. The police went to the Rainer home to investigate the complaint and, during their investigation, found drug paraphernalia in Tommy's bedroom. The current charge represented Tommy's fourth formal involvement with the judicial system; he had previous convictions on the charges of arson, assault, and violation of probation. Of note was that Tommy's assault charge had originated from an incident in which he and three of his friends had conspired to kill fellow classmates. The following statement is illustrative of his stated intent to follow through with the crime: "Good thing they caught me before I did it, because me and a few hundred people wouldn't be here." When asked about his involvement in illegal activities, Tommy stated that he had been involved in stealing, breaking into and entering dwellings, dealing drugs, and racing cars. He noted that he believed he was quite skilled at these activities, and bragged that he was one of only a few people who could get past home and business alarm systems.

From birth until 9 years of age, Tommy had resided with his mother, stepfather, and brother in a three-bedroom home in a middle-class neighborhood. When asked about Tommy's temperament and behavior, Mrs. Rainer stated that as a young child, her son was loving, quiet, and generally easygoing. Overtime, however, his temperament and behavior worsened—as evident by numerous instances of defiance and disrespect in multiple settings, and his history of illegal behavior (e.g., setting fire to an abandoned home, breaking into and entering homes and vehicles, stealing, and shooting at people with pellet guns). As a direct result, Tommy was sent out of state to live with his father, whom he had only had minimal contact throughout the course of his life.

Tommy's account of his life with his father suggested events that could be construed as child endangerment. According to Tommy, his father had severe alcoholism; he spent the majority of his time either drinking in bars or being intoxicated at home. Tommy also described his father as a violent individual with whom he argued and engaged in fist fights on a regular basis. Tommy further stated that he and his stepmother (also reported to have an alcohol abuse problem) argued frequently, and that he often threatened to harm her and her 5-year-old son, who also resided in the home.

A review of school records indicated that Tommy's grades and behavior during the early years of school (kindergarten through second grade) were good. In contrast, however, records from the third grade indicated that Tommy' grades fell over the course of that year. A note written by one teacher suggested that his poor grades were the direct result of his poor behavior in the classroom. Tommy completed the sixth grade and attended approximately 1 month of the seventh grade prior to his expulsion for conspiring to kill fellow classmates. Tommy's life history was therefore positive for witnessing violence in the home, frequent acts of violence toward others, and acts of violence toward himself. When discussing all events, he exhibited no distress, and in fact appeared amused by the outcome of some of these acts of violence. Tommy reported having an extensive history of using illicit drugs, which included marijuana, acid, cocaine, and Ecstasy.

With regard to mental health history, Tommy had received five diagnoses of major mental illness—specifically, attention-deficit/hyperactivity disorder, depressive disorder not otherwise specified, dysthymic disorder, impulse-control disorder not otherwise specified, and polysubstance dependence. Treatment recommendations included individual and family therapy, substance abuse treatment, residential treatment, pharmacological intervention, and enrollment in continuing education. At the time of the evaluation, Tommy was enrolled in court-ordered substance abuse rehabilitation and individual therapy. With regard to progress in treatment, his therapist described him as uninterested in change and nonresponsive to intervention. Tommy concurred with this assessment, and added that his involvement in substance abuse counseling did nothing but make him more interested in illicit substance use.

On the RST-I Risk for Dangerousness scale, Tommy's raw score was 29 (T-score = 73, 99th percentile), with scores of 10, 12, and 7 for the R-VAT, R-PEX, and R-PPF clusters, respectively. These scores reflected his extensive history of violence. Of particular concern were his exhibition of severe antisocial behavior, his premeditated crimes, and his leadership role in the commission of crimes. In addition, Tommy's attitude of superiority and flippant statements regarding criminal activity suggested that he showed little empathy for others and little remorse for his behavior.

On the RST-I Sophistication–Maturity scale, Tommy's raw score was 22 (T-score = 76, 98th percentile), with scores of 8, 10, and 4 for the S-AUT, S-COG, and S-EMO clusters, respectively. His behavior matched the sophistication–maturity description on numerous items. For example, the interview data indicated that he was high in autonomy, felt in control of his actions, used foresight, and could anticipate the consequences of his behavior. His awareness of the wrongfulness of his actions, his proactive cost–benefit analyses, and his decisions to commit crimes further elevated his score. Although Tommy demonstrated areas of emotional immaturity, for the most part he was able to regulate his emotions and delay gratification in order to commit his crimes.

On the RST-I Treatment Amenability scale, Tommy's raw score was 11 (T-score = 48, 46th percentile), with scores of 4, 4, and 3 for the T-PAT, T-RES, and T-CAT clusters, respectively. He expressed concern for himself, but little concern for society in relation to his criminal activities. Tommy did not view prior treatment attempts as having been useful, nor did he expect to make any changes in behavior or attitude via current attempts at rehabilitation. His therapist concurred with this opinion and did not hold out much hope that treatment attempts would be successful.

In closing, Tommy was a 16-year-old with multiple areas of concern. He exhibited problematic family relations; a history of violence toward others, animals, and himself; an extensive history of substance use problems; minimal attachment to others; and a long history of disrespectful and defiant behavior toward adults. Like many other individuals in the juvenile justice system, Tommy met criteria for CD, childhood-onset type, severe (determined, in part, from the results of a separate clinical instrument assessing disruptive behavior disorders). This disorder can present in a variety of different ways, but key components include frequent antisocial behavior, a tendency to violate the rights of others, failure to conform to social norms, lack of remorse, and indifference to the effects of his behavior on others. When this constellation of interpersonal, affective, and behavioral symptoms was considered in light of his history, there was concern about his potential for recidivism, both violent and nonviolent. In addition, if left unchanged, these risk factors placed Tommy at risk for academic, occupational, and interpersonal failure.

There was no indication that previous treatment attempts had been successful for Tommy, and at the time of the evaluation, he was complying with his treatment but was doing so in a mechanical and uninvolved manner. The following treatment plan was considered necessary: enrollment in general equivalency diploma classes; involvement in a mentorship model program, with the goal of developing a bond with a positive adult role model who could provide guidance and support; vocational and occupational guidance; external placement in a residential program; family counseling; and involvement in and close monitoring by the juvenile justice system.

REFERENCES

Anastasi, A. (1998). *Psychological testing* (7th ed.). Upper Saddle River, NJ: Prentice Hall.

Bar-On, R., & Parker, J. D. A. (2000). *Bar-On Emotional Quotient Inventory: Youth Version: Technical manual.* Toronto: Multi-Health Systems.

Clark, L. A., & Watson, D. (1995). Construct validity: Basic issues in objective scale development. *Psychological Assessment, 7,* 309–319.

Ewing, C. P. (1990). Juveniles or adults?: Forensic assessment of juveniles for considered for trial in criminal court. *Forensic Reports, 3,* 3–13.

Floyd, F. J., & Widaman, K. F. (1995). Factor analysis in the development and refinement of clinical assessment instruments. *Psychological Assessment, 7,* 286–299.

Forth, A. E., Kosson, D. S., & Hare, R. D. (2003). *The Hare Psychopathy Checklist: Youth Version.* Toronto: Multi-Health Systems.

Foster, S. L., & Cone, J. D. (1995). Validity issues in clinical assessment. *Psychological Assessment, 7,* 248–260.

Griffin, P. (2000). *National overviews: State juvenile justice profiles.* Pittsburgh, PA: National Center for Juvenile Justice.

Griffin, P., Torbet, P., & Szymanski, L. (1998). *Trying juveniles as adults in criminal* court: An analysis of state transfer provisions. Washington, DC: Office of Juvenile Justice and Delinquency Prevention.

Grisso, T. (1998). Forensic evaluation of juveniles. Sarasota, FL: Professional Resource Press.

Grisso, T., Tomkins, A., & Casey, P. (1986). Psychosocial concepts in juvenile law. Law and Human Behavior, 12, 403–437.

Haynes, S. N., Richard, D. C. S., & Kubany, E. S. (1995). Content validity in psychological assessment: A functional approach to concepts and methods. Psychological Assessment, 7, 238–247.

Heilbrun, K., Leheny, C., Thomas, L., & Huneycutt, D. (1997). A national survey of U.S. statutes on juvenile transfer: Implications for policy and practice. Behavioral Sciences and the Law, 15, 125–149.

Kaufman, A. S., & Kaufman, N. L. (1990). Kaufman Brief Intelligence Test (K-BIT) manual. Circle Pines, MN: American Guidance Service.

Kent v. United States, 383 U.S. 541 (1966).

Kruh, I. P., & Brodsky, S. L. (1997). Clinical evaluations for transfer of juveniles to criminal court: Current knowledge and future research. Behavioral Sciences and the Law, 15, 151–165.

Leistico, A. R. (2002). Juvenile transfer to adult court: Risk, sophistication–maturity, treatment amenability, and related constructs. Unpublished master's thesis, University of Alabama, Tuscaloosa.

Leistico, A. R., & Salekin, R. T. (2003). Testing the reliability and validity of the Risk, Sophistication–Maturity, and Treatment Amenability Inventory (RST-I): An assessment tool for juvenile offenders. International Journal of Forensic Mental Health, 2, 101–117.

Loeber, R. (1991). Antisocial behavior: More enduring than changeable? Journal of the American Academy of Child and Adolescent Psychiatry, 30, 393–397.

Melton, G. B., Petrila, J., Poythress, N. G., & Slobogin, C. (1997). Psychological evaluations for the courts: A handbook for mental health professionals and lawyers (2nd ed.). New York: Guilford Press.

Moffitt, T. E. (1993). Adolescence-limited and life-course-persistent antisocial behavior: A developmental taxonomy. Psychological Review, 100, 674–701.

Office of Juvenile Justice and Delinquency Prevention. (2002). Statistical briefing book. Retrieved http://ojjdp.ncjrs.org/ojstatbb/asp/ JAR_Display.asp?ID=qa220 1012002

Salekin, R. T. (1998). [Miami Juvenile Detention Center Project]. Unpublished raw data.

Salekin, R. T. (2000). [Tuscaloosa Juvenile Detention Center Project]. Unpublished raw data.

Salekin, R. T. (2001). Juvenile transfer to adult court: How can developmental and child psychology inform policy decision making? In B. L. Bottoms, M. B. Kovera, & B. D. McAuliff (Eds.), Children, social science, and U.S. law (pp. 203–232). New York: Cambridge University Press.

Salekin, R. T. (2002). Clinical evaluation of youth considered for transfer to adult criminal court: Refining practice and directions for science. Journal of Forensic Psychology Practice, 2, 55–72.

Salekin, R. T. (2004). Risk–Sophistication–Treatment Inventory: Professional manual. Lutz, FL: Psychological Assessment Resources.

Salekin, R. T., Rogers, R., & Ustad, K. L. (2001). Juvenile waiver to adult criminal courts: Prototypes for dangerousness, sophistication–maturity, and amenability to treatment. *Psychology, Public Policy, and Law, 7,* 381–408.

Salekin, R. T., Yff, R. M., Neumann, C., Leistico, A. R., & Zalot, A. A. (2002). Juvenile transfer to adult courts: A look at the prototypes for dangerousness, sophistication–maturity, and amenability to treatment through a legal lens. *Psychology, Public Policy, and Law, 8,* 373–410.

Sanborn, J. B., Jr. (1994). Certification to criminal court: The important policy questions of how, when, and why. *Crime and Delinquency, 40,* 262–281.

Sternberg, R. J. (1993). *Sternberg Triarchic Abilities Test, High School Level.* Unpublished manuscript.

Teplin, L., Abram, K., McClelland, G., Dulcan, M., & Mericle, A. (2002). Psychiatric disorders in youth in juvenile detention. *Archives of General Psychiatry, 59,* 1133–1143.

Trapnell, P. D., & Wiggins, J. S. (1990). Extension of the Interpersonal Adjective Scales to include the Big Five dimensions of personality. *Journal of Personality and Social Psychology, 59,* 781–790.

Zalot, A. A. (2002a). *How do dangerousness, sophistication–maturity, and amenability to treatment influence the juvenile transfer decision?* Unpublished master's thesis, University of Alabama, Tuscaloosa.

Zalot, A. A. (2002b). [Taylor Hardin Secure Medical Facility Project]. Unpublished raw data.

CHAPTER 22

Instruments for Assessing Understanding and Appreciation of *Miranda* Rights

Naomi E. Sevin Goldstein
Lois Oberlander Condie
Rachel Kalbeitzer

PURPOSE

The 1966 U.S. Supreme Court ruling *Miranda v. Arizona* (384 U.S. 436) established procedural safeguards to protect suspects from self-incrimination and police intimidation in custodial interrogations. The warnings inform suspects of their right to silence, the intent to use their statements against them in court, their right to an attorney, and their right to a court-appointed attorney if the suspects cannot afford one. A suspect may waive these rights, but the waiver is valid only if it is given knowingly, intelligently, and voluntarily. In other words, the suspect must understand the basic meaning of rights, appreciate the consequences of waiving rights, and provide the waiver without police coercion or intimidation (Grisso, 1981).

Guided by case law (see Goldstein, Condie, Kalbeitzer, Osman, & Geier, 2003; Grisso, 1998a; Oberlander & Goldstein, 2001), courts generally decide the validity of a suspect's waiver based on the *totality of the circumstances* in which the waiver was provided. Factors considered in the totality test include situational conditions of the interrogation (e.g., length of interrogation) and characteristics of the suspect (e.g., age, intelligence, prior experience with the justice system) (Grisso, 1998a). Attorneys and judges may retain forensic evaluators to provide information about these factors through assessment of personality, social development, and cognitive development, in order to decide the defendant's capacity to have provided a knowing, intelligent, and voluntary waiver of rights prior to having made a confession.

The Instruments for Assessing Understanding and Appreciation of *Miranda* Rights were initially developed as a standardized tool for researchers examining youths' capacities to understand and appreciate the significance of *Miranda* rights and to compare these capacities to those of adult offenders (Grisso, 1998b). Over the past three decades, the instruments have gained clinical utility as well. Forensic psychologists recognized the contribution that data from these instruments could make beyond those of the batteries of psychological tests performed to help courts decide juvenile defendants' capacities to understand and waive rights. The instruments were published and made available for clinical use in 1998 (Grisso, 1998b), approximately a quarter of a century after they were initially introduced for research. The instruments may be used for evaluations with juveniles or adults, but much of the research has focused on juveniles' capacities because of their developmental immaturity and vulnerability when dealing with the complexities of the justice system.

The Instruments for Assessing Understanding and Appreciation of *Miranda* Rights are currently the only standardized measures designed to assess defendants' understanding of *Miranda* rights. However, to maintain the instruments' utility, they are being revised (Condie, Goldstein, & Grisso, 2006). Preliminary research with the revised instruments, the *Miranda* Rights Comprehension Instruments–II (MRCI-II), is establishing psychometric properties and norms with several different populations—such as juvenile offenders, adult offenders with serious mental illness, and adults with mental retardation (Cooper, 2003; Goldstein et al., 2003; Goldstein, Condie, Mesiarik, Kalbeitzer, & Osman, 2004; O'Connell, 2004).

BASIC DESCRIPTION

A forensic assessment of a juvenile defendant's comprehension of the *Miranda* warning includes several basic features (Oberlander & Goldstein, 2001). Evaluators should determine what methods police officers used to deliver the warnings, whether a parent or another interested adult was present during the *Miranda* warnings, what role the adult (if present) assumed, and whether the adult offered any consultation to the youth. If there is evidence that the *Miranda* warning was delivered, the evaluator should determine when, how often, and under what circumstances it was delivered. It is useful to determine the detainee's previous warrant or arrest experience, although repeated experience does not necessarily improve *Miranda* comprehension (Grisso, 1981). Critical records for the assessment include relevant police, medical, educational, assessment, mental health, criminal justice, and probation records. The evaluator should review arrest records, confession transcripts, documentation of how and when the *Miranda* warning was issued, documentation that a waiver was agreed upon by the defendant, audiotapes or videotapes of the interrogation (if available/applicable), and translation procedures used for non-English-speaking detainees. Interviews of the youth and the interested adult (if an adult was present) should include relevant historical data and their accounts of the process from apprehension through confession. Questions and procedures related to potential malingering or lack of comprehension should be included (Oberlander & Goldstein, 2001).

The Instruments for Assessing Understanding and Appreciation of *Miranda* Rights consist of four instruments, each assessing a different aspect of understanding of *Miranda* rights and the significance of waiving those rights. The instruments are appropriate for delinquent and nondelinquent youths ages 10–17 and for offending and nonoffending adults. Administration time varies for each instrument. The following describes the four instruments.

Comprehension of *Miranda* Rights (CMR) assesses the examinee's understanding of the basic meaning of each of the four *Miranda* warnings. The examiner reads each warning aloud to the examinee, and the examinee is asked to paraphrase the meaning of each warning. Scoring criteria for the CMR are based on a large number of juveniles' responses that were independently reviewed by a collaborating panel of attorneys and psychologists across the United States. Responses to each item are assigned 0, 1, or 2 points for "inadequate," "questionable," or "adequate" understanding, respectively. Examiners are instructed to probe with standardized questions if inadequate or questionable responses are initially provided. Subscores on the CMR may range from 0 to 8 points. Administration typically requires 15 minutes.

Comprehension of *Miranda* Rights—Recognition (CMR-R) also assesses the examinee's understanding of *Miranda* warnings; however, to account for possible confounding educational and/or expressive difficulties, this instrument eliminates the need for verbal expressive skills. The protocol consists of 12 recognition items in which there are three preconstructed sentences for each of the four *Miranda* warnings. For each warning, the examinee must determine whether each of the three preconstructed sentences has the same meaning as the original warning provided. Incorrect responses are assigned 0 points, and correct responses are assigned 1 point. Subscale scores for the CMR-R may range from 0 to 12 points. Administration typically requires 5–10 minutes to complete.

Function of Rights in Interrogation (FRI) is used to assess the examinee's *appreciation* of the significance of his or her rights in interrogation and legal situations. The examinee is presented with four drawn pictures depicting relevant police, legal, and court proceedings, along with a brief vignette describing each scene. For instance, an examinee is shown a picture of a boy sitting at a table with an attorney, and is told that this boy has just been arrested and is meeting with his lawyer before he is interrogated. The FRI consists of a total of 15 standardized questions to assess the examinee's appreciation of three areas: the adversarial nature of police officers when interrogating suspects (NI subscale); the advocacy role of the attorney in client–attorney relationships (RC subscale); and the entitlement to the right to silence that cannot be revoked by any authority figure (RS subscale) (Grisso, 1998b). Scoring procedures and criteria for the FRI are similar to those of the CMR, and scores may range from 0 to 30. Administration typically requires approximately 15 minutes.

Comprehension of *Miranda* Vocabulary (CMV) was developed to assess understanding of six vocabulary words that are typically used in *Miranda* warnings: "consult," "attorney," "interrogation," "appoint," "entitled," and "right." Nine words were chosen initially by a panel of attorneys and psychologists; however, a pilot study revealed that nearly all of the participants adequately understood three of the words, so these were discarded. To administer the CMV, the examiner shows a vocabulary word to the examinee while reading it aloud, using it in a sentence, and then repeating it. The examinee is then asked to define the word. Scoring procedures are identical to those of the CMR and FRI, and scores may range from 0 to 12 points. Administration typically requires about 10 minutes.

There is no overall *Miranda* comprehension score. There are no "cutoff scores" signifying impaired or unimpaired performance. Scores should be evaluated individually for each instrument. The manual presents average scores of adult and juvenile samples for each instrument (Grisso, 1998b). The Instruments assess current capacity (at the time of the evaluation); they do not necessarily indicate the individual's understanding of the *Miranda* warnings at an earlier time, during police questioning, which might depend on a number of other factors involving the circumstances of the questioning.

HISTORY OF THE METHOD'S DEVELOPMENT

The Original Instruments

Research that led to the Instruments for Assessing Understanding and Appreciation of *Miranda* Rights was conducted in the late 1970s (Grisso, 1980, 1981) and funded by the National Institute of Mental Health. The Instruments were included in an appendix of the primary report of that research (Grisso, 1981) but were published as a separate manual in 1998 by Professional Resource Press. In 1998, Condie and colleagues (2006) began to update and revise the original instruments with funding from the Small Grants Program at the University of Massachusetts Medical School, leading to initial research with the MRCI-II. This research is ongoing (availability of the MRCI-II is anticipated in 2006); it is aimed at establishing updated psychometric properties and norms for the revised instruments with a variety of populations (Cooper, 2003; Goldstein et al., 2003, 2004; O'Connell, 2004).

The original Instruments were designed to fulfill several objectives. First, through the standardized administration and objective scoring procedures, they provide a reliable measurement of an examinee's basic understanding of *Miranda* rights and specific vocabulary words included in those rights, as well as a deeper appreciation of the significance of waiving the rights. In addition, to maximize the validity of the assessment tool, each instrument was individually developed to assess different capacities needed to make decisions about the waiver of *Miranda* rights. For instance, a youth may understand that he or she has the right to an attorney; however, the youth may not grasp that an attorney is a legal representative who advocates on the defendant's behalf, regardless of guilt. Although the youth may understand his or her right (thereby meeting the "knowing" requirement of a valid waiver), if he or she does not comprehend the attorney's role, the "intelligent" requirement is not met.

In the creation of the *Miranda* Instruments, both general adolescent development and problems that this specific population of youths may experience (e.g., educational difficulties) were kept in mind. Many items have visual stimuli to engage youths (e.g., the pictures of the scenarios for the FRI, cue cards with the preconstructed sentences written on them for the CMR-R). There is no minimum required reading level, as all of the items are read aloud by the examiner. In addition, since youths' levels of cognitive development vary (not all adolescents of the same age possess the same capacity for understanding), instruments were designed to give youths ample opportunity to express their understanding and appreciation of rights. For instance, a youth may understand his or her right to remain silent, but the youth may not be able to articulate the meaning of that right, as required by the CMR. However, he or she will be able to convey this understanding through the preconstructed sentences on the CMR-R and performance on the RS subscale of the FRI.

Revising the Instruments

Condie and colleagues (2006) are updating the Instruments for Assessing Understanding and Appreciation of *Miranda* Rights for several reasons. First, there is currently no standardized wording or method of delivering *Miranda* warnings across jurisdictions. The language used in the original instruments was based on the warnings used in St. Louis County, Missouri, in the 1970s, when the initial instruments were developed. In the past three decades, the language used in *Miranda* warnings in many jurisdictions has been simplified, and a fifth warning has been added informing suspects that they have the right to stop the interrogation process at any time to ask for an attorney (Oberlander, 1998). The updated instruments, the MRCI-II, have added this fifth warning to each of the relevant instruments (i.e., the CMR-II, CMR-R-II, and CMV-II) and simplified the wording to better reflect warnings read to youths in many jurisdictions today.

Second, a supplemental instrument, Perceptions of Coercion during Holding and Interrogation Procedures (P-CHIP), has been developed to assess confession behavior (i.e., self-reported likelihood of offering false confessions, self-reported likelihood of talking with police if guilty, and self-reported stress levels) in response to a selected variety of police interrogation tactics. Whereas the original four instruments assess juveniles' capacities related to the "knowing" and "intelligent" components of a valid waiver, the P-CHIP assesses self-report data related to the "voluntary" construct. Lastly, there are questions about whether the norms established in the 1970s are applicable to youths today. Thus, to maintain the utility and applicability of the instruments, norms for youths of the 21st century are being established from current research with the revised instruments.

RESEARCH EVIDENCE

The psychometric properties of the original Instruments for Assessing Understanding and Appreciation of *Miranda* Rights were based on data collected in an extensive study that culminated in 1980 (Grisso, 1980). Participants for this study included 431 white non-Hispanic (73%) and black (25%) girls and boys, ages 10–16 years, who had been adjudicated delinquent or were awaiting adjudication. The study also assessed 260 offending and nonoffending white and black adults ages 17–50 years for comparative purposes. Both offending and nonoffending adults were included, to examine any differences that might exist between adult offenders' understanding based on experience with the criminal justice system and intellectual skills associated with older age. Research with the revised instruments (the MRCI-II) is extending tests of generalizability to a broader sample of juvenile offenders that includes Hispanic and Asian youths (Goldstein et al., 2004).

Internal Consistency and Reliability

The Original Instruments

Grisso (1998b) reported the internal consistency of the CMR and CMV instruments, using item–total correlations from juvenile samples. Strong positive relationships were found between each item on the CMR and the total CMR score (r = .55 to .73), and between scores for each word and overall scores on the CMV (r = .51 to .72). Thus there is consistency between item scores within an instrument and overall scores on an instrument. No one has reported indexes of internal consistency for the CMR-R or the FRI.

Grisso (1998b) evaluated interrater reliability for the CMR, CMV, and FRI by using independently scored protocols from several pairs of trained raters, where one rater interviewed each subject and a second rater scored responses based on information documented on answer sheets. Raters received several months of training in the scoring procedures. Three research assistants independently scored the first 76 protocols, and two scorers independently scored the last 90 protocols in the study. In addition, an inexperienced trainee also scored the last 90 protocols, so that correlations with experienced scorers could be calculated.

Overall, interrater reliability was good to excellent between experienced scorers, with the CMV having the highest agreement (r = .89 to .98 for items, r = .97 to .98 for total scores), followed by the FRI (r = .72 to 1.00 for items, r = .80 to .94 for subscale scores, and r = .94 to .96 for total scores) and the CMR (r = .80 to .97 for items, r = .92 to .94 for total scores). High interrater reliability was found between experienced and inexperienced scorers on the CMV (r = .88 to 1.00 for items, r = .98 for totals) and CMR (r = .85 to .90 for items, r = .89 for totals) (these estimates were not conducted for the FRI). Strong interrater reliability was therefore found, regardless of raters' scoring experience and interview observations. Estimates of interrater reliability are not necessary for the CMR-R because of the objective nature of the scoring criteria.

Test–retest reliability is only available for the CMR. Grisso (1998b) reported a strong correlation (r = .84) for the CMR's 2-day test–retest reliability by correlating test scores from participants' first day in a detention center to the third day of their stay. Half the youths tested obtained the same scores on retest; nearly 38% obtained higher scores on retest; and the remaining 12% received lower scores on retest (Grisso, 1998b).

The MRCI-II

We (Goldstein et al., 2004) have identified comparable indexes of reliability for the MRCI-II. Item–total internal-consistency estimates demonstrated positive relationships for the CMR-II (r = .50 to .81) and the CMV-II (r = .06 to .61). The wider range of correlations on the CMV-II than the original CMV may be due to an increase in the number of items. Interrater agreement was also comparable to Grisso's findings for the CMR-II (r = .77 to 1.00 for items, r = .97 for totals), FRI (r = .81 to 1.00 for items, r = .99 to 1.00 for subscales, and r = .99 for totals), and CMV-II (r = .80 to 1.00 for items, r = .98 for totals). Test–retest reliability of the CMR-II was examined through repeat administrations to 47 youths over a period of 3 days to 1 month. No differences were found based on the time span (r = .61). In a finding similar to Grisso's, nearly half the participants obtained the same scores on retest.

Validity

The Original Instruments

Performance on the CMR, CMR-R, and CMV is positively related. Grisso (1981) reported strong positive relationships between the CMR and CMV (r = .67) and between the CMR and the CMR-R (r = .55). A much weaker association existed between the FRI and the other measures (CMR, r = .28; CMR-R, r = .32; CMV, r = .29; Grisso, 1998b). This was expected because the FRI was designed to assess youths' *appreciation*, rather than their *understanding*, of the significance of warnings.

Intelligence measures may serve as one test of the concurrent validity of the Instruments for Assessing Understanding and Appreciation of *Miranda* Rights, since intelligence should theoretically be related to capacity to understand rights. The measures share a strong positive correlation with IQ scores on an abbreviated version of the Wechsler Intelligence Scale for Children— Revised (WISC-R; Kaufman, 1979), ranging from $r = .47$ to $.59$ for the CMR, CMR-R, and CMV. A significant, but weaker, relationship ($r = .19$ to $.34$) exists between these measures and age, such that youths under age 15 years score much lower than youths ages 15 and older (Grisso, 1998b).

The 1970s research demonstrated that age and intelligence characteristics were most closely related to comprehension scores, but intelligence was a better predictor of understanding (Grisso, 1981). Generally, age was related to comprehension scores for youth ages 10–14 years, such that older youths performed better than younger ones. However, this pattern was dependent on intelligence among youths ages 15 and 16. Youths of these ages with intelligence scores of 80 and below performed similarly to younger youths, and those with intelligence scores of 81 and above performed similarly to older youths and adults. No differences were found in comprehension scores by gender (Grisso, 1981).

Miranda comprehension scores differed by race of the examinee (Grisso, 1981), such that comprehension scores were lower for black youths than for white non-Hispanic youths on average. Although black youths also had significantly lower intelligence scores on average, this difference continued to exist when age and intelligence were held constant, most notably among those in the lower intelligence categories (below 90). Black youths with intelligence scores below 90 performed lower than their white counterparts.

Prior experience with the justice system is not directly related to *Miranda* comprehension. In Grisso's (1981) study, both juveniles and adults who had rarely or never been detained demonstrated levels of understanding similar to those of individuals who had been detained many times. However, race moderated this relationship. For white youths, *Miranda* comprehension improved as the number of felony arrests increased, but comprehension among black youths declined as the number of prior felony arrests increased. Grisso suggested that because this pattern was evident across all intelligence levels, these group differences in understanding were not necessarily due to differences in intellectual ability.

The MRCI-II

The validity of the revised instruments is still being tested. However, these instruments, with the exception of the P-CHIP, are expected to prove as valid as Grisso's original instruments because of their striking consistency. Norms for the revised instruments exist for youth ages 10–17 years. Like with Grisso's (1998) research, these instruments revealed that age and IQ were the primary predictors of level of understanding of *Miranda* rights (Goldstein et al., 2003). Older youths generally had better understanding than younger youths, and more intelligent youths generally demonstrated better comprehension than those with lower IQs. Race also appears to moderate the relationship between prior arrests and *Miranda* comprehension, and between comprehension and the number of times youths recalled being detained and delivered the *Miranda* warning by police (Goldstein et al., 2003). Similar to the performance of black youths in Grisso's (1981) study, this generation's Hispanic youths demonstrated poorer understanding of rights with increased detainments and administrations of the *Miranda* warning. However, this pattern only held true for those reporting up to five detentions. Other comparisons based on racial/ethnic status were less robust. Preliminary data suggest that these instruments are suitable for use with individuals of different races, provided that examinees are fluent in English. Gender differences on the revised instruments are under investigation. For more information on the psychometric properties of the *MRCI-II*, see Goldstein and colleagues (2004).

There have been no comparisons made between scores on *Miranda* comprehension instruments and external criteria of capacity to waive rights, such as judicial decisions about the validity of a waiver in court. This would not be an accurate measure of validity for these instruments, because many factors in addition to individuals' *Miranda* Instruments or MRCI-II scores are likely to influence judicial decisions about waiver validity.

APPLICATION

The Instruments for Assessing Understanding and Appreciation of *Miranda* Rights (Grisso, 1998b) were designed initially for researchers to inform public policy. Now they are available from Professional Resource Press for clinical assessments of defendants' capacities to waive *Miranda* rights. The instruments are standardized, manualized, and recommended for use by licensed psychologists or psychiatrists who are forensic evaluators of criminal and delinquency cases, or by nonlicensed clinicians with proper supervision. As noted earlier, we anticipate that the revised instruments will be available from Professional Resource Press in 2006. The revisions should increase these instruments' current applicability, by modernizing the language and adding a test related to the voluntariness component of valid waivers.

These are the only tools for assessing capacity to waive *Miranda* rights available today; however, the frequency of their use is unknown. According to one survey of 64 board-certified forensic psychologists of the American Board of Professional Psychology, the *Miranda* instruments and the Wechsler Adult Intelligence Scale—Third Edition (WAIS-III) were the only assessment tools recommended for use in psycholegal contexts by the majority (Lally, 2003). (For many youths, especially younger or cognitively impaired ones, we would recommend one of the WAIS-III's child/youth counterparts, the WISC-III or WISC-IV.) In addition, several court cases have documented uses of the original research or the instruments for addressing legal issues related to capacities to provide valid waivers (see Grisso, 1998b).

Nevertheless, these instruments have several limitations. First, they measure an examinee's capacity to understand and appreciate the significance of rights at the time of the evaluation. Often evaluations are not requested until a matter of law is disputed regarding the validity of the waiver, which could be weeks, months, or years after an interrogation actually took place. Therefore, an examinee's understanding and appreciation of his or her rights may have improved as a result of exposure to the legal process, consultation with an attorney, and/or developmental maturation from the passing of time. In such instances, scores on the the instruments—based on performance during the evaluation—would probably provide an overestimation of the youth's understanding of rights at the time of past police questioning. This overestimation could be compounded by difficulties concentrating and reasoning as a result of the heightened stress of an interrogation compared to a forensic evaluation (Oberlander, Goldstein, & Goldstein, 2003).

These instruments are not to be used to answer the ultimate legal question pertaining to the validity of a waiver. Instead, they permit clinicians to inform courts about a youth's ability to understand the vocabulary and meaning of the warnings, as well as the capacity to understand the consequences of waiving rights. Information ascertained from the instruments should be presented to courts in conjunction with other factors outlined in the totality-of-circumstances test (see "Purpose," above) to draw conclusions about the admissibility of a waiver.

CASE EXAMPLE

John Doe, a 13½-year-old sixth grader detained and charged with murder in the first degree, was referred for a forensic evaluation by defense counsel. The evaluator began the forensic assessment with cognitive and educational testing to determine John's overall level of cognitive functioning, to provide information potentially related to *Miranda* comprehension, and to serve as a basis for judging the trustworthiness of John's responses to *Miranda* measures. John's Full Scale IQ on the WISC-III was 76, consistent with previous testing. He demonstrated no significant Verbal–Performance differences. Achievement tests (recent and historic) showed a persistent two-grade delay in most subjects, with more significant delays in reading and oral comprehension skills, which were at a second-grade level. John received special academic assistance, and his school grades were average to below average. He had been retained in fourth grade because of attendance and academic problems. His recent school attendance and school behavior were good.

Records and interviews showed that John had no history of physical illness or injury, or of substance use or abuse. John's father was deceased, and his mother was physically disabled and used a wheelchair. The child protective services department had questioned his mother's supervision, but she was not under the department's scrutiny at the time of evaluation. Outpatient mental health records revealed that John suffered from depression, judged to be at mild levels at both the time of arrest and forensic assessment.

With respect to the arrest, *Miranda* warnings, and confession, John said he was awoken from sleep after midnight and abruptly arrested. He and his mother both said that the officers yelled a warning that he would "face jail for life" if he did not confess, and they repeatedly told him that they "had firm evidence" that he had committed the crime. John reported that he was read the *Miranda* warning twice. Records revealed that he signed a waiver of his privilege to make a telephone call at 2:05 A.M. and a waiver of his *Miranda* rights at 2:10 A.M., after many interview questions had been asked. John's mother was permitted to consult with him prior to further interrogation. However, she waited silently at the other side of the room before and after the *Miranda* warning was issued, only once instructing, "You be a good boy and tell the truth!" She asked no questions and offered no other advice to John. At 2:25 A.M., she left the room and did not return. As described by John and his mother, the interrogation included a variety of techniques, ranging from soft-spoken and encouraging questions to a reminder of legal consequences in a loud voice. John was interrogated for a total of 5 hours, according to police interrogation records. He gave several confessions, the second of which implicated him as part of a group crime, and the third of which implicated him as primarily responsible for the murder.

During the forensic assessment, John was asked to read the *Miranda* warning used in his jurisdiction. Clinical observations were used to determine his ability to read the warning and to ascertain whether reading problems might have contributed to incomplete comprehension or miscomprehension of the warning. John read the *Miranda* warning and his typewritten confession in a slow and halting fashion, in a style consistent with his reading during the educational assessment. He could not decode, pronounce, or define many words that appeared in his confession.

The forensic evaluator then administered the four *Miranda* measures from the Instruments for Assessing Understanding and Appreciation of *Miranda* Rights. On the CMR measure, John obtained a score of 4 out of a possible 8 points. On the CMR-R measure, he obtained a score of 7 out of a possible 12 points. On the CMV measure, he obtained a score of 8 out of a possible 12 points. On the FRI measure, he obtained a score of 21 out of a possible 30 points. His scores and item responses suggested that John thought the *right* to remain silent meant he had a *duty* to remain silent until officers questioned him, and also that he thought he was *obligated* to speak to the police officers. Furthermore, he appeared to believe that the judge would require him to answer police questions if he declined to speak with police officers, and that his attorney would have no right to dispute the judge's order. He knew that he would be assigned a public defender, but, based on prior experience, he thought he would not be allowed to speak with his attorney until the morning after the police interrogation. He knew the attorney would be provided free of charge, despite his inability to define "afford." His account of the warnings and confession remained reasonably consistent across time. Interview data also revealed that the officers convinced John he had been blamed by his accomplice, would be viewed kindly by the judge for giving a confession, and would be allowed to return home after confessing.

The evaluator concluded that (1) John did not comprehend several components of the *Miranda* warning, (2) his poor comprehension was consistent with his level of intellect and educational achievement, (3) his depression had little bearing on his *Miranda* comprehension, and (4) he gave no responses suggestive of malingering. John seemed to make a deliberate effort to understand the *Miranda* warning during the evaluation; he was disappointed when he did not understand it, and he was embarrassed about his halting reading. At the hearing—based on the records; forensic evaluation report; and police, psychologist's, and teacher's testimony—the judge ruled that the waiver was not valid.

REFERENCES

Condie, L., Goldstein, N. E., & Grisso, T. (2006). *The Miranda Rights Comprehension Instruments–II*. Manuscript in preparation.

Cooper, V. G. (2003). *Waiver of Miranda rights in psychiatric patients*. Unpublished doctoral dissertation, University of Alabama, Tuscaloosa.

Goldstein, N. E., Condie, L., Kalbeitzer, R., Osman, D., & Geier, J. (2003). Juvenile offenders' *Miranda* rights comprehension and self-reported likelihood of offering false confessions. *Assessment, 10*(4), 359–369.

Goldstein, N. E., Condie, L., Mesiarik, C., Kalbeitzer, R., & Osman, D. (2004). Psychometric properties of the *Miranda Rights Comprehension Instruments–II*. Manuscript in preparation.

Grisso, T. (1980). Juveniles' capacities to waive *Miranda* rights: An empirical analysis. *California Law Review, 68*, 1134–1166.

Grisso, T. (1981). *Juveniles' waiver of rights: Legal and psychological competence*. New York: Plenum Press.

Grisso, T. (1998a). *Forensic evaluations of juveniles*. Sarasota, FL: Professional Resource Press.

Grisso, T. (1998b). *Instruments for Assessing Understanding and Appreciation of Miranda Rights*. Sarasota, FL: Professional Resource Press.

Kaufman, A. S. (1979). *Intelligent testing with the WISC-R*. New York: Wiley.

Lally, S. J. (2003). What tests are acceptable for use in forensic evaluations?: A survey of experts. *Professional Psychology: Research and Practice, 34*, 491–498.

Miranda v. Arizona, 384 U.S. 436 (1966).

Oberlander, L. (1998). *Miranda* comprehension and confessional competence. *Expert Opinion, 2*, 11–12.

Oberlander, L., & Goldstein, N. E. (2001). A review and update on the practice of evaluating *Miranda* comprehension. *Behavioral Sciences and the Law, 19*, 453–471.

Oberlander, L., Goldstein, N. E., & Goldstein, A. M. (2003). Competence to confess. In I. B. Weiner (Series Ed.) & A. M. Goldstein (Vol. Ed.), *Handbook of psychology: Vol. 11. Forensic psychology* (pp. 335–357). New York: Wiley.

O'Connell, M. J. (2004, March). The risk of false confessions for individuals with mental retardation. In N. E. Goldstein (Chair), *The Miranda Rights Comprehension Instruments–II: Related research and policy implications.* Symposium conducted at the annual convention of the American Psychology–Law Society, Scottsdale, AZ.

CHAPTER 23

MacArthur Competence Assessment Tool— Criminal Adjudication

Jennifer L. Woolard
Samantha Harvell

PURPOSE

Competence to stand trial is a fundamental tenet of the justice system, because it is essential for meeting the requirements of due process. Such competence requires that defendants have basic capacities to understand the proceedings against them and assist counsel before their case may go forward. The legal standard for competence to stand trial, defined by the U.S. Supreme Court in *Dusky v. United States* (1960) and *Drope v. Missouri* (1975), requires that courts determine "whether [the defendant] has sufficient present ability to consult with his lawyer with a reasonable degree of rational understanding— and whether he has a rational as well as factual understanding of the proceedings against him" (*Dusky v. United States*, 1960, p. 402).

Various interpretations of the *Dusky* standard have been set forth (e.g., Bonnie, 1992, 1993; Laboratory of Community Psychiatry, 1973; Melton, Petrila, Poythress, & Slobogin, 1997), but one of the more compelling suggests that relevant abilities fall into two categories (Bonnie, 1993): "competence to assist counsel," involving understanding the charges and system components, reasoning about and conveying case-related information to counsel, and appreciating the particular circumstances of one's own situation; and "decisional competence," involving the capacity to express choices about decisions in one's case. In adult (criminal) court, all states have established some variant of the *Dusky* criteria, sometimes stipulating that a finding of incompetence be based on mental illness or mental retardation (Grisso, 2003).

Historically, questions of competence have been raised for adult defendants when mental illness and/or mental retardation might significantly impair their capacities to participate (Barnum, 2000). Competence of young defendants was raised rarely during most of the 20th century, for several reasons: Few young adolescents were tried in adult court, and the lack of a coherent legal theory of competence in juvenile court, combined with a treatment-oriented approach, rendered the issue less salient (Bonnie & Grisso, 2000). Changes in court jurisdiction and sentencing practices over the past 25 years have directed increasing attention to the competence-relevant abilities of youths in criminal and juvenile courts (Grisso, 1997; Grisso, Miller, & Sales, 1987). Recent legal reforms in transfer, waiver, and sentencing schemes have resulted in greater numbers of youths facing criminal prosecution or punitive juvenile justice sentences. Unfortunately, youth-specific assessments and data are quite limited (Grisso, 1997).

The majority of juvenile justice jurisdictions that provide young offenders with the right to competence (currently more than half of the states in the United States; Bonnie & Grisso, 2000) have simply extended the adult standard explicitly or by default, despite the notion that traditional contributors to incompetence may operate differently among youths. As we discuss below, developmental factors that may affect competence have only recently been considered in research (Grisso, 1997; Scott, Reppucci, & Woolard, 1995; Steinberg & Cauffman, 1996) and are recognized by only a few states (e.g., Florida; Fla. Stat. Ann. § 985.223 (2)). The few studies that used the "first-generation" adult assessment instruments with juvenile samples generally found that on average, and all else being equal, adolescents ages 14 and under demonstrated greater deficits than adults, but youths over 14 years performed similarly to adults (Cooper, 1997; Cowden & McKee, 1995; McGaha, Otto, McClaren, & Petrila, 2001; McKee, 1998; Savitsky & Karras, 1984).

Unique assessment complications, combined with the need for clinicians to respond to increasing referrals for competence evaluations of youths in criminal and juvenile courts, have resulted in greatly increased attention to competence assessment practices with youths (Redding, 2000). The dearth of age-specific assessments raises the possibility of simply applying an adult assessment tool to juvenile defendants. Psychological assessment mechanisms for competence developed prior to the 1990s have offered clinicians a variety of techniques with limited connection to the *Dusky* criteria (Poythress, Bonnie, Monahan, Otto, & Hoge, 2002; see Grisso, 2003, for comprehensive reviews of competence-to-stand-trial instruments). Screening instruments, such as the Competency Screening Test (Lipsitt, Lelos, & McGarry, 1971) and the Georgia Court Competency Test (Wildman et al., 1978), use quantifiable scores to identify general impairment. Semistructured interview approaches, such as the Competence to Stand Trial Assessment Instrument (Laboratory of

Community Psychiatry, 1973), afford examiners more flexibility but less standardization and objectivity. The Evaluation of Competence to Stand Trial—Revised (Rogers, Tillbrook, & Sewell, 2004) allows both objectivity and flexibility, but, like most of these instruments, it emphasizes existing factual knowledge and does not address defendants' ability to learn about aspects of the adjudicative process (e.g., plea agreements) and other relevant capacities (e.g., reasoning, appreciation).

The authors of the MacArthur Competence Assessment Tool—Criminal Adjudication (MacCAT-CA; Poythress et al., 1999) have attempted to remedy the deficits in existing instrumentation. The MacCAT-CA represents a significant improvement in adult competence evaluations by extending the assessment process to reasoning, appreciation, and learning potential. This chapter discusses the complexities associated with juvenile competence assessments and the limits of existing instrumentation. We focus on the MacCAT-CA as a potentially useful but limited alternative for assessing competence in juveniles. This chapter provides a description of the development and properties of the MacCAT-CA, the complications of assessing competence in youths, and the strengths and limitations of the MacCAT-CA's use with juvenile defendants.

BASIC DESCRIPTION

The MacCAT-CA (Poythress et al., 1999) was developed for forensic assessments of capacities relevant to competence to stand trial among adult defendants. It is capable of producing quantifiable impairment scores that can be interpreted in reference to national adult norms (Otto et al., 1998), and has been validated for use with English-speaking adult misdemeanor and felony defendants in inpatient, outpatient, forensic, or correctional settings. The instrument is intended to serve as one aspect of comprehensive forensic evaluations, which may also include social histories, mental status exams, and personal interviews with a client and collateral informants, among other components.

The MacCAT-CA was designed for administration and interpretation by mental health professionals with specific training in assessment, as well as an understanding of the legal process and the construct of adjudicative competence. The 22-item measure is administered in a structured individual interview; the interviewer uses an instrument booklet with each item appearing on the right-hand page and scoring criteria on the left-hand page. Participant responses are recorded verbatim and scored 0 ("clinically significant impairment"), 1 ("mild impairment"), or 2 ("minimal or no impairment"). Objective scoring criteria are included for each item; scoring does not rely on subjective clinical judgment. Item scores are transferred to the Scoring Summary form and summed to yield three subscale scores: Understanding (the ability to understand general information related to the law and adjudicatory proceedings); Reasoning (the ability to discern the potential legal relevance of information, and capacity to reason about specific choices that confront a defendant in the course of adjudication); and Appreciation (rational awareness of the meaning and consequences of the proceedings in one's own case). See Table 23.1 for a brief overview of the MacCAT-CA and individual item content.

The Understanding (items 1–8) and Reasoning (items 9–16) sections of the MacCAT-CA are based on a short vignette of a hypothetical crime in which the defendant gets into a fight and causes serious injury to the victim.

TABLE 23.1. Brief Overview of the MacCAT-CA Item Content

Understanding

1. Roles of defense attorney and prosecutor
2. Elements of an offense
3. Elements of a lesser included offense
4. Role of the jury
5. Role of the judge at trial
6. Consequences of conviction
7. Pleading guilty
8. Rights waived in making a guilty plea

Reasoning

 9. Self-defense
10. Mitigating the prosecution's evidence of intent
11. Possible provocation
12. Fear as a motivator for one's behavior
13. Possible mitigating effects of intoxication
14. Seeking information: A defendant's ability to identify information that might inform Fred's choice
15. Weighing consequences: A defendant's ability to infer or think through the implications of a chosen course of action
16. Making comparisons: A defendant's ability to verbalize features (advantages–disadvantanges) of a chosen option, in contrast or comparison to features of the other option

Appreciation

17. Likelihood of being treated fairly
18. Likelihood of being assisted by defense counsel
19. Likelihood of fully disclosing case information to the defense attorney
20. Likelihood of being found guilty
21. Likelihood of punishment if convicted
22. Likelihood of pleading guilty

The Understanding items assess the defendant's capacity to understand the law and the legal process. In contrast to other competence assessment instruments, the MacCAT-CA uses a teaching mechanism in six of the eight items to assess preexisting knowledge and the capacity to learn relevant information. If an examinee provides an incomplete or inadequate response (i.e., scores a 0 or 1) to the initial factual question (Part A), an examiner reads a disclosure statement containing the relevant information and asks the defendant to paraphrase it (Part B). The final item score is the higher score of Part A or B. The eight items are summed to produce an Understanding subscale score ranging from 0 to 16.

The Reasoning items assess a defendant's ability to determine the legal relevance of information and to reason about choices confronted in the adjudication process. For items 9–13, a defendant is asked to choose the more relevant of two case facts and explain the reasons for that choice. Full points are assigned for correct identification of the more relevant fact and a reason that encompasses the legal relevance of the concept. For example, item 9 calls for weighing the relative importance of two facts: The defendant thought he saw the victim reaching for a knife, and the defendant went out to dinner with a friend prior to the fight. The examinee would receive a score of 2 for (1) recognizing that the first fact is more important, because it helps the lawyer understand the defendant's thoughts at the time of the fight; and (2) justifying the choice, because it suggests that the defendant may have acted in self-defense. Items 14–16 assess reasoning about the advantages and disadvantages of pleading guilty and going to trial. Respondents receive full credit for identifying additional relevant information helpful to the decision, identifying specific advantages, disadvantages, and comparative advantages of the choice. The Reasoning items are summed into a subscale score ranging from 0 to 16.

The six Appreciation items assess the ability to appreciate the legal process and how it will function in an examinee's case, as opposed to that of a hypothetical defendant. An examinee receives full credit for plausible reasoning and a score of 0 for not offering a reason or for implausible thinking that appears to be related to symptoms of a mental disorder (e.g., delusions). A score of 1 represents questionable thinking with an unclear link to mental disorder. Appreciation subscale scores range from 0 to 12.

Subscale scores are compared to cutoff scores presented in the manual and classified into one of three impairment levels, as noted earlier: "minimal or no impairment," "mild impairment," or "clinically significant impairment." For the Understanding and Reasoning subscales, clinically significant impairment is defined by scores 1.5 standard deviations or more below the mean of a sample of approximately 90% of jail inmates presumed competent. For the Appreciation subscale, clinically significant impairment is defined by scores of 0 on two or more items. Exceeding clinical impairment scores on any subscale is suggestive of impaired functioning. Mild impairment scores represent probable impairment, but should be evaluated in light of additional case specific and contextual information. Because significant impairment in any of the three abilities may be a sufficient contributor to incompetence, the instrument yields no overall competence score. As such, MacCAT-CA results are intended to serve as one set of data weighed in accordance with case-specific features of the clinician's full evaluation of competence-relevant capacities.

HISTORY OF THE METHOD'S DEVELOPMENT

Development of the MacCAT-CA was preceded by a multiphase study of adjudicative competence conducted by the MacArthur Foundation Research Network on Mental Health and the Law, with funding from the John D. and Catherine T. MacArthur Foundation. After delineating the meaning and purposes of legal competence, the group designed the seven-scale, 47-item MacArthur Structured Assessment of Competencies of Criminal Defendants (MacSAC-CD; Hoge et al., 1997). Advantages of the MacSAC-CD were that it (1) was based on a comprehensive legal theory of competence (Bonnie, 1992, 1993); (2) assessed capacities rather than mere current knowledge; (3) assessed discrete competence-related abilities; and (4) involved standardized administration and criterion-based scoring (Otto et al., 1998; Poythress et al., 1999). Hoge and colleagues (1997) developed and validated the MacSAC-CD on 472 adult pretrial detainees, jailed defendants receiving mental health services, and defendants found legally incompetent and referred to state hospitals for restoration. Although the instrument demonstrated adequate psychometric properties, was related in expected ways to measures of psychopathology and clinical competence assessments, and distinguished between the presumed competent and incompetent samples, its lengthy administration time (from 1.5 to 2 hours) precluded its use in the field.

By 1996, the developers condensed the MacSAC-CD into the brief (30-minute), clinical, and user-friendly MacCAT-CA, using standardized item-reduction techniques and considerations of face validity. From 1996 to 1998, the MacCAT-CA authors conducted a large-scale, multisite study in eight states with varying forensic systems, with support from the National Institute of Mental Health, to develop national norms and evaluate the new instrument's utility (Otto et al., 1998; Poythress et al, 1999). Data were collected from 729 pretrial felony defendants between the ages of 18 and 65 years from one of three groups: (1) a hospitalized group, adjudicated incompetent and committed to a forensic psychiatric unit for restoration; (2) a jail group of incarcerated inmates, presumed competent but receiving treatment for mental health problems; and (3) an unscreened jail group, presumed competent and randomly selected from the general jail population. The predominantly male (90%) sample included approximately 48% participants from racial minority groups (further detail was not reported). In addition to the MacCAT-CA, participants completed two subtests of the Wechsler Adult Intelligence Scale—Revised (Wechsler, 1981); the Brief Psychiatric Rating Scale—Anchored

(Overall & Gorham, 1962); and the Psychoticism scale of the Minnesota Multiphasic Personality Inventory–2 (Harkness, McNulty, & Ben-Porath, 1995). Researchers also obtained judgments of competence from mental health professionals familiar with individuals in the first group (those hospitalized and adjudicated incompetent). We describe the psychometric properties derived from these studies below.

RESEARCH EVIDENCE

Adult Samples

Internal Consistency and Reliability

The MacCAT-CA norming study reported good internal consistency for all three subscales, with alpha coefficients ranging from .81 (Reasoning) to .88 (Appreciation) (Otto et al., 1998; Poythress et al., 1999, 2002). The mean interitem correlations (Reasoning, .36; Understanding, .42; Appreciation, .54) confirmed appropriate consistency within each scale. Interrater reliability estimates, based on ratings from eight research assistants on 48 protocols, were also promising (intraclass correlations [ICCs] of .75 on Appreciation, .85 on Reasoning, and .90 on Understanding). Results from a more recent study in the United Kingdom using a slightly modified version of the instrument, the MacArthur Competence Assessment Tool—Fitness to Plead (Akinkunmi, 2002), yielded comparably strong evidence of internal consistency (ranging from .74 to .85) and interrater reliability (ranging from .73 to .99) (Akinkunmi, 2002).

Validity

Several studies of adults have demonstrated that the MacCAT-CA has acceptable validity. In the initial sample (Otto et al., 1998; Poythress et al., 1999, 2002), higher MacCAT-CA scores were associated with higher IQ scores and lower psychoticism scores. Subscale scores on the MacCAT-CA were moderately correlated with clinicians' ratings of competence ($r = .36$ for Understanding, $r = .42$ for Reasoning, and $r = .49$ for Appreciation). The hospitalized sample scored significantly lower than both jail samples, suggesting that the MacCAT-CA differentiated between incompetent and competent mentally ill defendants.

With respect to generalizability, there were modest but significant bivariate correlations between subscale scores and ethnicity ($r < .15$). However, the correlations were not significant after IQ was controlled for, suggesting that the associations could be explained by existing differences between the racial and ethnic groups in cognitive functioning. No gender-specific differences or considerations have been provided.

Youth Samples (with Caveats)

Because the MacCAT-CA has not been validated with youths, use of the measure with this population should be undertaken cautiously. The first issue is whether the instrument provides *accurate* information about youths' capacities. The second issue rests on how *well* it captures the relevant issues for assessment of youths' capacities. More substantive problems arise here, because important developmental differences that implicate youths' capacities as defendants are not captured by the MacCAT-CA.

Several recent published and unpublished studies have used the MacCAT-CA to examine age-based differences in competence-related abilities, but few have reported psychometric data on juveniles. In a study of 320 juvenile and adult male defendants detained before trial, Woolard and colleagues (Woolard, 1998; Woolard, Fried, & Reppucci, 2001) reported that adolescents aged 15 and younger scored significantly lower on Reasoning than older adolescents, but neither group differed from adults, whose scores fell slightly below those of older adolescents. Rutherford (2000) compared 70 predispositional delinquent youths, 40 community youths, and the national norm study sample of adult inmates presumed competent. Relative to adults, youths aged 16 and under had significantly lower Understanding and Reasoning scores, and youths aged 14 and under also had significantly lower Appreciation scores. Conversely, a study of 126 juvenile male inpatients found that age did not make significant contributions to predictions of MacCAT-CA subscale scores (Lexcen, 2000). A study of community juveniles and adults (Redlich, Silverman, & Steiner, 2003) reported inconsistent age-based differences, but these conclusions may be limited by the small sample size ($n = 35$).

Grisso and colleagues (2003) reported the most extensive data, generated from a study of approximately 1,400 adolescents and adults from four states who fell into one of four groups: youths in pretrial detention ($n = 453$), detained adults ($n = 233$), community youths ($n = 474$), and community adults ($n = 233$). The majority of participants were male (58%) and black (40%), while 23% were Hispanic and 35% were white non-Hispanic. In addition to the MacCAT-CA, the interview protocol included measures of intelligence (the Wechsler Abbreviated Scale of Intelligence; Psychological Corporation, 1999), psychological disturbance (the Massachusetts Youth Screening Instrument—Version 2; Grisso & Barnum, 2003) and judgment (the MacArthur Judgment Evaluation [MacJEN]; Woolard, Reppucci, Steinberg, Grisso, & Scott, 2003). The MacCAT-CA's interrater reliability was assessed at the early and final phases of data collection. Interrater agreement on Understanding (ICC = .63) and Reasoning (ICC = .60) from youths' protocols were somewhat low during the early phase, but improved by the final phase (ICC = .91 and .80, respectively) and were comparable to those from adults' protocols (ICC = .88 and .70, respectively). Interrater agreement was considerably lower for Appreciation, regardless of the sample and phase (ranging from .17 to

.88); perhaps this was due to truncated scoring within some age groups (e.g., few 0 responses among young adults).

Average MacCAT-CA subscale scores and degree of impairment varied by age, even after intelligence and socioeconomic status were controlled for. Youths ages 15 and younger performed more poorly than adults on the Understanding and Reasoning subscales. Approximately 30% of 11- to 13-year-olds and 19% of 14- to 15-year-olds demonstrated clinically significant impairment on one or both scales, compared to only 12% of older adolescents and adults. These age differences did not vary by gender, ethnicity, or justice system status. Juveniles and adults with lower IQs had a higher likelihood of scoring in the impaired range than those with IQ scores that were average or higher. For the most part, there were few differences in MacCAT-CA scores in relation to mental health problems, but this may have been due to samples that did not include persons with serious mental disorders.

THE ROLE OF DEVELOPMENTAL IMMATURITY IN YOUTH COMPETENCE ASSESSMENTS

Beyond the practical limitations, recent theoretical and empirical work raises serious concerns about whether the adult competence standards and corresponding assessment instruments capture developmental constructs that affect adolescents' capacities to participate in their trials. Several authors have argued that developmental differences in maturity of judgment could differentially affect adolescents' decision making during the trial process (Scott, 1992; Scott et al., 1995; Steinberg & Cauffman, 1996). Three of the primary judgment factors are *risk perception and preference, temporal perspective*, and *susceptibility to influence*. Youths' risk perception differs from that of adults, in that adolescents are less likely to identify certain actions as entailing personal risk to health or safety, but are more likely to engage in activities that pose those risks. Temporal perspective is different in youths as well: Short-term consequences are more salient than long-term consequences for adolescents. Finally, susceptibility to peer influences peaks in midadolescence and tapers off into young adulthood. As they progress to adulthood, adolescents predictably become more aware of and more sensitive to risk, more future-oriented, and less susceptible to influence by their peers. These factors implicate decisional competence—the capacities to make important decisions about waiver of rights that go beyond understanding and reasoning (Bonnie, 1992, 1993).

Psychosocial factors are not included in the legal definition of competence, but two studies indicate that adolescents and adults do make different choices, partly as a function of the youths' immaturity of judgment (Grisso et al., 2003; Woolard et al., 2001). These two studies used structured interviews and vignettes about police interrogation, attorney consultation, and consideration of a plea agreement to investigate the relation between decision choices and psychosocial factors. Both studies produced consistent findings, despite some instrumentation differences (the MacJEN was based in part on the earlier Woolard et al. measure). Grisso and colleagues (2003) found that adolescents and adults made different choices in two of the three MacJEN decision contexts: confession and acceptance of a plea agreement (both choices that involve compliance with authority, which decreased linearly with age). Almost 50% of the youngest adolescents (11 to 13 years) chose confessions over remaining silent or lying about crime involvement, compared to 20% of the adults. Furthermore, 75% of the 11- to 13-year-olds recommended a plea agreement over going to trial, compared to only 50% of adults.

Adolescents also differed from adults in the psychosocial factors constituting judgment. Adolescents were less likely to identify risks, to rate risks as likely to occur, or to view risks as having a serious impact. The youngest adolescents also identified fewer long-range consequences than older groups. The age-related impact of peer influence on decision choices was dependent on each examinee's original choice in the vignettes. However, results suggested that adolescents may have been more susceptible than adults to peer influence under some, but not all, legal situations tested.

Although these psychosocial judgment factors are not explicitly included in the commonly used legal standard for competence to stand trial, the results of these studies suggest that developmental factors may differentially affect adolescents' decisions during the trial process. These important developmental differences are not captured by the MacCAT-CA. Although significant age differences in the MacCAT-CA have been found, an assessment limited to the cognitive factors of understanding, reasoning, and appreciation would fail to provide a complete picture of potential age-based differences in capacity to participate effectively.

APPLICATION

The MacCAT-CA is a promising development in the assessment of competence-relevant capacities among adult defendants. For this purpose, the MacCAT-CA manual (Poythress et al., 1999) and test materials are available from a commercial publisher (Psychological Assessment Resources, Inc.; *http://www.parinc.com*). The MacCAT-CA is designed for use by mental health professionals with specific training in assessment (i.e., a bachelor's degree in psychology or a related field with coursework in test statistics, psychometrics, or test interpretation, or licensure that requires appropriate training in psychological testing), as well as an understanding of the legal process and the construct of adjudicative competence. The instrument has not been validated for individuals with an IQ under 60.

Developmental and clinical researchers agree that an assessment tool designed specifically for youths is needed (Grisso et al., 2003; Poythress et al., 2002). In the meantime, some suggest that the MacCAT-CA represents a reasonable alternative for juvenile assessments, in part because forensic assessment guidelines (including those provided with the MacCAT-CA) consistently recommend that this type of instrument should represent only one component of a larger assessment protocol (Poythress et al., 2002). This advice notwithstanding, the research reviewed above implies that adolescent defendants, particularly those in early adolescence, may differ from adults in meaningful ways that are not captured by adult instruments.

Although the review above has described several studies indicating that the MacCAT-CA can be successfully administered to adolescents, this use of the MacCAT-CA suffers from significant limitations. Three aspects of its current status raise cautions about its accuracy for youth (Poythress et al., 2002). First, norms for scoring and interpretation of adolescent performance are nonexistent. The research studies reviewed above applied the MacCAT-CA scoring scheme for identifying impairment that was based on the adult normative sample. It is possible that an age-based norming scheme would be more accurate for youths. Second, some items and scoring techniques are less relevant or potentially incomplete for use with adolescents in juvenile court. For example, items about the role of the jury, findings of guilt, or going to prison are irrelevant for youths in juvenile court.

Third, the emphasis on mental illness as the basis for impairment in the design and scoring system of the Appreciation subscale, in particular, may lead to misidentification or misinterpretation of adolescents' scores. As the editors of this handbook have mentioned in Chapter 2, mental illness and psychopathology can manifest themselves differently during adolescence, complicating the determination of whether disturbances are operating as stable traits or transient states (Barnum, 2000). It is unclear whether manifestations during adolescence would or should result in deficits in Appreciation scores, which are designed to detect impairment primarily through delusional thought processes. Also, adolescents may be more likely to achieve low Appreciation scores because they cannot or do not provide reasons for their choices. For example, Grisso and colleagues (2003) found that virtually all of the 0-credit Appreciation responses in their juvenile samples were due to "I don't know" responses, rather than delusional thought processes.

Research into developmental immaturity of judgment and decision making indicates that adolescents often differ from adults in important ways that implicate their effectiveness as defendants, but are not included in adult assessment instruments or protocols. Forensic evaluators should consider incompetence due to developmental immaturity and the implications of immaturity for assessment and remediation (see Grisso, 1998). To do so, evaluators must recognize the strengths and weakness of the MacCAT-CA and other assessment tools in the context of a developmentally sensitive assessment. Clinicians should consider the MacCAT-CA as one component of a comprehensive clinical assessment of adults' abilities relevant to competence to stand trial.

REFERENCES

Akinkunmi, A. (2002). The MacArthur Competence Assessment Tool—Fitness to plead: A preliminary evaluation of a research instrument for assessing fitness to plead in England and Wales. *Journal of the American Academy of Psychiatry and the Law, 30*(4), 476–482.

Barnum, R. (2000). Clinical and forensic evaluation of competence to stand trial in juvenile defendants. In T. Grisso & R. Schwartz (Eds.), *Youth on trial: A developmental perspective on juvenile justice* (pp. 193–224). Chicago: University Press.

Bonnie, R. (1992). The competence of criminal defendants: A theoretical reformulation. *Behavioral Sciences and the Law, 10*(3), 291–316.

Bonnie, R. (1993). The competence of criminal defendants: Beyond *Dusky* and *Drope*. *University of Miami Law Review, 47*, 539–601.

Bonnie, R. J., & Grisso, T. (2000). Adjudicative competence and youthful offenders. In T. Grisso & R. Schwartz (Eds.), *Youth on trial: A developmental perspective on juvenile justice* (pp. 73–104). Chicago: University of Chicago Press.

Cauffman, E., & Steinberg, L. (2000). Researching adolescents' judgment and culpability. In T. Grisso & R. Schwartz (Eds.), *Youth on trial: A developmental perspective on juvenile justice* (pp. 325–343). Chicago: University Press.

Cooper, D. (1997). Juveniles' understanding of trial-related information: Are they competent defendants? *Behavioral Sciences and the Law, 15*, 167–180.

Cowden, V., & McKee, G. (1995). Competence to stand trial in juvenile delinquency proceedings: Cognitive maturity and the attorney–client relationship. *Journal of Family Law, 33*, 629–660.

Drope v. Missouri, 420 U.S. 162 (1975).

Dusky v. United States, 362 U.S. 402 (1960).

Grisso, T. (1997). The competence of adolescents as trial defendants. *Psychology, Public Policy, and Law, 3*, 3–32.

Grisso, T. (1998). *Forensic evaluation of juveniles*. Sarasota, FL: Professional Resource Press.

Grisso, T. (2003). *Evaluating competencies: Forensic assessments and instruments* (2nd ed.). New York: Kluwer Academic/Plenum.

Grisso, T., & Barnum, R. (2003). *Massachusetts Youth Screening Instrument—Version 2: User's manual and technical report*. Sarasota, FL: Professional Resource Press.

Grisso, T., Miller, M., & Sales, B. (1987). Competency to stand trial in juvenile court. *International Journal of Law and Psychiatry, 10*, 1–20.

Grisso, T., Steinberg, L., Woolard, J., Cauffman, E., Scott, E., Graham, S., et al. (2003). Juveniles' competence to stand trial: A comparison of adolescents' and adults' capacities as trial defendants. *Law and Human Behavior, 27*(4), 333–363.

Harkness, A., McNulty, J., & Ben-Porath, Y. (1995). The Personality Psychopathology Five (PSY-5): Constructs and MMPI-2 scales. *Psychological Assessment, 7*(1), 104–114.

Hoge, S., Bonnie, R., Poythress, N., Monahan, J., Feucht-Haviar, T., & Eisenberg, M. (1997). The MacArthur adjudicative competence study: Development and validation of a research instrument. *Law and Human Behavior, 21*, 141–179.

Laboratory of Community Psychiatry, Harvard Medical School. (1973). *Competency to stand trial and mental illness* (DHEW Publication No. ADM 77-103). Rockville, MD: Department of Health, Education and Welfare.

Lexcen, F. (2000). *Factors associated with juvenile competence to stand trial: Neuropsychological, psychopathological and psychosocial variables.* Unpublished doctoral dissertation, University of Virginia.

Lipsitt, P., Lelos, D., & McGarry, A. (1971). Competency for trial: A screening instrument. *American Journal of Psychiatry, 128,* 105–109.

McGaha, A., Otto, R., McClaren, M. D., & Petrila, J. (2001). Juveniles adjudicated incompetent to proceed: A descriptive study of Florida's competence restoration program. *Journal of the American Academy of Psychiatry and the Law, 29,* 427–437.

McKee, G. (1998). Competence to stand trial in pre-adjudicatory juveniles and adults. *Journal of the American Academy of Psychiatry and the Law, 26,* 89–99.

Melton, G. B., Petrila, J., Poythress, N. G., & Slobogin, C. (1997). *Psychological evaluations for the courts: A handbook for mental health professionals and lawyers* (2nd ed.). New York: Guilford Press.

Otto, R., Poythress, N., Edens, N., Nicholson, R., Monahan, J., Bonnie, R., et al. (1998). Psychometric properties of the MacArthur Competence Assessment Tool—Criminal Adjudication. *Psychological Assessment, 10,* 435–443.

Overall, J., & Gorham, D. (1962). The Brief Psychiatric Rating Scale. *Psychological Reports, 10,* 799–812.

Poythress, N. G., Bonnie, R. J., Monahan, J., Otto, R., & Hoge, S. K. (2002). *Adjudicative competence: The MacArthur studies.* New York: Kluwer Academic/ Plenum.

Poythress, N. G., Nicholson, R., Otto, R., Edens, J., Bonnie, R., Monahan, J., & Hoge, S. (1999). *The MacArthur Competence Assessment Tool—Criminal Adjudication: Professional manual.* Lutz, FL: Psychological Assessment Resources.

Psychological Corporation. (1999). *Wechsler Abbreviated Scale of Intelligence.* San Antonio, TX: Author.

Redding, R. E. (2000). *Adjudicative competence in juveniles: Legal and clinical issues* (Juvenile Justice Fact Sheet). Charlottesville: Institute of Law, Psychiatry, and Public Policy, University of Virginia.

Redlich, A., Silverman, M., & Steiner, H. (2003). Pre-adjudicative and adjudicative competence in juveniles and young adults. *Behavioral Sciences and the Law, 21*(3), 393–410.

Rogers, R., Tillbrook, C., & Sewell, K. W. (2004). *Evaluation of Competency to Stand Trial—Revised (ECST-R).* Lutz, FL: Psychological Assessment Resources.

Rutherford, D. (2000). Evaluation of competency to stand trial among adolescents. *Adolescence, 19,* 349–359.

Savitsky, J., & Karras, D. (1984). Competency to stand trial among adolescents. *Adolescence, 19*(74), 349–358.

Scott, E. (1992). Judgment and reasoning in adolescent decision making. *Villanova Law Review, 37,* 1607–1669.

Scott, E., Reppucci, N., & Woolard, J. (1995). Evaluating adolescent decisionmaking in legal contexts. *Law and Human Behavior, 19,* 221–244.

Steinberg, L., & Cauffman, E. (1996). Maturity of judgment in adolescence: Psychosocial factors in adolescent decision-making. *Law and Human Behavior, 20,* 249–272.

Wechsler, D. (1981). *Manual for the Wechsler Adult Intelligence Scale—Revised (WAIS-R)*. New York: Psychological Corporation.

Wildman, R., Batchelor, E., Thompson, L., Nelson, F., Moore, J., Patterson, M., et al. (1978). *The Georgia Court Competence Test: An attempt to develop a rapid, quantitative measure for fitness for trial*. Unpublished manuscript, Forensic Services Division, Central State Hospital, Milledgeville, GA.

Woolard, J. (1998). *Competence and judgment in serious juvenile offenders*. Unpublished manuscript, University of Virginia.

Woolard, J. L., Fried, C. S., & Reppucci, N. D. (2001). Toward an expanded definition of adolescent competence in legal contexts. In R. Roesch, R. Corrado, & R. Dempster (Eds.), *Psychology in the courts: International advances in knowledge* (pp. 21–40). London: Routledge.

Woolard, J. L., Reppucci, N. D., Steinberg, L., Grisso, T., & Scott, E. S. (2003). *Judgment in Legal Contexts Instrument manual*. Unpublished manuscript.

Index